Environmental and Chemical Toxins and Psychiatric Illness

Environmental and Chemical Toxins and Psychiatric Illness

James S. Brown Jr., M.D.

Director, Mental Health Clinic
McGuire Veterans Affairs Medical Center
Assistant Professor of Psychiatry
Medical College of Virginia
Richmond, Virginia

American Psychiatric Publishing, Inc.

Washington, DC
London, England

Note: The author has worked to ensure that all information in this book concerning drug dosages, schedules, and routes of administration is accurate as of the time of publication and consistent with standards set by the U.S. Food and Drug Administration and the general medical community. As medical research and practice advance, however, therapeutic standards may change. For this reason and because human and mechanical errors sometimes occur, we recommend that readers follow the advice of a physician who is directly involved in their care or the care of a member of their family. A product's current package insert should be consulted for full prescribing and safety information.

Books published by American Psychiatric Publishing, Inc., represent the views and opinions of the individual authors and do not necessarily represent the policies and opinions of APPI or the American Psychiatric Association.

Manufactured in the United States of America on acid-free paper
06 05 04 03 02 5 4 3 2 1
First Edition

American Psychiatric Publishing, Inc.
1400 K Street, N.W.
Washington, DC 20005
www.appi.org

Library of Congress Cataloging-in-Publication Data
Brown, James S., 1951–
Environmental and chemical toxins and psychiatric illness / James S. Brown, Jr.—1st ed. p. ; cm.
Includes bibliographical references and index.
ISBN 0-88048-954-5 (alk. paper)
1. Mental illness—Environmental aspects. 2. Mental health—Environmental aspects. 3. Environmental psychology. 4. Mental illness—Etiology. I. Title.
[DNLM: 1. Environmental Illness—etiology. 2. Neurotoxicity Syndromes. 3. Mental Disorders—etiology. 4. Neurotoxins—adverse effects. WL 140 B878e 2002]
RC455.4.E58 B764 2002
616.8′0471—dc21 2001056177

British Library Cataloguing in Publication Data
A CIP record is available from the British Library.

Contents

Part II
Pesticides

Part III
Metals

Introduction

Beginning in the twentieth century, chemical exposures became part of life. We use personal care products, take prescription drugs, spray defroster on the car windshield, purchase gasoline, work at a chemical plant, use typewriter correction fluid, drink alcohol, spray insecticides, and strip lead-based paint from old furniture. These events occur millions of times per day. Many people, especially children, experience toxic exposures that cause symptoms and require treatment. Poison control centers owe their existence to these events. Some persons have daily exposures to neurotoxic chemicals. Significant exposures to the chemicals described in this book can cause central nervous system damage that causes psychiatric illness.

Public awareness of neurotoxic chemicals comes from media descriptions of mass chemical disasters involving hundreds, if not thousands, of victims. Many mass chemical disasters fueled environmental movements, forced legislation of new laws, changed public perceptions of government and industry, and caused adverse health outcomes for many individuals. Most of my "top 10" mass chemical disasters of psychiatric importance listed on p. xii (see box) produced significant psychosocial effects on communities, regions, nations, and even international relations. Other events affected fewer individuals but showed the importance of psychiatric assessment and treatment of chemical exposures. In some disasters, stress caused the

"Top 10" mass chemical disasters of psychiatric importance

1. Hiroshima
2. Nagasaki
3. World War I
4. Chernobyl
5. Bhopal, India
6. Three Mile Island
7. Love Canal, New York
8. Gulf War
9. Vietnam War/Agent Orange
10. Minamata, Japan

Other important events

"Ginger Jake paralysis," United States, 1930
Thallium poisoning epidemic, California, 1932
Stalinon (tin) epidemic, France, 1950s
Tri-ortho-cresyl phosphate mass poisoning, Morocco, 1959
Polychlorinated biphenyl poisoning, Japan, 1968
Methyl mercury epidemic, Iraq, 1971
Toxic oil epidemic, Spain, 1981
Kepone poisoning, Hopewell, Virginia, 1970s

major psychiatric symptoms; in others, neurotoxic injury defined the outcomes. Best-selling books, television programs, and major movies portrayed some of these events to the public.

Profound controversy surrounds many chemicals. This makes objective analysis nearly impossible. Special economic interest groups argue against, and even sue, researchers of pesticides, radiation, solvents, lead, and other toxins. Military, economic, and political issues mire discussion of the Agent Orange and Gulf War syndromes. Intense professional differences exist between mainstream medicine and so-called ecological medicine over multiple chemical sensitivities and sick building syndrome, the latter more acceptable to the mainstream than the former. Persons claiming disability from exposures, sometimes included in case reports or cohort studies, confound the analysis of toxic properties of chemicals.

The awareness of industrial exposures causing psychiatric illness traces to the nineteenth century, when the psychiatric effects of carbon disulfide in French rubber workers became known. Many years passed before American medicine recognized the dangers of carbon disulfide. Eventually, American medical journals carried frequent reports about chemicals with psychiatric risks. Several landmark articles appeared that identified the hazards of carbon monoxide, thallium, mercury, radiation, and others. By the 1960s, psychiatric texts (Hoff 1967; Kolb 1968) summarized psychiatric symptoms from chemical poisonings, a practice no longer followed in general psychiatry texts despite the growing body of literature attributing psychiatric disorders to chemical exposures published since the 1970s.

Before 1970, most clinicians recognized lead, mercury, carbon disulfide, carbon monoxide, and bromine as causes of psychiatric illness (Landrigan 1983; Randle 1997). Psychiatric awareness of pesticides, nerve gases, other solvents, and metals emerged in later decades following the development of behavioral toxicology by psychologists and occupational physicians. The first international symposium on behavioral toxicology, sponsored by the National Institute for Occupational Safety and Health, took place in 1973 after the "formal debut" of the field the previous year (Johnson 1993). Important early contributions by psychiatrists, neurotoxicologists, and psychologists identified deficits in children with elevated dentine lead levels, mechanisms of neurotoxicity, delayed neurotoxicity, and occupational exposure guidelines. Early work included efforts to develop adequate assessment techniques to quantify neurotoxicity (Hanninen 1985). Landmark articles of psychiatric applications soon appeared (Damstra 1978; Dembert 1991; Landrigan 1981, 1983).

Why should we remain familiar with rare, often no longer existent, syndromes produced by banned chemicals? Reports of occupational exposures causing psychiatric illness have markedly declined since the 1930s, a trend noted more than 30 years ago (Sutton 1969). Recent terrorist attacks on the United States highlight the need to prepare for both physical and psychological injuries from chemical and/or biological agents. Chemical and/or biological attacks, such as the recent attack on the United States with anthrax, not only cause physical injuries but also induce stress-related syndromes in victims and communities. The increasing number of mass chemical disasters, the threat of chemical warfare, and new chemicals with poorly defined neurotoxicities require unceasing attention to these matters. Despite the reduction of occupational exposures, as a result of laws governing the maximum allowable exposures to many chemicals, the bulk of *mass* poisonings with psychiatric sequelae has occurred since the 1960s.

Chemicals come and go, but their dangers may remain; sometimes these dangers appear later without warning or time for preparation. The case of pentaborane illustrates the point. The military discontinued use of pentaborane, a neurotoxin and a new and exotic rocket fuel, in the 1960s. In the 1980s, a construction crew in Virginia unearthed 21 cylinders of the substance. When a process to detoxify the material went awry, pentaborane caused death, neurotoxic injury, and other problems in workers, ambulance crews, and emergency department personnel.

Other reasons require the constant monitoring of chemical developments by physicians, environmental scientists, and other professionals. Failure of premarketing testing led to the poisoning of many workers by 2-t-butylazo-2-hydroxy-5-methylhexane (Horan et al. 1985; Johnson 1993). The rapid development of Third World countries, many with nonexistent environmental and work laws, replicates the early industrial era of the Western world, when constant exposures of workers and consumers required psychiatric attention (National Research Council 1991). The absence of child labor laws in some countries compounds the problem (Harari et al. 1997). Finally, poor industrial hygiene led to individual injury by chemicals in the first half of the twentieth century, whereas entire community and regional exposures marked the latter half. An estimated 6,000 persons live near each of the 32,000 hazardous waste sites estimated to exist in the United States (Amler and Lybarger 1993). Approximately 2 million children, women of childbearing age, and elderly live near high-priority waste sites containing heavy metals and solvents (Amler and Lybarger 1993).

The psychiatric recognition and treatment of exposures relies on knowledge of the signs and symptoms of poisoning, the occupational and environmental circumstances of exposure, the psychiatric outcomes from stress and physiological effects of exposure, and the recommended medical and psychiatric interventions. This book compiles literature from numerous medical sources. It serves as a bridge between psychiatry, public health, neurotoxicology, neurobehavioral toxicology, occupational medicine, and neurology. The final hope for this book rests with those who refer to it during future chemical disasters, both accidental and intentional. This might correct the universal problem, noted especially in radiation accidents, that lack of knowledge about the physical and psychological effects of exposure exacerbates the psychological injuries of victims and rescuers.

REFERENCES

Amler RW, Lybarger JA: Research program for neurotoxic disorders and other adverse health outcomes at hazardous chemical sites in the United States of America. Environ Res 61:279–284, 1993

Damstra T: Environmental chemicals and nervous system dysfunction. Yale J Biol Med 51:457–468, 1978

Dembert ML: Occupational chemical exposures and psychiatric disorders. Jefferson Journal of Psychiatry 9:57–69, 1991

Hanninen H: Twenty-five years of behavioral toxicology within occupational medicine: a personal account. Am J Ind Med 7:19–30, 1985

Harari R, Forastiere F, Axelson O: Unacceptable "occupational" exposure to toxic agents among children in Ecuador. Am J Ind Med 32:185–189, 1997

Hoff EC: Brain syndromes associated with drug or poison intoxication, in Comprehensive Textbook of Psychiatry. Edited by Freedman AM, Kaplan HI. Baltimore, MD, Williams & Wilkins, 1967, pp 759–775

Horan JM, Kurt TL, Landrigan PJ, et al: Neurologic dysfunction from exposure to 2-t-butylazo-2-hydroxy-5-methylhexane (BHMH): a new occupational neuropathy. Am J Public Health 75:513–517, 1985

Johnson BL: Neurobehavioral toxicology in the 21st century: a future or a failure? Environ Res 62:114–124, 1993

Kolb LC: Noyes' Modern Clinical Psychiatry, 7th Edition. Philadelphia, PA, WB Saunders, 1968

Landrigan PJ: Toxic exposures and psychiatric disease: an epidemiologic approach, in Proceedings of the Third World Congress of Biological Psychiatry, June 28 to July 3, 1981, Stockholm, Sweden. Edited by Perris C, Struwe G, Jansson B. Amsterdam, Elsevier/North-Holland Biomedical Press, 1981, pp 108–113

Landrigan PJ: Toxic exposures and psychiatric disease—lessons from the epidemiology of cancer. Acta Psychiatr Scand Suppl 303:6–15, 1983

National Research Council: Environmental Epidemiology: Public Health and Hazardous Wastes. Washington, DC, National Academy Press, 1991

Randle HW: Suntanning: differences in perceptions throughout history. Mayo Clin Proc 72:461–466, 1997

Sutton WL: Psychiatric disorders and industrial toxicology. International Psychiatry Clinics 6:339–351, 1969

I

Military, Terrorist, and Disaster Incidents

1

Military and Terrorist Incidents

CHEMICAL WEAPONS

German scientists developed organophosphate (OP) warfare chemicals or nerve gases just before and during World War II (Chambers 1992; Costa 1988; Ecobichon 1982; Maynard and Beswick 1992; O'Brien 1960). The first OP warfare agents—named tabun and sarin, or GA and GB, respectively—entered the German arsenal in 1937 (Maynard and Beswick 1992). Production of soman began in 1944, followed by the V-agents such as VX in the 1950s (Maynard and Beswick 1992).

Two major events during the 1990s highlighted the importance of understanding the symptoms of OP poisoning. First, the Department of Defense notified 20,000 soldiers that they were possibly exposed to low levels of nerve gas in the Gulf War (Presidential Advisory Committee on Gulf War Veterans' Illnesses 1997). Second, in Tokyo, Japan, a religious cult poisoned 5,000 civilians in a terrorist attack with nerve gas in the subway system (Okumura et al. 1996). A smaller terrorist release of nerve agent occurred in Matsumoto, Japan, causing 200 poisonings (Okumura et al. 1996). Emergency department personnel were exposed when the victims arrived at hospitals for treatment (Nozaki et al. 1995; Okudera et al. 1997). The necessity of psychiatric interventions for both physiological and stress-induced symptoms from nerve gases increases in importance with the growing threat from domestic terrorist incidents (DiGiovanni 1999).

The persistence of psychiatric symptoms after symptomatic nerve gas exposure appears undisputed. Symptomatic exposures were evaluated in the 1950s when the United States Army Chemical Warfare Service contracted physicians in Colorado near the Rocky Mountain Arsenal to evaluate persons exposed to nerve gases and OP pesticides (Holmes and Gaon 1956). In a group of several hundred men with histories of acute exposure, approximately one-third experienced severe dreams, poor sleep, nervousness, irritability, or mood changes. Some of the victims developed chronic symptoms. Three years after the terrorist attack with sarin in Matsumoto, a study of victims and nonvictims found a positive correlation between chronic symptoms and grades of sarin exposure (Nakajima et al. 1999). The physical and psychiatric signs and symptoms of OP chemical weapons are the same as those of OP insecticide poisoning. These are listed in Tables 1–1 and 1–2, respectively. More detailed discussion of the symptoms is presented in Chapter 4. The diagnostic workup and recognized diagnoses from OP exposure may be found in Tables 1–3 and 1–4, respectively.

A question remains as to whether the onset of acute symptoms from OP exposure is necessary for the development of chronic symptoms. Similar debate surrounds experimental data obtained from animal exposures to OPs (Clark 1971). Some reviewers claim that acute central nervous system effects, including electroencephalogram (EEG) and psychiatric changes, resolve over a period of weeks (Brown 1971; Namba et al. 1971). Other studies have had different findings. As a follow-up to a study of primates with extended EEG changes after OP exposure, investigators performed EEGs on 77 industrial workers with histories of accidental, acute exposures to sarin (Burchfiel et al. 1976a, 1976b; Duffy and Burchfiel 1980; Duffy et al. 1979). The study, code-named Project Leache (Late Effects of Anticholinesterase Exposure), resulted from the United States government's growing awareness of psychiatric effects of OP exposure (Duffy and Burchfiel 1980). No exposures occurred in the year before the EEGs were performed. Compared with a control group, exposed workers had statistically significant changes, including increased

TABLE 1–1. Physical signs and symptoms of organophosphate nerve gas exposure

Acute	Chronic
Gastrointestinal	
Nausea, vomiting, abdominal pain diarrhea, fecal incontinence, tenesmus, anorexia, abdominal tightness	Same if chronically exposed
Glands	
Salivation, tearing or lacrimation, perspiration	Same if chronically exposed
Eyes	
Miosis, ptosis, blurred vision, conjunctival congestion, "bloody tears," eye pain	Same if chronically exposed
Bladder	
Urinary frequency and incontinence	Same if chronically exposed
Respiratory	
Bronchorrhea, rhinitis, pulmonary edema, chest tightness, wheezing, bronchoconstriction, cough, dyspnea, bronchospasms	Same if chronically exposed
Cardiovascular	
Bradycardia or tachycardia, dysrhythmias, heart block, hypertension or hypotension	Same if chronically exposed
Musculoskeletal	
Muscle fasciculations, cramps, weakness, loss of reflexes, paralysis, flacid or rigid tone, restlessness, generalized motor activity, tremulousness	Same if chronically exposed
Neurological	
Headache, coma, loss of reflexes, Cheyne-Stokes respiration, seizures, electroencephalogram abnormalities	Organophosphate-induced delayed polyneuropathy manifested by flaccidity or paralysis of extremities, paresthesias, footdrop, gait ataxia, spasticity; develops 1–2 weeks after exposure Intermediate syndrome: 1–4 days after exposure; manifested by weakness of proximal limb and respirator muscles loss of knee reflexes, cranial nerve palsy, death

TABLE 1–2. Psychiatric signs and symptoms attributed to organophosphate nerve gases

Mood	Mood lability, anxiety, irritability, depression, giddiness
Behavior	Apathy, restlessness, suicidal ideation, hyperactivity
Cognitive	Confusion, poor concentration, memory loss, academic decline
Perceptual	Hallucinations, paranoia
Other	Dissociation, nightmares, insomnia, excessive dreaming, fatigue, poor appetite, somatic complaints, change in libido

TABLE 1–3. Recommended tests for psychiatric evaluation of organophosphate nerve gas exposure

Complete blood count, electrolytes, liver and renal function tests
Red blood cell count and plasma cholinesterase
Urinalysis and urine pesticide/metabolite screen—if recent exposure
Lymphocyte and platelet NTE assay
Neurology evaluation
Neuropsychological testing
Electroencephalogram

TABLE 1–4. DSM-IV-TR diagnoses attributed to organophosphate nerve gas exposure

Substance-induced delirium
Substance-induced psychotic disorder
Substance-induced mood disorder
Substance-induced persisting amnestic disorder
Substance-induced anxiety disorder

beta activity, increased delta and theta slowing, decreased alpha activity, and increased rapid eye movement sleep. Additional reports emerged suggesting that EEG and emotional changes persisted significantly longer than a few weeks after exposure (Taneda 1974). Recent electrocortigraphic (EcoG) studies of soman-exposed animals, including monkeys, demonstrated that power shifts toward the delta band during soman-induced seizures predict cerebral lesions and neuronal loss to follow (Carpentier et al. 2001).

Other Chemical Warfare Agents

Several histories of chemical warfare describe the chemicals available in the world's arsenals (Fullerton et al. 1996; Harris and Paxman 1982; Heller 1984; Newhouse 1987; Shemer and Danon 1994). World War I combatants saw the introduction of cyanide, chlorine, phosgene, mustard gas, and arsenic (Newhouse 1987). With the use of such fear-inducing weapons, separating true poisoning symptoms from "gas hysteria," now called "acute stress disorder" or, in some cases, malingering, became difficult (Gilchrist 1928; Heller 1984; Hulbert 1920; Newhouse 1987).

Cyanide

The World War I chemical arsenal included cyanide. Other potential cyanide exposures in the twentieth century came from medicinal and industrial sources. Thiocyanate, a medicine in the early twentieth century prescribed for hypertension, caused severe psychosis (Barnett et al. 1951). Hamilton and Hardy (1974) reviewed two cases of chronic occupational exposure to cyanide that caused intellectual impairment in one case and nervousness in the other.

Survivors of the massive methyl isocyanate leak in Bhopal, India, where more than 2,000 died in 1984, experienced no increased risk for psychosis (Sethi et al. 1987). Cases of depression and anxiety resulted mostly from posttraumatic stress disorder or acute stress disorder. In the 200,000 exposed and 10,700 hospitalized, symptoms included weakness, apathy, hypersomnolence, tremor, tetany, and coma (Misra et al. 1987).

Aliphatic nitriles metabolize to cyanide in humans, causing in vivo exposures to workers exposed to these chemicals (O'Donoghue 1985). Workers exposed to dimethylaminopropionitrile (DMAPN), an aliphatic nitrile, experienced urinary tract problems with concurrent libido changes, irritability, and insomnia (Keogh et al. 1980; O'Donoghue 1985). The authors attributed the symptoms to either DMAPN or other nitriles used in the production process.

BZ

Several unclassified and declassified sources mention a chemical warfare agent named "BZ" or "QNB." The military designed BZ, believed to be a phenylglycolate ester of an aminoalcohol with anticholinergic blocking effects, to produce psychiatric casualties (Sidell 1990). Chosen as a "psychochemical" over lysergic acid diethylamide (LSD), BZ disrupts higher cortical functions of memory, problem solving, attention, and comprehension (Hassett 1963; World Health Organization 1970). Additional symptoms from exposure could include sedation, confusion, hallucinations, disorientation, and incoherent speech (Sidell 1990). Supplies of BZ no longer exist (Harris and Paxman 1982; Sidell 1990), but certain aggressor nations or terrorists could have BZ or similar weapons.

Stress Reactions to Chemical Warfare

Psychiatric casualties from combat, especially from chemical weapons, have significant military importance (Augerson 1988; Brooks et al. 1983; Gilstead 1988). Significant numbers of Israeli civilians experienced psychiatric injury during the Gulf War. When Iraq attacked with missiles, civilians had instructions to put on gas masks, enter sealed rooms, and, if exposed to nerve gas, inject themselves with atropine (Carmeli et al. 1994). Of 1,059 total casualties, 230 resulted from false atropine injections, 544 from acute anxiety reactions, 7 from suffocation by improperly used gas masks, and 40 from injuries sustained rushing to "sealed rooms" (Karsenty et al. 1994).

The intensity of the chemical and biological warfare environment causes psychiatric casualties even during training simulations (Brooks et al. 1983; Carter and Cammermeyer 1985a, 1985b; Fullerton and Ursano 1994; Ursano 1988). In addition to the fear of bodily harm, the invisible nature of many chemicals causes additional terror from fear of the unknown, uncanny, or unnatural (Fullerton et al. 1996; World Health Organization 1970). Sensory deprivation associated with wearing of protective gear accentuates the terror (Brooks et al. 1983).

AGENT ORANGE AND OTHER HERBICIDES

Epidemiology of Agent Orange Exposure

Little information exists about human neurotoxicity of the several classes of herbicides, except for the phenoxy herbicides and their dioxin contaminants. The first phenoxy herbicides developed in the 1940s and 1950s had both agricultural and chemical warfare purposes (Ecobichon 1996). Agent Orange, a herbicide used in the Vietnam War as a defoliant, consisted of a mixture of the phenoxy herbicides 2,4-dichlorophenol (2,4-D) and 2,4,5-trichlorophenol (2,4,5-T) (Korgeski and Leon 1983). The Agent Orange controversy developed in the mid-1970s when Vietnam veterans claimed that Agent Orange caused a variety of symptoms, including physical complaints, mood changes, loss of sex drive, and weakness (Holden 1979). The controversy involved a toxic contaminant of Agent Orange, 2,3,7,8-tetrachlorodibenzo-*p*-dioxin (TCDD) (Shepard and Young 1983). One of several molecular forms of dioxin, TCDD forms as a toxic by-product during the production of 2,4,5-T (Ecobichon 1996; Lavy 1987).

Exposures to TCDD also resulted from industrial wastes or accidents that contaminated entire communities such as Times Beach, Missouri, and Seveso, Italy. Although TCDD is no longer commercially available, it remains a hazard for several occupations and occupants of certain geographical localities (Table 1–5). Cocaine abusers can encounter cocaine derived from coca plants treated with phenoxy herbicides in countries without herbicide regulation (Elsohly et al. 1984).

TABLE 1–5. Occupations and locations at risk for herbicide poisoning

Occupations	Firefighters (transformer/capacitor fires)
	Hazardous waste cleanup crews
	Manufacturers of chlorinated herbicides, germicides, and organic solvents
	Municipal/waste incinerator workers
	Utility workers working in or spraying herbicides along rights-of-way
	Vietnam War veterans
Residence	Herbicide-sprayed utility or other right-of-way
	Municipal/waste incinerators
	Other agricultural spraying areas
Others	Breast-fed children of exposed women
	Cocaine users

Signs and Symptoms of TCDD Poisoning

TCDD, the most toxic of the 75 dioxin isomers and possibly the most toxic manufactured chemical, contaminates phenoxy herbicides during the production process (Demers and Perrin 1995; Klaassen 1985). Conflicting literature addresses TCDD lethality in humans. Some reviews deny that human deaths result from systemic effects of TCDD (Demers and Perrin 1995). Others describe successful suicides with phenoxy herbicides (Nielsen et al. 1965). Despite extensive reports of numerous medical conditions from TCDD, the literature confirms only chloracne and transient mild hepatotoxicity in humans. Table 1–6 lists the various, but unconfirmed, signs and symptoms associated with human poisonings. Table 1–7 lists the unconfirmed psychiatric symptoms attributed to TCDD exposure.

TABLE 1–6. Signs and symptoms attributed to TCDD poisoning

Neurological	Headache, dizziness, weakness, fatigue, cold intolerance, peripheral neurotoxicity
Gastrointestinal	Nausea, vomiting, diarrhea, transient hepatotoxicity
Musculoskeletal	Aching and tender muscles
Skin	Chloracne and other dermatological complaints
Other	Skin, eye, respiratory tract irritation; various cancers; renal dysfunction

Note. TCDD = 2,3,7,8-tetrachlorodibenzo-*p*-dioxin.

TABLE 1–7. Psychiatric signs and symptoms attributed to TCDD poisoning

Mood	Anger/rage, irritability, depression, anxiety
Behavior	Hypomania, suicidality
Cognitive	Poor concentration and memory
Other	Insomnia, loss of libido, fatigue

Note. TCDD = 2,3,7,8-tetrachlorodibenzo-*p*-dioxin.

Psychiatric Signs and Symptoms Attributed to Agent Orange

Industry- and government-sponsored studies directly contradict the clinical findings of worker- and Vietnam veteran–sponsored studies, even of the same patient groups (Moses et al. 1984; Suskind and Hertzberg 1984). One study of phenoxy herbicide applicators found increased mortality from suicide, whereas another did not (Asp et al. 1994; Green 1987). The most important study, by the Institute of Medicine (IOM), found that existing but inadequate studies could not determine whether an association exists between exposure and neuropsychiatric outcomes (Goetz et al. 1994). The presence of large uncertainties in epidemiological studies and the lack of control for numerous confounders formed the basis of this opinion.

One confounder of the effects of Agent Orange is that several defoliants were used during the Vietnam War. Stellman et al. (1988a, 1988b) studied the exposure data for Agents Blue and White. Agent Blue contained dimethylarsinic acid, an arsenic-based herbicide. Agent White was picloram, or 4-amino-3,5,6-trichloropicolinic acid. Not knowing the exact exposures experienced by any given solider makes the effects of Agent Orange difficult to isolate.

Other Herbicides

Bidstrup (1952) described a case in 1952 of 3,5-dinitro-ortho-cresol, used as a herbicide, causing a feeling of well-being and "abounding energy" in one agricultural worker.

Diagnosis and Treatment of TCDD/ Agent Orange Exposure

Expensive biological measures, including blood and adipose levels of TCDD, do not correlate with clinical symptoms (Demers and Perrin 1995). Elevated liver function tests in the presence of chloracne indicate exposure. Dioxin has no antidote, and most symptoms require supportive management. No specific literature addresses psychiatric treatment issues of dioxin poisoning. In most exposures to an unknown herbicide, fumigant, or pesticide, the clinical evaluation should proceed as described in Chapter 4.

GULF WAR SYNDROME

In August 1990, Iraq invaded Kuwait, an event that forced a United Nations response and the rapid deployment of American troops to Operation Desert Shield. Operation Desert Storm began 5 months later in January 1991 with a 39-day air war followed by a ground war in February 1991 (Persian Gulf Veterans Coordinating Board 1995). The war ended 100 hours later. Before the fighting began, commanders expected large numbers of casualties. About 697,000 American men and women served in the Persian Gulf War, of which 148 died in combat, 145 died from disease or unintentional injury, and 467 were wounded (Lashof and Cassells 1998; Presidential Advisory Committee on Gulf War Veterans' Illnesses 1996a, 1996b). When military personnel arrived home, many complained of diverse gastrointestinal, musculoskeletal, neurological, and dermal symptoms, forming a clinical picture eventually called the "Gulf War syndrome" (GWS). Spouses and other family members of returning military personnel also complained of new ailments. British and Australian troops reported similar problems (Beale 1994; Tattam 1999). Many physicians suspected that the troops had some form of chemical, biological, or infectious exposure.

Several incidents during the war fueled these suspicions. When Iraqi troops retreated from the ground war in February 1991, they set fire to 749 oil field facilities in Kuwait. This environmental disaster exposed hundreds of thousands of soldiers to smoke-filled air containing hydrocarbons, hydrogen sulfide, and sulfur dioxide (Bullman and Kang 1994). Nerve and mustard gases were detected in some areas, and United States personnel destroyed 8.5 metric tons of the nerve gas sarin in a bunker in Khamisiyah in southern Iraq (Presidential Advisory Committee on Gulf War Veterans' Illnesses 1996a, 1996b). Other troops had exposures to modern artillery shells containing depleted uranium. Many took pyridostigmine bromide (PB) for prophylaxis against nerve gas and received anthrax and botulinum toxoid vaccines in case of biological weapon attack. They also experienced extremes of heat and cold, blowing dust, infectious diseases, and psychological and physiological stress (Landrigan 1997).

To study the problem, the government created the Persian Gulf War Registry. The Comprehensive Clinical Evaluation Program (CCEP) then examined the health of 20,000 veterans who enrolled. Numerous expert panels, including the Presidential Advisory Committee on Gulf War Veterans' Illnesses, investigated and reported on the syndrome. Investigators and veterans alike noted the similarity of their symptoms to chronic fatigue syndrome, fibromyalgia, and multiple chemical sensitivities. Many symptoms reported by veterans lacked objective findings (Presidential Advisory Committee on Gulf War Veterans' Illnesses 1996a, 1996b).

Characteristics of Gulf War Syndrome

Table 1–8 lists the common symptoms reported by Gulf War veterans. Virtually all studies that examined the epidemiology of the syndrome found that deployed veterans complained of more symptoms than did nondeployed military counterparts. With some important exceptions, investigative panels found no Gulf War chemical or biological exposures that could explain the syndrome (Presidential Advisory Committee on Gulf War Veterans' Illnesses 1996a, 1996b). Analysis of the Persian Gulf War Registry found no evidence of a new disease or a consistent set of symptoms (Joseph 1997). Some questions lingered concerning the extent and effect of low-level chemical warfare exposures and the possible synergistic effects of PB with other chemical exposures. In 2000, the Institute of Medicine's Committee on Health Effects Associated With Exposures During the Gulf War concluded that because of the lack of exposure data on Gulf War veterans, the committee could not assess the health impacts of depleted uranium, sarin, pyridostigmine bromide, and vaccines on the veterans (Institute of Medicine 2000).

TABLE 1–8.	Most common symptoms of Gulf War syndrome
Gastrointestinal	Diarrhea, gas, bloating, cramps, abdominal pain
Neurological	Headache, fatigue
Musculoskeletal	Muscle pain, joint pain, stiffness
Psychiatric	Memory problems, sleep disturbances, trouble finding words, irritability, moodiness, depression
Other	Skin rash, shortness of breath, chest pain, cough, sinus problems

Gulf War Syndrome Committees and Panels

The Presidential Advisory Committee issued interim, special, and final reports on the GWS (Presidential Advisory Committee on Gulf War Veterans' Illnesses 1996a, 1996b, 1997). Table 1–9 summarizes the major recommendations and conclusions of this and other committees and panels.

The Persian Gulf Veterans Coordinating Board (1995) concluded that no consistent physical or laboratory abnormalities could be identified and that local inhabitants in Kuwait did not complain of GWS. The National Institutes of Health Technology Assessment Workshop Panel (1994) found little evidence for an association between chemical exposures and GWS, alluding to an important role of stress. Various federally sponsored studies reached similar conclusions (Doebbeling et al. 2000; Engel et al. 2000; Kang and Bullman 2001; Storzbach et al. 2001). While noting the important role of stress in GWS, the Institute of Medicine concluded that inadequate medical record keeping during the war constituted the single greatest problem in analyzing GWS (Committee to Review the Health Consequences of Service During the Persian Gulf War 1996). The IOM cautioned against using the results from the self-selected CCEP for epidemiological research. None of the foregoing investigative bodies rated the deficiencies of current research significant enough to discount the conclusion that stress was the single most significant factor associated with GWS.

Since the Civil War, soldiers have returned home with syndromes similar to GWS (Hyams et al. 1996). Civil War veterans complained of "irritable heart" from "nostalgia," World War I veterans endured "soldier's heart," World War II and Korean War veterans experienced "effort syndrome" and "battle fatigue," and Vietnam War veterans developed posttraumatic stress disorder and "Agent Orange" syndrome (Hyams et al. 1996). The surprise and terror ex-

TABLE 1–9. Recommendations and conclusions of investigative panels and committees regarding Gulf War syndrome

1. Many Gulf War veterans have illnesses connected with their service in the Persian Gulf.
2. The link between exposures and Gulf War syndrome are as follows:

Pesticides	No evidence
Chemical warfare agents	No evidence
Biological warfare agents	No evidence
Vaccines	No evidence
Pyridostigmine bromide	No evidence
Infectious diseases	No or some evidence
Depleted uranium	No evidence
Oil well fires	No evidence
Petroleum products	No or possible evidence
Sand/dust	Unlikely
Chemical-resistant coatings	Responsible for some cases
Stress	Good evidence

3. Substantial evidence exists for site-specific, low-level exposures to chemical weapons; more research is needed to clarify.
4. The Comprehensive Clinical Evaluation Program adequately assessed the health of Gulf War veterans.
5. A serious lack of adequate medical record keeping occurred during the war.
6. The health effects of certain exposures, including stress, pyridostigmine bromide, and low-level chemical weapon exposures, need more research.

pected from Iraqi chemical weapons in the Gulf War produced extreme levels of stress (Fullerton et al. 1996). Adjustment reactions, posttraumatic stress disorder, and other mental disorders from various traumas constituted a significant percentage of the diagnoses reported by the CCEP (Joseph 1997; Roy et al. 1998). The Gulf War Health Center at Walter Reed Army Medical Center used multidisciplinary evaluations and treatments to successfully treat many veterans with these disorders (Engel et al. 1998).

Dissenting Opinions Concerning Gulf War Syndrome

Veterans who believed that they were neither adequately diagnosed nor treated distrusted the findings of investigative panels. In addition to the possible exposures listed in Table 1–9, alternative explanations for GWS include beef allergy secondary to aggressive military immunizing that sensitized personnel to beef protein and Al Eskan disease, a previously unreported condition caused by fine sand dust (Hollander 1995; Korenyi-Both and Juncer 1997). Other deficiencies in studies of GWS that support alternative hypotheses include poor medical record keeping during the war, the warning by the IOM not to use the CCEP for epidemiological research, the chemical weapon destruction at Khamisiyah, and the exposures of certain personnel to oil-well fires and pesticides.

Non-fire-fighting personnel near the Kuwaiti oil fires did not have elevated levels of petroleum products, but firefighters had 10 times the normal blood levels of ethylbenzene and twice the normal levels of benzene, xylene, styrene, and toluene (Etzel and Ashley 1994). The burning oil in Kuwait contained nickel and vanadium that were not measured in exposed military personnel (Madany and Raveendran 1992). Gulf War veterans had additional exposures to several pesticides, especially chlorpyrifos and malathion (Persian Gulf Veterans Coordinating Board 1995). A recent study by Haley et al. (1999) correlated their subjects' symptoms with genetic variations in the paraoxonase/arylesterase 1 gene, which influences sensitivity to nerve gases. A study of Gulf War veterans from the United Kingdom found statistically significantly lower levels of paraoxon hydrolysis and paraoxonase serum levels (Mackness et al. 2000).

The strongest evidence suggesting an organic basis to GWS comes from studies of 249 Gulf War veterans by Haley et al. (1997b). This study attributed six syndromes, derived from factor analysis, to neurological injury. Syndromes 1 through 3 correlated with specific exposures and objective findings. Table 1–10 summarizes the syndromes proposed by this and other studies. Proton magnetic resonance spectroscopy studies of syndromes 1 through 3 found evidence of basal ganglia and/or brain stem damage (Haley et al. 2000; Steele 2000).

Controversy exists over the possible role of PB. Large doses of PB can cause bromide psychosis (Rothenberg et al. 1990). The literature is conflicted as to whether a genetic variation of butyrylcholinesterase can cause a severe reaction to PB (Loewenstein-Lichtenstein et al. 1995; Lotti and Moretto 1995; Senecal and Osterloh 1990). PB also may act synergistically with *N,N*-diethyl-*m*-toluamide, or DEET, an insect repellent, and permethrin, a pyrethroid insecticide. DEET, PB, and permethrin in various combinations are more neurotoxic to hens than are these agents when administered alone (Abou-Donia et al. 1996).

TABLE 1–10. Summary of findings by Haley and Kurt 1997 and Haley et al. 1997a, 1997b

Syndrome 1	
Symptoms	Impaired cognition; decreased attention, memory, and reasoning; insomnia; depression; daytime somnolence; headache
Exposure	Wearing flea collars
Findings	Impaired brain stem auditory evoked potentials
Syndrome 2	
Symptoms	Confusion, ataxia, problems with thinking, disorientation, balance problems, vertigo, impotence
Exposure	Increased adverse effects from pyridostigmine bromide, belief in exposure to chemical weapons while in northeastern sector of Saudi Arabia on day 4 of the air war
Findings	Impaired Halstead Impairment Index, rotational testing, asymmetry of saccadic velocity, and somatosensory evoked potentials
Syndrome 3	
Symptoms	Joint or muscle pain, fatigue, weakness, paresthesias
Exposure	Increased frequency and amount of *N,N*-diethyl-*m*-toluamide (DEET) and pyridostigmine bromide
Findings	Impaired caloric stimulation
Syndrome 4	
Symptoms	Phobia, apraxia
Exposure	Not identified
Findings	Not identified
Syndrome 5	
Symptoms	Fever, adenopathy
Exposure	Not identified
Findings	Not identified
Syndrome 6	
Symptoms	Weakness, incontinence
Exposure	Not identified
Findings	Not identified

Recommendations for Evaluating and Treating Gulf War Syndrome

GWS presents significant challenges for psychiatric assessment and management. Based on CCEP findings, a thorough evaluation of GWS should rule out any preexisting psychiatric conditions or secondary conditions resulting from exposure to stress. Veterans presenting with so-called multiple chemical sensitivities should receive treatment as described in Chapter 18. As with multiple chemical sensitivities, disagreement over the etiology of GWS does not alter the necessity or efficacy of conventional psychiatric treatment.

DEET

DEET, an insect repellent, is included in this chapter because some researchers attribute GWS to the combined use of DEET and other chemicals. The first case of acute toxic encephalopathy from dermal application of DEET on a child occurred in 1961 (Gryboski et al. 1961). Other exposures ended in death preceded by lethargy, mood changes, nightmares, agitation, screaming, and combativeness that simulated an emotional disorder (Heick et al. 1980; Zadikoff 1979). Several poisoning cases have occurred in many countries (Briassoulis et al. 2001; Edwards and Johnson 1987; Petrucci and Sardini 2000; Pronczuk de Garbino et al. 1983; Roland et al. 1985). In many cases, illness followed the dermal application of copious amounts of spray or lotion on children because of numerous mosquitoes in the children's environments. At least four cases of psychosis, mania, or encephalopathy have occurred in adults following application of DEET (Hampers et al. 1999; Leo et al. 2001; Poe et al. 1987; Snyder et al. 1986).

In another setting of heavy DEET use, National Park Service employees in the Everglades National Park used heavy applications of DEET (McConnell et al. 1986). A government study of the workers found that high DEET exposure correlated with insomnia, muscle cramps, mood disturbances, and skin and urinary problems. A second study of the group with neurobehavioral testing correlated heavy DEET use with sleep disturbances, "psychic distress," and impaired cognitive function (McConnell et al. 1986; Robbins and Cherniack 1986).

The role of DEET, and of compounds used with it, in generating psychiatric symptoms is suggestive but unclear. The combined exposure of DEET and chloroquine, for example, may result in mental retardation (Sesline and Jackson 1994). Considering the exposure of troops in the Gulf War to the potentially toxic combination of DEET, PB, and permethrin, researchers hypothesized that GWS resulted from such combinations (Abou-Donia et al. 1996).

REFERENCES

Abou-Donia MB, Wilmarth KR, Jensen KF, et al: Neurotoxicity resulting from coexposure to pyridostigmine bromide, DEET, and permethrin: implications of Gulf War chemical exposures. J Toxicol Environ Health 48:35–56, 1996

American Psychiatric Association: Diagnostic and Statistical Manual of Mental Disorders, 4th Edition, Text Revision. Washington, DC, American Psychiatric Association, 2000

Asp S, Riihimaki V, Hernberg S, et al: Mortality and cancer morbidity of Finnish chlorophenoxy herbicide applicators: an 18-year prospective follow-up. Am J Ind Med 26:243–253, 1994

Augerson W: Behavioral aspects of chemical and biological warfare, in Performance and Operations in Toxic Environments. Bethesda, MD, Uniformed Services University of the Health Sciences, 1988, pp 1–13

Barnett HJM, Jackson MV, Spaulding WB: Thiocyanate psychosis. JAMA 147:1554–1558, 1951

Beale P: Gulf illness (letter). BMJ 308:1574, 1994

Bidstrup PL: Clinical aspects of poisoning by dinitro-ortho-cresol. Proceedings of the Royal Society of Medicine 45:574–575, 1952

Briassoulis G, Narlioglou M, Hatzis T: Toxic encephalopathy associated with use of DEET insect repellents: a case analysis of its toxicity in children. Hum Exp Toxicol 20:8–13, 2001

Brooks FR, Ebner DG, Xenakis SN, et al: Psychological reactions during chemical warfare training. Mil Med 148:232–235, 1983

Brown HW: Electroencephalographic changes and disturbance of brain function following human organophosphate exposure. Northwestern Medicine 70:845–846, 1971

Bullman TA, Kang HK: The effects of mustard gas, ionizing radiation, herbicides, trauma, and oil smoke on US military personnel: the results of veteran studies. Annu Rev Public Health 15:69–90, 1994

Burchfiel JL, Duffy FH, Sim VM: Persistent effects of organophosphate exposure as evidenced by electroencephalographic measurements, in Pesticide Induced Delayed Neurotoxicity. Edited by Baron RL. Research Triangle Park, NC, U.S. Environmental Protection Agency, 1976a, pp 102–151

Burchfiel JL, Duffy FH, Sim VM: Persistent effects of sarin and dieldrin upon the primate electroencephalogram. Toxicol Appl Pharmacol 35:365–379, 1976b

Carmeli A, Liberman N, Mevorach L: Anxiety-related somatic reactions during missile attacks, in Chemical Warfare Medicine: Aspects and Perspectives From the Persian Gulf War. Edited by Danon YL, Shemer J. Jerusalem, Gefen, 1994, pp 186–190

Carpentier P, Foquin A, Dorandeu F, et al: Delta activity as an early indicator for soman-induced brain damage: a review. Neurotoxicology 22:299–315, 2001

Carter BJ, Cammermeyer M: Biopsychological responses of medical unit personnel wearing chemical defense ensemble in a simulated chemical warfare environment. Mil Med 150:239–249, 1985a

Carter BJ, Cammermeyer M: Emergence of real casualties during simulated chemical warfare training under high heat conditions. Mil Med 150:657–665, 1985b

Chambers HW: Organophosphorus compounds: an overview, in Organophosphates: Chemistry, Fate and Effects. Edited by Chambers JE, Levi PE. San Diego, CA, Academic Press, 1992, pp 3–17

Clark G: Organophosphate insecticides and behavior, a review. Aerospace Medicine 42:735–740, 1971

Committee to Review the Health Consequences of Service During the Persian Gulf War: Health Consequences of Service During the Persian Gulf War: Recommendations for Research and Information Systems. Washington, DC, National Academy Press, 1996

Costa LG: Organophosphorous compounds, in Recent Advances in Nervous System Toxicology. Edited by Galli CL, Manzo L, Spencer PS. New York, Plenum, 1988, pp 203–245

Demers R, Perrin E: Dioxin toxicity, in Environmental Medicine: Integrating a Missing Element Into Medical Education. Edited by Pope AM, Rall DP. Washington, DC, National Academy Press, 1995, pp 332–348

DiGiovanni C Jr: Domestic terrorism with chemical or biological agents: psychiatric aspects. Am J Psychiatry 156:1500–1505, 1999

Doebbeling BN, Clarke WR, Watson D, et al: Is there a Persian Gulf War syndrome? Evidence from a large population-based survey of veterans and nondeployed controls. Am J Med 108:695–704, 2000

Duffy FH, Burchfiel JL: Long term effects of the organophosphate sarin on EEGs in monkeys and humans. Neurotoxicology 1:667–689, 1980

Duffy FH, Burchfiel JL, Bartels PH, et al: Long-term effects of an organophosphate upon the human electroencephalogram. Toxicol Appl Pharmacol 47:161–176, 1979

Ecobichon DJ: Organophosphorus ester insecticides, in Pesticides and Neurological Diseases. Edited by Ecobichon DJ, Joy RM. Boca Raton, FL, CRC Press, 1982, pp 151–203

Ecobichon DJ: Toxic effects of pesticides, in Casarett and Doull's Toxicology: The Basic Science of Poisons. Edited by Klaassen CD. New York, McGraw-Hill, 1996, pp 643–689

Edwards DL, Johnson CE: Insect-repellent-induced toxic encephalopathy in a child. Clin Pharm 6:496–498, 1987

Elsohly MA, Arafat ES, Jones AB, et al: Study of the concentration of the herbicide (2,4-dichlorophenoxy)-acetic acid in coca leaves and paste obtained from plants treated with this herbicide. Bull Narc 36:65–77, 1984

Engel CC, Roy M, Kayanan D, et al: Multidisciplinary treatment of persistent symptoms after Gulf War service. Mil Med 163:202–208, 1998

Engel CC Jr, Liu X, McCarthy BD, et al: Relationship of physical symptoms to posttraumatic stress disorder among veterans seeking care for Gulf War–related health concerns. Psychosom Med 62:739–745, 2000

Etzel RA, Ashley DL: Volatile organic compounds in the blood of persons in Kuwait during the oil fires. Int Arch Occup Environ Health 66:125–129, 1994

Fullerton CS, Ursano RJ: Health care delivery in the high-stress environment of chemical and biological warfare. Mil Med 159:524–528, 1994

Fullerton CS, Brandt GT, Ursano RJ: Chemical and biological weapons: silent agents of terror, in Emotional Aftermath of the Persian Gulf War. Edited by Ursano RJ, Norwood AE. Washington, DC, American Psychiatric Press, 1996, pp 111–142

Gilchrist HL: A Comparative Study of World War Casualties From Gas and Other Weapons. Washington, DC, U.S. Government Printing Office, 1928

Gilstead D: Biobehavioral aspects of low dose exposure to chemical agents, in Performance and Operations in Toxic Environments. Bethesda, MD, Uniformed Services University of the Health Sciences, 1988, pp 39–58

Goetz CG, Bolla KI, Rogers SM: Neurologic health outcomes and Agent Orange: Institute of Medicine report. Neurology 44:801–809, 1994

Green LM: Suicide and exposure to phenoxy acid herbicides (letter). Scand J Work Environ Health 13:460, 1987

Gryboski J, Weinstein D, Ordway NK: Toxic encephalopathy apparently related to the use of an insect repellent. N Engl J Med 264:289–291, 1961

Haley RW, Kurt TL: Self-reported exposure to neurotoxic chemical combinations in the Gulf War: a cross-sectional epidemiologic study. JAMA 277:231–237, 1997

Haley RW, Hom J, Roland PS, et al: Evaluation of neurologic function in Gulf War veterans: a blinded case-control study. JAMA 277:223–230, 1997a

Haley RW, Kurt TL, Hom J: Is there a Gulf War syndrome? Searching for syndromes by factor analysis of symptoms. JAMA 277:215–222, 1997b

Haley RW, Billecke S, La Du BN: Association of low PON1 Type Q (Type A) arylesterase activity with neurologic symptom complexes in Gulf War veterans. Toxicol Appl Pharmacol 157:227–233, 1999

Haley RW, Fleckenstein JL, Marshall WW, et al: Effect of basal ganglia injury on central dopamine activity in Gulf War syndrome: correlation of proton magnetic resonance spectroscopy and plasma homovanillic acid levels. Arch Neurol 57:1280–1285, 2000

Hamilton A, Hardy HL: Cyanides, in Industrial Toxicology. Edited by Hamilton A, Hardy HL. Acton, MA, Publishing Sciences Group, 1974, pp 221–228

Hampers LC, Oker E, Leikin JB: Topical use of DEET insect repellent as a cause of severe encephalopathy in a healthy adult male. Acad Emerg Med 6:1295–1297, 1999

Harris R, Paxman J: A Higher Form of Killing: The Secret Story of Chemical and Biological Warfare. New York, Hill & Wang, 1982

Hassett CC: Study of Long-Term Human and Ecological Effects of Chemical Weapons Systems (CRDL Special Publication 2-52). Edgewood Arsenal, MD, U.S. Army Chemical Research & Development Laboratories, 1963

Heick HMC, Shipman RT, Norman MG, et al: Reye-like syndrome associated with use of insect repellent in a presumed heterozygote for ornithine carbamoyl transferase deficiency. Pediatric Pharmacology and Therapeutics 97:471–473, 1980

Heller CE: Chemical Warfare in World War I: The American Experience, 1917–1918. Fort Leavenworth, KS, U.S. Army Command & General Staff College Combat Studies Institute, 1984

Holden C: Agent Orange furor continues to build: for Vietnam veterans, the herbicide has become a symbol for everything that was wrong about the war (news). Science 205:770–772, 1979

Hollander DH: Beef allergy and the Persian Gulf syndrome. Med Hypotheses 45:221–222, 1995

Holmes JH, Gaon M: Observations on acute and multiple exposure to anticholinesterase agents. Trans Am Clin Climatol Assoc 68:86–103, 1956

Hulbert HS: Gas neurosis syndrome. American Journal of Insanity 77:213–216, 1920

Hyams KC, Wignall FS, Roswell R: War syndromes and their evaluation: from the U.S. Civil War to the Persian Gulf War. Ann Intern Med 125:398–405, 1996

Institute of Medicine: Gulf War and Health, Vol 1: Depleted Uranium, Sarin, Pyridostigmine Bromide, and Vaccines. Washington, DC, National Academy Press, 2000

Joseph SC: A comprehensive clinical evaluation of 20,000 Persian Gulf War veterans. Mil Med 162:149–155, 1997

Kang HK, Bullman TA: Mortality among US veterans of the Persian Gulf War: 7-year follow-up. Am J Epidemiol 154:399–405, 2001

Karsenty E, Shemer J, Alshech I, et al: Medical aspects of the Iraqi missile attacks on Israel, in Chemical Warfare Medicine: Aspects and Perspectives From the Persian Gulf War. Edited by Danon YL, Shemer J. Jerusalem, Gefen, 1994, pp 38–44

Keogh JP, Pestronk A, Wertheimer D, et al: An epidemic of urinary retention caused by dimethylaminopropionitrile. JAMA 243:746–749, 1980

Klaassen CD: Nonmetallic environmental toxicants: air pollutants, solvents and vapors, and pesticides, in The Pharmacological Basis of Therapeutics. Edited by Gilman AG, Goodman LS, Rall TW, et al. New York, Macmillan, 1985, pp 1628–1650

Korenyi-Both A, Juncer DJ: Al Eskan disease: Persian Gulf syndrome. Mil Med 162:1–13, 1997

Korgeski GP, Leon GR: Correlates of self-reported and objectively determined exposure to Agent Orange. Am J Psychiatry 140:1443–1449, 1983

Landrigan PJ: Illness in Gulf War veterans (editorial). JAMA 277:259–261, 1997

Lashof JC, Cassells JS: Illness among Gulf War veterans: risk factors, realities, and future research (editorial). JAMA 280:1010–1011, 1998

Lavy TL: Human Exposure to Phenoxy Herbicides. Washington, DC, Veterans Administration Central Office, 1987

Leo RJ, Del Regno PA, Gregory C, et al: Insect repellant toxicity associated with psychosis. Psychosomatics 42:78–80, 2001

Loewenstein-Lichtenstein Y, Schwarz M, Glick D, et al: Genetic predisposition to adverse consequences of anti-cholinesterases in "atypical" BCHE carriers (abstract). Nat Med 10:1082–1085, 1995

Lotti M, Moretto A: Cholinergic symptoms and Gulf War syndrome (letter). Nat Med 1:1225–1226, 1995

Mackness B, Durrington PN, Mackness MI: Low paraoxonase in Persian Gulf War veterans self-reporting Gulf War syndrome. Biochem Biophys Res Commun 276: 729–733, 2000

Madany IM, Raveendran E: Polycyclic aromatic hydrocarbons, nickel and vanadium in air particulate matter in Bahrain during the burning of oil fields in Kuwait. Sci Total Environ 116:281–289, 1992

Maynard RL, Beswick FW: Organophosphorus compounds as chemical warfare agents, in Clinical and Experimental Toxicology of Organophosphates and Carbamates. Edited by Ballantyne B, Marrs TC, Aldridge WN. Oxford, UK, Butterworth Heinemann, 1992, pp 373–385

McConnell R, Fidler AT, Chrislip D: Health Hazard Evaluation Report: NTIS, HETA 83-085-1757, Everglades National Park, Everglades, Florida. Cincinnati, OH, Hazard Evaluations and Technical Assistance Branch, National Institute for Occupational Safety and Health, U.S. Department of Health and Human Services, 1986

Misra NP, Pathak R, Gaur KJBS, et al: Clinical profile of gas leak victims in acute phase after Bhopal episode. Indian J Med Res 86 (suppl):11–19, 1987

Moses M, Lilis R, Crow KD, et al: Health status of workers with past exposure to 2,3,7,8-tetrachlorodibenzo-p-dioxin in the manufacture of 2,4,5-trichlorophenoxyacetic acid: comparison of findings with and without chloracne. Am J Ind Med 5:161–182, 1984

Nakajima T, Ohta S, Fukushima Y, et al: Sequelae of sarin toxicity at one and three years after exposure in Matsumoto, Japan. J Epidemiol 9:337–343, 1999

Namba T, Nolte CT, Jackrel J, et al: Poisoning due to organophosphate insecticides. Am J Med 50:475–492, 1971

National Institutes of Health Technology Assessment Workshop Panel: The Persian Gulf experience and health. JAMA 272:391–396, 1994

Newhouse P: Neuropsychiatric aspects of chemical warfare, in Contemporary Studies in Combat Psychiatry. Edited by Belenky G. New York, Greenwood Press, 1987, pp 185–202

Nielsen K, Kaempe B, Jensen-Holm J: Fatal poisoning in man by 2,4-dichlorophenoxyacetic acid (2,4-D): determination of the agent in forensic materials. Acta Pharmacologica et Toxicologica 22:224–234, 1965

Nozaki H, Hori S, Shinozawa Y, et al: Secondary exposure of medical staff to sarin vapor in the emergency room. Intensive Care Med 21:1032–1035, 1995

O'Brien RD: Toxic Phosphorus Esters: Chemistry, Metabolism, and Biological Effects. New York, Academic Press, 1960

O'Donoghue JL: Cyanide, nitriles and isocyanates, in Neurotoxicity of Industrial and Commercial Chemicals, Vol II. Edited by O'Donoghue JL. Boca Raton, FL, CRC Press, 1985, pp 25–37

Okudera H, Morita H, Iwashita T, et al: Unexpected nerve gas exposure in the city of Matsumoto: report of rescue activity in the first sarin gas terrorism. Am J Emerg Med 15:527–528, 1997

Okumura T, Takasu N, Ishimatsu S, et al: Report on 640 victims of the Tokyo subway sarin attack. Ann Emerg Med 28:129–135, 1996

Persian Gulf Veterans Coordinating Board: Unexplained illnesses among Desert Storm veterans. Arch Intern Med 155:262–268, 1995

Petrucci N, Sardini S: Severe neurotoxic reaction associated with oral ingestion of low-dose diethyltoluamide-containing insect repellent in a child. Pediatr Emerg Care 16:341–342, 2000

Poe RO, Snyder JW, Stubbins JF, et al: Psychotic reaction to an insect repellent (letter). Am J Psychiatry 144:1103–1104, 1987

Presidential Advisory Committee on Gulf War Veterans' Illnesses: Presidential Advisory Committee on Gulf War Veterans' Illnesses: Interim Report. Washington, DC, U.S. Government Printing Office, 1996a

Presidential Advisory Committee on Gulf War Veterans' Illnesses: Presidential Advisory Committee on Gulf War Veterans' Illnesses: Final Report. Washington, DC, U.S. Government Printing Office, 1996b

Presidential Advisory Committee on Gulf War Veterans' Illnesses: Special Report. Washington, DC, U.S. Government Printing Office, 1997

Pronczuk de Garbino J, Laborde A, Fogel de Korc E: Toxicity of an insect repellent: N-N-diethyltoluamide. Vet Hum Toxicol 25:422–423, 1983

Robbins PJ, Cherniack MG: Review of the biodistribution and toxicity of the insect repellent N,N-diethyl-m-toluamide (DEET). J Toxicol Environ Health 18:503–525, 1986

Roland EH, Jan JE, Rigg JM: Toxic encephalopathy in a child after brief exposure to insect repellents. Canadian Medical Association Journal 132:155–156, 1985

Rothenberg DM, Berns AS, Barkin R, et al: Bromide intoxication secondary to pyridostigmine bromide therapy. JAMA 263:1121–1122, 1990

Roy MJ, Koslowe PA, Kroenke K, et al: Signs, symptoms, and ill-defined conditions in Persian Gulf War veterans: findings from the comprehensive clinical evaluation program. Psychosom Med 60:663–668, 1998

Senecal P-E, Osterloh J: Confusion from pyridostigmine bromide: was there bromide intoxication? (letter) JAMA 264:454–455, 1990

Sesline DH, Jackson RJ: The effects of prenatal exposure to pesticides, in Prenatal Exposure to Toxicants: Developmental Consequences. Edited by Needleman HL, Bellinger D. Baltimore, MD, Johns Hopkins University Press, 1994, pp 233–248

Sethi BB, Sharma M, Trivedi JK, et al: Psychiatric morbidity in patients attending clinics in gas affected areas in Bhopal. Indian J Med Res 86 (suppl):45–50, 1987

Shemer J, Danon YL: Eighty years of the threat and use of chemical warfare: the medical-organizational challenge, in Chemical Warfare Medicine: Aspects and Perspectives From the Persian Gulf War. Edited by Danon YL, Shemer J. Jerusalem, Gefen, 1994, pp 19–25

Shepard BM, Young AL: Dioxins as contaminants of herbicides: the U.S. perspective, in Human and Environmental Risks of Chlorinated Dioxins and Related Compounds. Edited by Tucker RE, Young AL, Gray AP. New York, Plenum, 1983, pp 3–16

Sidell FR: What to do in case of an unthinkable chemical warfare attack or accident. Postgrad Med 88:70–84, 1990

Snyder JW, Poe RO, Stubbins JF, et al: Acute manic psychosis following the dermal application of N,N-diethyl-m-toluamide (DEET) in an adult. J Toxicol Clin Toxicol 24:429–439, 1986

Steele L: Prevalence and patterns of Gulf War illness in Kansas veterans: association of symptoms with characteristics of person, place, and time of military service. Am J Epidemiol 152:992–1002, 2000

Stellman SD, Stellman JM, Sommer JF Jr: Combat and herbicide exposures in Vietnam among a sample of American legionnaires. Environ Res 47:112–128, 1988a

Stellman SD, Stellman JM, Sommer JF Jr: Health and reproductive outcomes among American legionnaires in relation to combat and herbicide exposure in Vietnam. Environ Res 47:150–174, 1988b

Storzbach D, Rohlman DS, Anger WK, et al: Neurobehavioral deficits in Persian Gulf veterans: additional evidence from a population-based study. Environ Res 85:1–13, 2001

Suskind RR, Hertzberg VS: Human health effects of 2,4,5-T and its toxic contaminants. JAMA 251:2372–2380, 1984

Taneda M: [The electroencephalogram and psychoneurotic symptoms in chronic organophosphorus intoxication]. Pesticides Abstracts 7:448–449, 1974

Tattam A: Gulf War syndrome admission in Australia (news). Lancet 353:2136, 1999

Ursano RJ: Combat stress in the chemical and biological warfare environment. Aviat Space Environ Med 59:1123–1132, 1988

World Health Organization: Health Aspects of Chemical and Biological Weapons. Geneva, World Health Organization, 1970

Zadikoff CM: Toxic encephalopathy associated with use of insect repellant. J Pediatr 95:140–142, 1979

ADDITIONAL READINGS

Chemical Weapons

Bleich A, Kron S, Margalit C, et al: Israeli psychological casualties of the Persian Gulf War: characteristics, therapy, and selected issues. Isr J Med Sci 27:673–676, 1991

Bowers MB, Goodman E, Sim VM: Some behavioral changes in man following anticholinesterase administration. J Nerv Ment Dis 138:383–389, 1964

Burchfiel JL, Duffy FH: Organophosphate neurotoxicity: chronic effects of sarin on the electroencephalogram of monkey and man. Neurobehavioral Toxicology and Teratology 4:767–778, 1982

Ecobichon DJ: Organophosphorus ester insecticides, in Pesticides and Neurological Diseases. Edited by Ecobichon DJ, Joy RM. Boca Raton, FL, CRC Press, 1982, pp 151–203

Ecobichon DJ, Ozere RL, Reid E, et al: Acute fenitrothion poisoning. Canadian Medical Association Journal 116:377–379, 1977

Finesinger JE: Psychological Studies on the Effects of CW Agents/Defense Technical Information Center AD 144023. Fort Belvoir, VA, Defense Technical Information Center, 1950

Fullerton CS, Ursano RJ, Kao T-C, et al: The chemical and biological warfare environment: psychological responses and social supports in a high-stress environment. Journal of Applied Social Psychology 22:1608–1624, 1992

Grob D, Harvey JC: Effects in man of the anticholinesterase compound sarin (isopropyl methyl phosphonofluoridate). J Clin Invest 37:350–368, 1958

Kaplan Z, Singer Y, Lichtenberg P, et al: Post-traumatic stress disorder in Israel during the Gulf War, in Chemical Warfare Medicine: Aspects and Perspectives From the Persian Gulf War. Edited by Danon YL, Shemer J. Jerusalem, Gefen, 1994, pp 191–196

Korsak RJ, Sato MM: Effects of chronic organophosphate pesticide exposure on the central nervous system. Clinical Toxicology 11:83–95, 1977

Murata K, Araki S, Yokoyama K, et al: Asymptomatic sequelae to acute sarin poisoning in the central and autonomic nervous system 6 months after the Tokyo subway attack. J Neurol 244:601–606, 1997

Murphy JM: War stress and civilian Vietnamese: a study of psychological effects. Acta Psychiatr Scand 56:92–108, 1977

Nozaki H, Aikawa N, Fujishima S, et al: A case of VX poisoning and the difference from sarin (letter). Lancet 346:698–699, 1995

Perold JG, Bezuidenhout DJJ: Chronic organophosphate poisoning. S Afr Med J 57:7–9, 1980

Rodezno RA, Lundberg I, Escalona E: Development of a questionnaire in Spanish on neurotoxic symptoms. Am J Ind Med 28:505–520, 1995

Sidell FR: Soman and sarin: clinical manifestations and treatment of accidental poisoning by organophosphates. Clinical Toxicology 7:1–17, 1974

Solomon Z, Margalit C, Waysman M, et al: In the shadow of the Gulf War: psychological distress, social support and coping among Israeli soldiers in a high risk area, in Chemical Warfare Medicine: Aspects and Perspectives From the Persian Gulf War. Edited by Danon YL, Shemer J. Jerusalem, Gefen, 1994, pp 197–209

Stockholm International Peace Research Institute: Delayed Toxic Effects of Chemical Warfare Agents. Stockholm, Almqvist & Wiksell International, 1975

Ursano RJ: Combat stress in the chemical and biological warfare environment. Aviat Space Environ Med 59:1123–1132, 1988

Agent Orange Exposure in Vietnam

Barrett DH, Morris RD, Akhtar FZ, et al: Serum dioxin and cognitive functioning among veterans of Operation Ranch Hand. Neurotoxicology 22:491–502, 2001

Bogen G: Symptoms in Vietnam veterans exposed to Agent Orange (letter). JAMA 242:2391, 1979

Boyle CA, Decoufle P, Delaney RJ, et al: Postservice Mortality Among Vietnam Veterans. Atlanta, GA, U.S. Department of Health and Human Services, 1987

Decoufle P, Holmgreen P, Boyle CA, et al: Self-reported health status of Vietnam veterans in relation to perceived exposure to herbicides and combat. Am J Epidemiol 135:312–323, 1992

Fleck H: An Agent Orange: case history. Mil Med 150:103–104, 1985

Lawrence CE, Reilly AA, Quickenton P, et al: Mortality patterns of New York State Vietnam veterans. Am J Public Health 75:277–279, 1985

Levy CJ: Agent Orange exposure and posttraumatic stress disorder. J Nerv Ment Dis 176:242–245, 1988

Robinowitz R, Dolan MP, Patterson ET, et al: Carcinogenicity and teratogenicity vs. psychogenicity: psychological characteristics associated with self-reported Agent Orange exposure among Vietnam combat veterans who seek treatment for substance abuse. J Clin Psychol 45:718–728, 1989

Thomas TL, Kang HA: Mortality and morbidity among army chemical corps Vietnam veterans: a preliminary report. Am J Ind Med 18:665–673, 1990

Visintainer PF, Barone M, McGee H, et al: Proportionate mortality study of Vietnam-era veterans of Michigan. J Occup Environ Med 37:423–428, 1995

Industrial Exposures to TCDD

Alderfer R, Sweeney M, Fingerhut M, et al: Measures of depressed mood in workers exposed to 2,3,7,8-tetrachlorodibenzo-p-dioxin (TCDD). Chemosphere 25:247–250, 1992

Bond GG, McLaren EA, Cartmill JB, et al: Cause-specific mortality among male chemical workers. Am J Ind Med 12:353–383, 1987

Bond GG, Wetterstroem NH, Roush GJ, et al: Cause specific mortality among employees engaged in the manufacture, formulation, or packaging of 2,4-dichlorophenoxyacetic acid and related salts. British Journal of Industrial Medicine 45: 98–105, 1988

Bond GG, McLaren EA, Lipps TE, et al: Update of mortality among chemical workers with potential exposure to the higher chlorinated dioxins. Journal of Occupational Medicine 31:121–123, 1989

Gilioli R, Genta P, Cotroneo L, et al: Electroencephalographic spectral analysis in chemical and engineering workers, in Neurobehavioral Methods in Occupational Health. Edited by Gilioli R, Cassitto MG, Foa V. Oxford, UK, Pergamon, 1983, pp 219–229

Green LM: Suicide and exposure to phenoxy acid herbicides (letter). Scand J Work Environ Health 13:460, 1987

Green LM: A cohort mortality study of forestry workers to phenoxy acid herbicides. British Journal of Industrial Medicine 48:234–238, 1991

Neuberger M, Rape C, Bergek S, et al: Persistent health effects of dioxin contamination in herbicide production. Environ Res 81:206–214, 1999

O'Donoghue JL: Cyclic halogenated hydrocarbons and related substances, in Neurotoxicity of Industrial and Commercial Chemicals, Vol II. Edited by O'Donoghue JL. Boca Raton, FL, CRC Press, 1985, pp 155–168

Oliver RM: Toxic effects of 2,3,7,8 tetrachlorodibenzo 1,4 dioxin in laboratory workers. British Journal of Industrial Medicine 32:49–53, 1975

Ott MG, Holder BB, Olson RD: A mortality analysis of employees engaged in the manufacture of 2,4,5-trichlorophenoxyacetic acid. Journal of Occupational Medicine 22:47–50, 1980

Ott MG, Olson RA, Cook RR, et al: Cohort mortality study of chemical workers with potential exposure to the higher chlorinated dioxins. J Occup Environ Med 29:422–429, 1987

Pazderova-Vejlupkova J, Nemcova M, Pickova J, et al: The development and prognosis of chronic intoxication by tetrachlorodibenzo-p-dioxin in men. Arch Environ Health 36:5–11, 1981

Poland AP, Smith D, Metter G, et al: A health survey of workers in a 2,4-D and 2,4,5-T plant. Arch Environ Health 22:316–327, 1971

Thiess AM, Frentzel-Beyme R, Link R: Mortality study of persons exposed to dioxin in a trichlorophenol-process accident that occurred in the BASF AG on November 17, 1953. Am J Ind Med 3:179–189, 1982

Zober A, Messerer P, Huber P: Thirty-four-year mortality follow-up of BASF employees exposed to 2,3,7,8-TCDD after the 1953 accident. Int Arch Occup Environ Health 62:139–157, 1990

Zober A, Ott MG, Messerer P: Morbidity follow up study of BASF employees exposed to 2, 3, 7, 8-tetrachlorodibenzo-p-dioxin (TCDD) after a 1953 chemical reactor incident. Occup Environ Med 51:479–486, 1994

Community/Environmental Exposures to TCDD

Hoffman RE, Stehr-Green PA, Webb KB, et al: Health effects of long-term exposure to 2,3,7,8-tetrachlorodibenzo-p-dioxin. JAMA 255:2031–2038, 1986

Peper M, Klett M, Frentzel-Beyme R, et al: Neuropsychological effects of chronic exposure to environmental dioxins and furans. Environ Res 60:233–244, 1993

Gulf War Syndrome

Axelrod BN, Milner IB: Neuropsychological findings in a sample of Operation Desert Storm veterans. J Neuropsychiatry Clin Neurosci 9:23–28, 1997

Cherry N, Creed F, Silman A, et al: Health and exposures of United Kingdom Gulf War veterans, Part II: the relation of health to exposure. Occup Environ Med 58:299–306, 2001

Cook JE, Kolka MA, Wenger CB: Chronic pyridostigmine bromide administration: side effects among soldiers working in a desert environment. Mil Med 157:250–254, 1992

Enserink M: Gulf War illness: the battle continues (news). Science 291:812–817, 2001

Etzel RA, Ashley DL: Volatile organic compounds in the blood of persons in Kuwait during the oil fires. Int Arch Occup Environ Health 66:125–129, 1994

Fukuda K, Nisenbaum R, Stewart G, et al: Chronic multisymptom illness affecting air force veterans of the Gulf War. JAMA 280:981–988, 1998

Gillert DJ: Internet has info on veterans' illnesses (news). The Mercury (U.S. Army Medical Department, Houston, TX), July 4, 1997

Goldstein G, Beers SR, Morrow LA, et al: A preliminary neuropsychological study of Persian Gulf veterans. J Int Neuropsychol Soc 2:368–371, 1996

Gray GC, Coate BD, Anderson CM, et al: The postwar hospitalization experience of U.S. veterans of the Persian Gulf War. N Engl J Med 335:1505–1513, 1996

Hom J, Haley RW, Kurt TL: Neuropsychological correlates of Gulf War syndrome. Archives of Clinical Neuropsychology 12:531–544, 1997

Hyams KC, Wignall FS: Identification of Gulf War syndrome: methodological issues and medical illnesses (letter). JAMA 278:384, 1997

The Iowa Persian Gulf Study Group: Self-reported illness and health status among Gulf War veterans. JAMA 277:238–245, 1997

Jamal GA, Hansen S, Apartopoulos F, et al: The "Gulf War syndrome": is there evidence of dysfunction in the nervous system? J Neurol Neurosurg Psychiatry 60: 449–451, 1996

Kang HK, Bullman TA: Mortality among U.S. veterans of the Persian Gulf War. N Engl J Med 335:1498–1504, 1996

Keeler JR, Hurst CG, Dunn MA: Pyridostigmine used as a nerve agent pretreatment under wartime conditions. JAMA 266:693–695, 1991

Labbate LA, Snow MP: Posttraumatic stress symptoms among soldiers exposed to combat in the Persian Gulf. Hospital and Community Psychiatry 43:831–833, 1992

Newmark J, Clayton WL: Persian Gulf illnesses: preliminary neurological impressions. Mil Med 160:505–507, 1995

Nicolson GL, Bruton DM, Nicolson NL: Chronic fatigue illness and Operation Desert Storm (letter). J Occup Environ Med 38:14–16, 1996

Sharabi Y, Danon YL, Berkenstadt H, et al: Survey of symptoms following intake of pyridostigmine during the Persian Gulf War. Isr J Med Sci 27:656–658, 1991

Simon TR, Hickey DC, Fincher CE, et al: Single photon emission computed tomography of the brain in patients with chemical sensitivities. Toxicol Ind Health 10:573–577, 1994

Southwick SM, Morgan A, Nagy LM, et al: Trauma-related symptoms in veterans of Operation Desert Storm: a preliminary report. Am J Psychiatry 150:1524–1528, 1993

Southwick SM, Morgan CAI, Nicolaou AL, et al: Consistency of memory for combat-related traumatic events in veterans of Operation Desert Storm. Am J Psychiatry 154:173–177, 1997

Stretch RH, Bliese PD, Marlowe DH, et al: Physical health symptomatology of Gulf War–era service personnel from the states of Pennsylvania and Hawaii. Mil Med 160:131–136, 1995

Stretch RH, Bliese PD, Marlowe DH, et al: Psychological health of Gulf War-era military personnel. Mil Med 161:257–261, 1996

White RF, Proctor SP, Heeren T, et al: Neuropsychological function in Gulf War veterans: relationships to self-reported toxicant exposures. Am J Ind Med 40:42–54, 2001

2

Community and Individual Stress Reactions

The first major recognition of individual stress reactions from the exposure to chemicals occurred during World War I. Combat casualties included "gas neurosis," an acute stress reaction to the perception of exposure to chemical weapons. In the ranks of battle-tested troops, an individual could give the alarm for gas, and without gas present, hundreds of soldiers would develop physical complaints of gassing (*One Hundred Years of American Psychiatry* 1944). Even today, the individual stress response to chemical weapons may lead to tragic results. During the Gulf War, seven Israeli citizens died when they suffocated in their improperly applied gas masks, perhaps thinking that their shortness of breath was caused by nerve gas (Karsenty et al. 1994). Such tragedy highlights the public's fear of chemicals revealed by Orson Welles's 1938 Halloween broadcast of H. G. Wells's *War of the Worlds.* This science fiction story depicted a Martian attack on the world, and the broadcast portrayed the attack occurring in New Jersey. Public hysteria erupted after the announcer said that the Martians had released poison gas that was moving toward New

York City. The public's fear of poison gas exceeded their fear of extraterrestrial beings (Cantril 1940).

The recognition of the community as victim of toxic contamination emerged after the Love Canal incident in the 1970s. Love Canal, a community of Niagara Falls, New York, became a pivotal event in the environmental movement and spurred environmental legislation controlling hazardous waste dumps. To many, Love Canal symbolized abandonment by government and institutional authorities, a general belief reported by victims of other mass chemical and radiation disasters (Edelstein and Wandersman 1987).

Following media publicity of Love Canal, the community became anxious, and government agencies ordered the evacuation of children and pregnant women. The largely "blue collar" neighborhood shunned the local mental health center's offer of help to avoid being "branded as crazy" (Gibbs 1983; Holden 1980). With the exception of some individuals, most residents did not experience symptoms severe enough to warrant formal diagnoses. Although the diagnoses did not reach clinical thresholds, the event changed people's lives and eliminated the community, an outcome of many community chemical disasters.

CHRONIC COMMUNITY EXPOSURE

Hazardous Waste Sites

Stress reactions to occupational and community chemical exposures occur in both acute and chronic forms. Much of the literature pertaining to community reactions to chronic chemical exposures involves hazardous waste sites. By 1988, the Environmental Protection Agency (EPA) identified 29,300 sites needing cleanup. The EPA listed 950 of them on the National Priorities List, also known as the Superfund sites (*Health Aspects of the Disposal of Waste Chemicals* 1986; Upton et al. 1989). Several sources review the medical and environmental aspects of hazardous waste sites (Andelman and Underhill 1987; Committee on Environmental Epidemiology 1991; Epstein et al. 1982; *Health Aspects of the Disposal of Waste Chemicals* 1986; Petts 1994; Weisaeth 1984). The most common chemicals in these sites include trichloroethylene, lead, toluene, benzene, chloroform, polychlorinated biphenyls, and miscellaneous solvents (Upton et al. 1989).

Hazardous waste sites affected the communities of Legler Township, New Jersey, and Woburn, Massachusetts, the latter being the basis of a movie and best-selling book (Harr 1995). In another case called "the phantom dump," residents of a Memphis, Tennessee, neighborhood in the 1980s developed severe stress reactions and staged a sit-in in the governor's regional office before investigators determined that a waste site never existed (Harris 1983).

Other Major Chronic Community Exposures

Additional chronic community exposures resulted from accidental, unknowing, or illegal activities. Health agencies in Mississippi during 1996 determined that indoor use of methyl parathion (MP) had contaminated more than 1,800 homes and businesses during a 10-year period. This incident was one of several involving the illegal shipment and use of MP in numerous states during the 1990s. Recovery required extensive restoration, and in some cases, there was total loss of the home (Rehner et al. 2000). A company sprayed dioxin-contaminated oil on roads as a dust suppressant in Times Beach, Missouri, followed by a flood during which thousands of Times Beach residents evacuated and became homeless. The dioxin contamination resulted in a federal "buyout" and abandonment of the town (Solomon and Smith 1994). In Spain, contaminated rapeseed oil intended for industrial use poisoned 20,000, leaving 350 dead and thousands needing psychiatric referral (Lopez-Ibor et al. 1985).

ACUTE MASS DISASTERS

The earliest reports of acute environmental incidents were of air pollution emergencies. In the Meuse Valley of Belgium during 1930, 63 persons died and thousands became ill from sulfur dioxide and sulfuric acid air pollution (French 1989). The Donora, Pennsylvania, smog disaster in 1948 left 20 dead and more than 5,000 ill (French 1989).

Certain chemical disasters have prominent places in medical history. In 1976, a chemical reactor explosion in Seveso, Italy, released 2,3,7,8-tetrachlorodibenzo-*p*-dioxin, which contaminated thousands of acres, killed 100,000 animals, and caused the evacuation of hundreds of people (Melius and Binder 1989). In 1984 in Bhopal, India, a carbamate pesticide plant released 30 tons of methyl isocyanate, causing more than 3,000 deaths and 50,000–300,000 injuries (Melius and Binder 1989). The Three Mile Island and Chernobyl nuclear accidents during the 1980s were the culmination of a string of eight nuclear accidents since 1952 (Melius and Binder 1989). Other chemical disasters severely affected local communities but did not generate widespread attention (De La Paz 1997; Withers 1988).

ORIGINS OF STRESS RESPONSES TO CHEMICAL EXPOSURES

Natural Versus Technological Disasters

Recognition of stress from technological disasters emerged only in recent decades. Major differences exist between the origins of stress from technological disasters and those from natural disasters. Stress from technological disasters, such as Three Mile Island and Chernobyl, is greater than stress from natural disasters in severity and duration. These differences, listed in Table 2–1, result in greater threat to and loss of control in victims.

Roles of Perception and Interpretation

The severity of symptoms depends on the perceived level of danger or harm. Especially in suggestible individuals, the perception of "bad odor" induces the perception of harm (Lees-Haley and Brown 1992). Community perceptions may lead to mass hysteria in the absence of actual exposure, or they may induce the collective response to a truly life-threatening disaster. In the latter case, individuals may present with symptoms of chemical injury, others may present with acute stress reactions, and the remainder may present with both. The community reaction in Memphis, Tennessee, to the inaccurate perception of a nonexistent toxic waste site showed how perceived exposure instills fear (Harris 1983). Following the perception of risk, the community interpreted all unanswered health problems as caused by the imaginary waste site (Harris 1983). Based on ignorance and poor communication with information agencies, the public developed distrust in government health authorities and became overwhelmed by the threat. Media distortion, a virtually universal event in chemical or radiation disasters, promoted the stress response.

Informing workers of chemical risks may have no effect on psychiatric complaints (Houts and McDougall 1988). Most victims initially respond with denial of both exposure and consequences. When asbestos workers with malignant mesothelioma learned of the apparent role of asbestos in their illness, most denied a causal link, denied personal responsibility, and denied anger at the asbestos industry (Lebovits et al. 1983). Michigan women with breast milk contaminated by polybrominated biphenyls refused testing and denied any effect of the chemical on their breast-fed children; some developed the

TABLE 2–1. Differences between technological and natural disasters

- Technological disasters "pollute, befoul, and taint," not just damage (Krol-Smith and Couch 1991).
- Belief systems concerning toxins may not be reality-based compared with those concerning natural disasters (Kroll-Smith and Couch 1991).
- Technological disasters are expected to have perpetrators, whereas natural disasters are interpreted as "acts of God" (Baum 1986; Reko 1984). Litigation often follows a technological disaster that perpetrates symptoms.
- Assistance offered in technological disaster may be tinged with responsibility (Reko 1984).
- Technological damage may be invisible; natural damage usually is visible. Invisible danger produces greater terror or horror (Baum 1986; Reko 1984).
- Technological disasters usually have no precedent for recovery compared with recovery expectations for natural disasters (Reko 1984).
- Technological disasters may be gradual or sporadic with no agreement on course of action to remedy (Couch and Kroll-Smith 1985; Kasperson and Pijawka 1985).
- The poorer information flow in technological disasters causes greater stress, and information itself is a stressor (Couch and Kroll-Smith 1985; Green et al. 1994).
- Hazard from technological disaster may become persistent and cause victims to experience chronic loss of control; natural disasters usually end rapidly (Baum 1986; Baum et al. 1983; Couch and Kroll-Smith 1985; Green et al. 1994; Kasperson and Pijawka 1985).
- Technological disaster may affect a lower-class community exploited by corporations or government; local leadership and communities may not have the financial ability to respond; "cultural specialization" (e.g., employment at polluting factory) may inhibit response to disaster (Couch and Kroll-Smith 1985).
- Technological disasters are less predictable and less familiar to the public (Baum 1986; Green et al. 1994; Kasperson and Pijawka 1985).
- Technological disasters may symbolize abandonment (Edelstein and Wandersman 1987).
- Technological breakdown is not expected (Baum et al. 1983).
- The "low point" in natural disasters usually is identifiable; it is not always recognized in technological disasters (Baum et al. 1983).

belief that the chemical brought them closer to their babies (Hatcher 1982). A study of daughters' responses when learning from their mothers of being exposed in utero to diethylstilbestrol reported the finding repeatedly seen in mass exposures—that optimal coping results when information comes from trusted sources (Schwartz and Stewart 1977).

Role of Bias

Recall bias occurs some time after an exposure and distorts the measurement of stress. The victim retrospectively reports more symptoms than would be recalled within 24–48 hours of the exposure (Hopwood and Guidotti 1988). The media can induce biased reporting by victims, and investigators using symptom checklists may suggest symptoms to victims. Bias also may result from victims' skepticism about the veracity of manufacturers' reports of the "known" toxic properties of commercial chemicals (Lees-Haley and Brown 1992).

Role of Litigation

Physicians learned many years ago that litigation affects the development and prognosis of symptoms, especially after head and back injuries. Certain medical theories of the nineteenth and early twentieth centuries gave physiological credibility to disability claims later believed to be psychological in origin. Some physicians believed that "railway spine," a common nineteenth-century workers' claim, resulted from "concussion of the spine." Before World War I, medical theory held that "battle neurosis" resulted from microstructural brain lesions (Trimble 1981). Other schools of thought ascribed the psychogenic development of posttraumatic symptoms to imbalances of pretraumatic personality and unconscious desires for compensation and dependency (Keiser 1968). Such opinions defined "compensation neurosis" as "a state of mind, born out of fear, kept alive by avarice, stimulated by lawyers, and cured by a verdict" (Levy 1992, p. 401).

A study of 70 individuals who had no organic findings but were in litigation for injury from noxious fumes identified two "pathways" to symptom development (Brodsky 1983). One group experienced the acute event and developed symptoms. These individuals attributed bodily changes from normal aging to the intoxication or believed that intentional poisoning had occurred. Work stress, secondary gains from sick roles, vindication, and compensation played major roles in generating symptoms. The second group recalled intoxications in the past but did not have acute reactions. They experienced a gradual onset of symptoms, searched for physicians who gave acceptable diagnoses, claimed that they had multiple chemical sensitivities, and showed symptoms of anxiety or psychosis. Keiser (1968) described a third pathway for symptoms. Individuals may recover uneventfully but realize that the accident could lead to financial assistance. The conflict between filing a claim and not filing a claim leads to stress symptoms.

More than 30 different diagnostic terms exist for "compensation neurosis." By current DSM-IV-TR (American Psychiatric Association 2000) criteria, the broad spectrum of these disorders usually includes criteria for somatoform, factitious, or conversion disorders; "other conditions"; or malingering. Symptoms rarely resolve during litigation and frequently do not resolve afterward. Many litigants have real and permanent injuries (Buxton and Hayward 1967; LeQuesne et al. 1976). Risk factors for a poor prognosis following litigation include overprotection by relatives, "total belief" by family members, stress of the legal process, older age, and loss of libido (Tarish and Royston 1985; Weissman 1990). Psychological testing does not always provide sufficient information to rule out malingering in alleged chemical exposures (Lees-Haley 1989a, 1989b, 1989c, 1990).

SYMPTOMS OF STRESS

Regardless of the chemical or radiation involved, acute and chronic stress reactions to perceived exposures have universal similarities (Table 2–2). The array of acute responses to such events was shown after a chemical disaster at Norway's largest paint factory in 1976 (Weisaeth 1989). Many victims completely lost the capacity to think and perceive. Some became stupified, torpid, and completely motionless. Others ran in uncontrolled flight or developed stereotyped actions. A few became leaders and led terrified victims to safety.

Disaster victims may show symptoms of acute stress disorder as defined by DSM-IV-TR. Some individuals develop acute responses when they learn of past chronic exposure. Others may attribute stress symptoms to physiological effects of the chemical agent (Weisaeth 1994). Symptoms also can result from ordinary stressful events following a major disaster (Soloman and Canino 1990). The acute phase of stress may lead to posttraumatic stress disorder or other mood disorder symptoms. Outcome varies with the degree of disaster training, the severity of the threat, and the amount of control experienced by the individual (Weisaeth 1994). Predictors of poorer outcomes include lack of community involvement and poor social supports and communication (Weisaeth 1994). Self-blaming for the trauma predicts better outcome by maintaining the illusion of control (Solomon and Smith 1994).

Nonclinical responses also can develop. These responses consist of changes in attitudes, beliefs, values, or lifestyle. Such responses

TABLE 2–2. Acute and chronic stress reactions to chemical exposures

Acute	*Immediate:* shaking, hyperventilation, breathing problems, palpitations, sweating, nausea, vomiting, diarrhea, motoric paralysis, uncontrolled flight, stereotypical behaviors, helplessness, anxiety, labile emotions
	Acute stress disorder: numbing, detachment, lack of emotional response, reduced awareness of environment, derealization, depersonalization, dissociative amnesia, recurrent thoughts, dreams, flashbacks, anxiety, insomnia, poor concentration, hypervigilance, exaggerated startle response, restlessness
Chronic	*Posttraumatic stress disorder:* similar but persistent symptoms as those described for acute stress disorder
Other	Bereavement, occupational problems, relational problems, malingering, stress-related physiological factors affecting medical condition (American Psychiatric Association 2000)
Quality-of-life changes	Loss of sense of community
	Loss of friends fearful to visit contaminated residences or communities
	Fear of early death or death of family
	Distrust of government or other authorities
	Stigma of being contaminated
	Fear of the destroyed area
	Increased smoking and eating
	Other lifestyle changes (e.g., unable to use local water for extended periods)

affect quality of life but evade quantitative measurement. Nonclinical responses lead to cultural changes, such as the loss of community cohesion. "Grass roots" organizations may replace or oppose economic or political agencies perceived as unable to help or threatening to the community (Gibbs 1983; Kasperson and Pijawka 1985).

The comprehensive picture of combined clinical and nonclinical responses was seen in a disaster in Ohio in 1985 near the Feed Materials Production Center. Residents believed that the center produced livestock feed, only to learn that "feed" referred to nuclear fuel that now contaminated their properties (Green et al. 1994). The "informed of radioactive contamination syndrome" described the combination of chronic clinical responses accompanied by quality-of-life changes.

MASS HYSTERIA

For this chapter, epidemic or mass hysteria or anxiety refers to mass illnesses mimicking outbreaks of toxic chemical exposures or infectious diseases but later attributed to psychogenic origins. A large review of epidemic hysteria found 78 outbreaks in the world's medical literature from 1872 to 1972 (Sirois 1974). Most occurred in schools or villages, but eight outbreaks took place in factories. Before the 1970s, only a few cases of mass hysteria in any setting appeared in American medical literature (Colligan and Smith 1978; Sirois 1974, 1982). The largest event in the United States resulted from the 1938 radio broadcast of H. G. Wells's *War of the Worlds* (Cantril 1940). Another large event occurred in 1954 in Seattle, Washington, during the "windshield pitting epidemic," when hundreds of residents reported damage to thousands of automobile windshields (Medalia and Larsen 1958). Residents attributed the nonexistent damage to radioactive fallout from hydrogen bomb tests in the Pacific Ocean. The first industrial report in the United States appeared in the book *The June Bug,* which described an outbreak attributed to the bites of insects (Kerckhoff and Back 1968). The medical literature contains increasing numbers of industrial outbreaks, possibly from increased awareness of and interest in these events.

Symptoms of Mass Hysteria

Sirois (1974, p. 27) described mass hysteria well:

> The classical outbreak involves a small group of segregated young females; it appears, spreads and subsides rapidly, occasionally re-

> curs, and is easily controlled with the dismemberment of the group. It is manifested by anxious and conversion reactions, sanctioned by the affected group. It is brought about by the activation of latent conflicts relevant to the formation, task and maintenance of the group.

At least 10 different names exist for mass hysteria, reflecting the many hypothesized causes of the illness rather than a variation of symptoms (Boxer 1985). In almost all cases, symptoms have similar characteristics of onset and transmission (Table 2–3). Symptoms in most incidents include headache, dizziness, nausea, dry mouth, and eye, nose, or throat irritation. Two classifications of the symptoms observed in mass hysteria describe the onset of the symptoms and the actual symptoms, respectively. The latter classification differentiates "mass anxiety hysteria" from "mass motor hysteria" (Wessely 1987). In mass anxiety hysteria, panic symptoms of chest tightness, dizziness, fainting, headache, nausea, and palpitations predominate. Seizures, "drop attacks," running, laughing, trances, agitation, and twitching characterize mass motor hysteria. The other classification uses "sudden onset explosive," "explosive with an identifiable prodromal stage," "cumulative outbreak," "rebound outbreak," and "large diffuse outbreak" to identify five types of onset (Sirois 1974). Cumulative outbreaks include "second waves" of hysteria following the initial onset. Rebound outbreaks vary with group dynamics and sizes. Large diffuse outbreaks involve entire communities.

TABLE 2–3. Symptom characteristics in mass hysteria
Diverse symptoms with few objective findings
Absence of usual symptoms produced by putative toxin
Transmission of symptoms not consistent with ventilation flow
Benign morbidity
Recurrence when affected group congregates
Transmission of illness by sight, sound, or both
Epidemic curve indicating "person-to-person" rather than "common-source" transmission
Frequent presence of hyperventilation or syncope
Rapid spread followed by rapid remission with dispersion of group

Table 2–4 lists the environmental factors most often identified in industrial mass hysteria. No specific personality types become involved more frequently (Colligan and Murphy 1979; Olkinuora 1984; Sirois 1974). An accepted mechanism of symptom induction begins with a sense of threat to the group that creates arousal (Olkinuora 1984). The group usually has a generalized belief in the presence of a toxic chemical in the workplace. This is followed by a precipitating event such as an individual fainting. Physiological arousal then develops in other group members. A new belief forms that gives meaning to the arousal that spreads within the group (Olkinuora 1984).

Several factors may induce, define, propagate, or confound mass hysteria. Prior episodes of actual chemical poisonings may sensitize the workforce. Two reports described shops in which a lingering fear of a previous carbon monoxide poisoning induced mass anxiety during a nontoxic event (Sinks et al. 1989; Smith et al. 1978). The transmission of belief in the toxic agent also can flow from an "external group," such as parents who believe a toxic substance poisoned their children, although the children do not hold the belief themselves. These events may represent "mass (hysteria) sociogenic illness by proxy" (Philen et al. 1989).

Cultural beliefs may define the interpretation of arousal experienced by a group. In several episodes of mass hysteria in Singapore factories, Malay females showed symptoms they attributed to "possession" by "jin," or spirits (Chew et al. 1976; Phoon 1982). Treatment of these cases often required help from a "bomoh," or medicine man, believed by the women to rule demons and exorcise spirits (Chew 1978).

TABLE 2–4. Environmental circumstances associated with industrial mass hysteria

Boring, repetitive, monotonous, noisy work
Production pressure/forced overtime
Physical stress or discomfort at the workplace
Poor labor-management relationships
Poor communication between victims
Assembly line/piecework
Poor job security
Unskilled or semiskilled female work force
High degree of management control of workers
High psychosocial stress or lack of social supports
Low wages

Several reports confirmed the power of the media to propagate hysteria (Hefez 1985; Philen et al. 1989; Sparks et al. 1990). In 1944 in Illinois, a woman reported that a man opened her bedroom window and sprayed her with a gas that paralyzed her and made her ill (Johnson 1945). The local newspaper ran the headline "Anesthetist Prowler on Loose," followed by "Mad Anesthetist Strikes Again" after more incidents occurred following the first headline. Many citizens armed themselves, some formed roving bands, and others waited for the phantom anesthetist on their porches and claimed that they could hear the assailant pumping his spray gun.

Although some authors argue not to look for environmental causes (Glotfelty et al. 1987), the majority opinion suggests not to readily attribute psychogenic causes to outbreaks. The precipitating event to mass hysteria may actually be a real poisoning (Aldous et al. 1994; Faust and Brilliant 1981; Troisi 1950). The best example of this involved a group of female workers who were poisoned with mercury (Benning 1958). The psychiatric manifestations of mercury poisoning, such as mood lability, predisposed the poisoned workers to develop additional symptoms of mass hysteria when another group of women collapsed.

Treatment of Mass Hysteria

Treatment consists of managing acute symptoms while ruling out organic causes. Once the diagnosis of mass hysteria is made, it is helpful to speak with employees as a group and review all findings, including the evidence used to rule out toxic and infectious agents (Boxer 1985). The clinician should avoid prescribing medications that have significant side effects so that victims will not confuse the side effects with symptoms from the epidemic. The evaluator should avoid labeling the epidemic psychogenic (Boxer 1985). The psychogenic origins of outbreaks should not be confused with individual "neurosis" or "psychopathology." The events usually result from group process rather than particular personality traits (Colligan 1981). Improvements in the environmental circumstances in Table 2–4 could prevent further incidents.

REFERENCES

Aldous JC, Ellam GA, Murray V, et al: An outbreak of illness among schoolchildren in London: toxic poisoning not mass hysteria. J Epidemiol Community Health 48: 41–45, 1994

American Psychiatric Association: Diagnostic and Statistical Manual of Mental Disorders, 4th Edition, Text Revision. Washington, DC, American Psychiatric Association, 2000

Andelman JB, Underhill DW: Health Effects From Hazardous Waste Sites. Chelsea, MI, Lewis, 1987

Baum A: Toxins, technology, and natural disasters, in Cataclysms, Crises, and Catastrophes: Psychology in Action. Edited by VandenBos GR, Bryant BK. Washington, DC, American Psychological Association, 1986, pp 9–53

Baum A, Fleming R, Davidson LM: Natural disaster and technological catastrophe. Environment and Behavior 15:333–354, 1983

Benning D: Outbreak of mercury poisoning in Ohio. Industrial Medicine and Surgery 27:354–363, 1958

Boxer PA: Occupational mass psychogenic illness: history, prevention, and management. Journal of Occupational Medicine 27:867–872, 1985

Brodsky CM: Psychological factors contributing to somatoform diseases attributed to the workplace. Journal of Occupational Medicine 25:459–464, 1983

Buxton PH, Hayward M: Polyneuritis cranialis associated with industrial trichloroethylene poisoning. J Neurol Neurosurg Psychiatry 30:511–518, 1967

Cantril H: The Invasion From Mars: A Study in the Psychology of Panic. Princeton, NJ, Princeton University Press, 1940

Chew PK: How to handle hysterical factory workers. Occup Health Saf 47:50–53, 1978

Chew PK, Phoon WH, Mae-Lim HA: Epidemic hysteria among some factory workers in Singapore. Singapore Med J 17:10–15, 1976

Colligan MJ: Mass psychogenic illness: some clarification and perspectives. Journal of Occupational Medicine 23:635–638, 1981

Colligan MJ, Murphy LR: Mass psychogenic illness in organizations: an overview. Journal of Occupational Psychology 52:77–90, 1979

Colligan MJ, Smith MJ: A methodological approach for evaluating outbreaks of mass psychogenic illness in industry. Journal of Occupational Medicine 20:401–402, 1978

Committee on Environmental Epidemiology: Environmental Epidemiology: Public Health and Hazardous Wastes. Washington, DC, National Academy Press, 1991

Couch SR, Kroll-Smith JS: The chronic technical disaster: toward a social scientific perspective. Social Science Quarterly 66:564–575, 1985

De La Paz MP: Diet and food contaminants, in Topics in Environmental Epidemiology. Edited by Steenland K, Savitz DA. New York, Oxford University Press, 1997, pp 64–88

Edelstein MR, Wandersman A: Community dynamics in coping with toxic contaminants, in Neighborhood and Community Environments. Edited by Altman I, Wandersman A. New York, Plenum, 1987, pp 69–112

Epstein SS, Brown LO, Pope C: Hazardous Waste in America. San Francisco, CA, Sierra Club, 1982

Faust HS, Brilliant LB: Is the diagnosis of "mass hysteria" an excuse for incomplete investigation of low-level environmental contamination? Journal of Occupational Medicine 23:22–26, 1981

French JG: Air pollution, in The Public Health Consequences of Disasters 1989. Atlanta, GA, Centers for Disease Control, Public Health Service, 1989, pp 91–96

Gibbs LM: Community response to an emergency situation: psychological destruction and the Love Canal. Am J Community Psychol 11:116–125, 1983

Glotfelty DE, Seiber J, Liljedahl LA: Pesticides in fog. Nature 325:602–605, 1987

Green BL, Lindy JD, Grace MC: Psychological effects of toxic contamination, in Individual and Community Responses to Trauma and Disaster: The Structure of Human Chaos. Edited by Ursano RJ, McCaughey BG, Fullerton CS. Cambridge, MA, Cambridge University Press, 1994, pp 154–176

Harr J: A Civil Action. New York, Vintage, 1995

Harris JS: Toxic waste uproar: a community history. J Public Health Policy 4:181–201, 1983

Hatcher SL: The psychological experience of nursing mothers upon learning of a toxic substance in their breast milk. Psychiatry 45:172–181, 1982

Health Aspects of the Disposal of Waste Chemicals. New York, Pergamon, 1986

Hefez A: The role of the press and the medical community in the epidemic of "mysterious gas poisoning" in the Jordon West Bank. Am J Psychiatry 142:833–837, 1985

Holden C: Love Canal residents under stress. Science 208:1242–1244, 1980

Hopwood DG, Guidotti TL: Recall bias in exposed subjects following a toxic exposure incident. Arch Environ Health 43:234–237, 1988

Houts PS, McDougall V: Effects of informing workers of their health risks from exposure to toxic materials. Am J Ind Med 13:271–279, 1988

Johnson DM: The "phantom anesthetist" of Mattoon: a field study of mass hysteria. J Abnorm Soc Psychol 40:175–186, 1945

Karsenty E, Shemer J, Alshech I, et al: Medical aspects of the Iraqi missile attacks on Israel, in Chemical Warfare Medicine: Aspects and Perspectives From the Persian Gulf War. Edited by Danon YL, Shemer J. Jerusalem, Gefen, 1994, pp 38–44

Kasperson RE, Pijawka KD: Societal responses to hazards and major hazard events: comparing natural and technological hazards. Public Administration Review 45:7–18, 1985

Keiser L: The Traumatic Neurosis. Philadelphia, PA, JB Lippincott, 1968

Kerckhoff AC, Back KW: The June Bug: A Study of Hysterical Contagion. New York, Appleton-Century-Crofts, 1968

Kroll-Smith JS, Couch SR: As if exposure to toxins were not enough: the social and cultural system as a secondary stressor. Environ Health Perspect 95:61–66, 1991

Lebovits AH, Chahinian P, Holland JC: Exposure to asbestos: psychological responses of mesothelioma patients. Am J Ind Med 4:459–466, 1983

Lees-Haley PR: Malingering emotional distress on the SCL-90-R: toxic exposure and cancerphobia. Psychol Rep 65:1203–1208, 1989a

Lees-Haley PR: Malingering post-traumatic stress disorder on the MMPI. Forensic Reports 2:89–91, 1989b

Lees-Haley PR: Malingering traumatic mental disorder on the Beck Depression Inventory: cancerphobia and toxic exposure. Psychol Rep 65:623–626, 1989c

Lees-Haley PR: Malingering mental disorder on the Impact of Event Scale (IES): toxic exposure and cancerphobia. J Trauma Stress 3:315–321, 1990

Lees-Haley PR, Brown RS: Biases in perception and reporting following a perceived toxic exposure. Percept Mot Skills 75:531–544, 1992

LeQuesne PM, Axford AT, McKerrow CB, et al: Neurological complications after a single severe exposure to toluene di-isocyanate. British Journal of Industrial Medicine 33:72–78, 1976

Levy A: Compensation neurosis rides again. Brain Inj 6:401–410, 1992

Lopez-Ibor JJ Jr, Soria J, Canas F, et al: Psychopathological aspects of the toxic oil syndrome catastrophe. Br J Psychiatry 147:352–365, 1985

Medalia NZ, Larsen ON: Diffusion and belief in a collective delusion: the Seattle windshield pitting epidemic. Am Sociol Rev 23:180–186, 1958

Melius J, Binder S: Industrial disasters, in The Public Health Consequences of Disasters 1989. Atlanta, GA, Centers for Disease Control, Public Health Service, 1989, pp 97–102

Olkinuora M: Psychogenic epidemics and work. Scand J Work Environ Health 10:501–504, 1984

One Hundred Years of American Psychiatry. New York, Columbia University Press, 1944

Petts J: Stress and public concern over hazardous waste, in Human Stress and the Environment: Health Aspects. Edited by Rose J. Yverdon, Switzerland, Gordon & Breach Science Publishers, 1994, pp 181–208

Philen RM, McKinley TW, Kilbourne EM, et al: Mass sociogenic illness by proxy: parentally reported epidemic in an elementary school. Lancet 2:1372–1376, 1989

Phoon WH: Outbreaks of mass hysteria at workplaces in Singapore: some patterns and modes of presentation, in Mass Psychogenic Illness: A Social Psychological Analysis. Edited by Colligan MJ, Pennebaker JW, Murphy LR. Hillsdale, NJ, Lawrence Erlbaum, 1982, pp 21–31

Rehner TA, Kolbo JR, Trump R, et al: Depression among victims of south Mississippi's methyl parathion disaster. Health Soc Work 25:33–40, 2000

Reko K: The psychosocial impact of environmental disasters. Bull Environ Contam Toxicol 33:655–661, 1984

Schwartz RW, Stewart NB: Psychological effects of diethylstilbestrol exposure. JAMA 237:252–254, 1977

Sinks T, Kerndt PR, Wallingford KM: Two episodes of acute illness in a machine shop. Am J Public Health 79:1024–1028, 1989

Sirois F: Epidemic hysteria. Acta Psychiatr Scand Suppl 252:1–45, 1974

Sirois F: Perspectives on epidemic hysteria, in Mass Psychogenic Illness: A Social Psychological Analysis. Edited by Colligan MJ, Pennebaker JW, Murphy LR. Hillsdale, NJ, Lawrence Erlbaum, 1982, pp 217–236

Smith MJ, Colligan MJ, Hurrell JJ Jr: Three incidents of industrial mass psychogenic illness: a preliminary report. Journal of Occupational Medicine 20:399–400, 1978

Soloman SD, Canino GJ: Appropriateness of DSM-III-R criteria for posttraumatic stress disorder. Compr Psychiatry 31:227–237, 1990

Solomon SD, Smith EM: Social support and perceived control as moderators of responses to dioxin and flood exposure, in Individual and Community Responses to Trauma and Disaster: The Structure of Human Chaos. Edited by Ursano RJ, McCaughey BG, Fullerton CS. Cambridge, MA, Cambridge University Press, 1994, pp 179–200

Sparks PJ, Simon GE, Katon WJ, et al: An outbreak of illness among aerospace workers. West J Med 153:28–33, 1990

Tarish MJ, Royston C: A follow-up study of accident neurosis. Br J Psychiatry 146:18–25, 1985

Trimble MR: Post-Traumatic Neurosis: From Railway Spine to the Whiplash. Chichester, UK, Wiley, 1981

Troisi FM: Chronic intoxication by ethylene glycol vapour. British Journal of Industrial Medicine 7:65–69, 1950

Upton AC, Kneip T, Toniolo P: Public health aspects of toxic chemical disposal sites. Annu Rev Public Health 10:1–25, 1989

Weisaeth L: Stress Reactions to an Industrial Disaster. Oslo, University of Oslo and the Joint Norwegian Armed Forces Medical Services, 1984

Weisaeth L: A study of behavioral responses to an industrial disaster. Acta Psychiatr Scand Suppl 355:13–24, 1989

Weisaeth L: Psychological and psychiatric aspects of technological disasters, in Individual and Community Responses to Trauma and Disaster: The Structure of Human Chaos. Edited by Ursano RJ, McCaughey BG, Fullerton CS. Cambridge, MA, Cambridge University Press, 1994, pp 72–102

Weissman HN: Distortions and deceptions in self presentation: effects of protracted litigation in personal injury cases. Behav Sci Law 8:67–74, 1990

Wessely S: Mass hysteria: two syndromes? Psychol Med 17:109–120, 1987

Withers J: Major Industrial Hazards: Their Appraisal and Control. New York, Halsted Press, 1988

ADDITIONAL READINGS

Chronic Community Exposure

Bachrach KM, Zautra AJ: Coping with a community stressor: the threat of a hazardous waste facility. J Health Soc Behav 26:127–141, 1985

Bachrach KM, Zautra AJ: Assessing the impact of hazardous waste facilities: psychology, politics, and environmental impact statements, in Advances in Environmental Psychology. Edited by Lebovits AH, Baum A, Singer JE. Hillsdale, NJ, Lawrence Erlbaum, 1986, pp 71–88

Baker DB, Greenland S, Mendlein J, et al: A health study of two communities near the Stringfellow waste disposal site. Arch Environ Health 43:325–334, 1988

Bowler RM, Mergler D, Huel G, et al: Psychological, psychosocial, and psychophysiological sequelae in a community affected by a railroad chemical disaster. J Trauma Stress 7:601–624, 1994

Deane M, Sanders G: Health effects of exposure to community odors from pulp mills, Eureka, 1971. Environ Res 14:164–181, 1977

Dunne MP, Burnett P, Lawton J, et al: The health effects of chemical waste in an urban community. Med J Aust 152:592–597, 1990

Fowle SE, Constantine CE, Fone D, et al: An epidemiological study after a water contamination incident near Worcester, England in April 1994. J Epidemiol Community Health 50:18–23, 1996

Gibbs MS: Psychopathological consequences of exposure to toxins in the water supply, in Advances in Environmental Psychology, Vol 6: Exposure to Hazardous Substances: Psychological Parameters. Edited by Lebovits AH, Baum A, Singer JE. Hillsdale, NJ, Lawrence Erlbaum, 1986, pp 47–70

Harris RH, Rodricks JV, Clark CS, et al: Adverse health effects at a Tennessee hazardous waste disposal site, in Health Effects From Hazardous Waste Sites. Edited by Andelman JB, Underhill DW. Chelsea, MI, Lewis Publishers, 1987, pp 221–240

Hertzman C, Hayes M, Singer JE, et al: Upper Ottawa street landfill site health study. Environ Health Perspect 75:173–195, 1987

Horowitz J, Stefanko M: Toxic waste: behavioral effects of an environmental stressor. Behav Med 15:23–28, 1989

Jonsson E, Deane M, Sanders G: Community reactions to odors from pulp mills: a pilot study in Eureka, California. Environ Res 10:249–270, 1975

Lavie P, Carmeli A, Mevorach L, et al: Sleeping under the threat of the Scud: war-related environmental insomnia, in Chemical Warfare Medicine: Aspects and Perspectives From the Persian Gulf War. Edited by Danon YL, Shemer J. Jerusalem, Gefen, 1994, pp 179–185

Logue JN, Fox JM: Residential health study of families living near the Drake Chemical Superfund site in Lock Haven, Pennsylvania. Arch Environ Health 41:222–228, 1986

Logue JN, Stroman RM, Reid D, et al: Investigation of potential health effects associated with well water chemical contamination in Londonderry Township, Pennsylvania, U.S.A. Arch Environ Health 40:155–160, 1985

Neutra R, Lipscomb J, Satin K, et al: Hypotheses to explain the higher symptom rates observed around hazardous waste sites. Environ Health Perspect 94:31–38, 1991

Ozonoff D, Colten ME, Cupples A, et al: Health problems reported by residents of a neighborhood contaminated by a hazardous waste facility. Am J Ind Med 11:581–597, 1987

Paigen B, Goldman LR: Lessons from Love Canal: the role of the public and the use of birth weight, growth, and indigenous wildlife to evaluate health risk, in Health Effects From Hazardous Waste Sites. Edited by Andelman JB, Underhill DW. Chelsea, MI, Lewis Publishers, 1987, pp 177–192

Paigen BJ, Goldman LR, Highland JH, et al: Growth and health in children living near a hazardous waste site (abstract). Pediatr Res 17:179A, 1983
Roht LH, Vernon SW, Weir FW, et al: Community exposure to hazardous waste disposal sites assessing reporting bias. Am J Epidemiol 122:418–433, 1985
Schechter MT, Spitzer WO, Hutcheon ME, et al: Cancer downwind from sour gas refineries: the perception and the reality of an epidemic. Environ Health Perspect 79:283–290, 1989
Shusterman D, Lipscomb J, Neutra R, et al: Symptom prevalence and odor-worry interaction near hazardous waste sites. Environ Health Perspect 94:25–30, 1991
Stephens RD: Integration of government resources in assessment of hazards, in Health Effects From Hazardous Waste Sites. Edited by Andelman JB, Underhill DW. Chelsea, MI, Lewis Publishers, 1987, pp 193–207
Swan SH, Robins JM: Comment. Journal of the American Statistical Association 81:604–609, 1986

Acute Mass Disasters

Ames RG, Howd RA, Doherty L: Community exposure to a paraquat drift. Arch Environ Health 48:47–52, 1993
Campbell D, Cox D, Crum J, et al: Initial effects of the grounding of the tanker Braer on health in Scotland. The Shetland Health Study Group. BMJ 307:1251–1255, 1993
Campbell D, Cox D, Crum J, et al: Later effects of grounding of tanker *Braer* on health in Shetland. BMJ 309:773–774, 1994
Dayal HH, Baranowski T, Li YH, et al: Hazardous chemicals: psychological dimensions of the health sequelae of a community exposure in Texas. J Epidemiol Community Health 48:560–568, 1994
Holden C: Love Canal residents under stress. Science 208:1242–1244, 1980
Hopwood DG, Guidotti TL: Recall bias in exposed subjects following a toxic exposure incident. Arch Environ Health 43:234–237, 1988
Kreutzer RA, Hewitt DJ, Sun R, et al: A community-based epidemiologic study of acute health effects from a metam-sodium spill on California's Sacramento River. Toxicol Ind Health 12:267–275, 1996
Lopez-Ibor JJ Jr, Soria J, Canas F, et al: Psychopathological aspects of the toxic oil syndrome catastrophe. Br J Psychiatry 147:352–365, 1985
Lyons RA, Temple JMF, Evans D, et al: Acute health effects of the Sea Empress oil spill. J Epidemiol Community Health 53:306–310, 1999
Markowitz JS, Gutterman EM: Predictors of psychological distress in the community following two toxic chemical incidents, in Advances in Environmental Psychology, Vol 6: Exposure to Hazardous Substances: Psychological Parameters. Edited by Lebovits AH, Baum A, Singer JE. Hillsdale, NJ, Lawrence Erlbaum, 1986, pp 89–107
Palinkas LA, Petterson JS, Russell J, et al: Community patterns of psychiatric disorders after the Exxon Valdez oil spill. Am J Psychiatry 150:1517–1523, 1993
Robins LN, Fischbach RL, Smith EM, et al: Impact of disaster on previously assessed mental health, in Disaster Stress Studies: New Methods and Findings. Edited by Shore JH. Washington, DC, American Psychiatric Press, 1986, pp 21–48
Sethi BB, Sharma M, Trivedi JK, et al: Psychiatric morbidity in patients attending clinics in gas affected areas in Bhopal. Indian J Med Res 86 (suppl):45–50, 1987
Smith EM, Robins LN, Przybeck TR, et al: Psychosocial consequences of a disaster, in Disaster Stress Studies: New Methods and Findings. Edited by Shore JH. Washington, DC, American Psychiatric Press, 1986, pp 49–76
Soloman SD, Canino GJ: Appropriateness of DSM-III-R criteria for posttraumatic stress disorder. Compr Psychiatry 31:227–237, 1990

Solomon SD, Smith EM: Social support and perceived control as moderators of responses to dioxin and flood exposure, in Individual and Community Responses to Trauma and Disaster: The Structure of Human Chaos. Edited by Ursano RJ, McCaughey BG, Fullerton CS. Cambridge, MA, Cambridge University Press, 1994, pp 179–200

Acute Individual Exposures

Brodsky CM: Psychological factors contributing to somatoform diseases attributed to the workplace. Journal of Occupational Medicine 25:459–464, 1983

Furst JB, Cooper A: Failure of systematic desensitization in 2 cases of obsessive-compulsive neurosis marked by fears of insecticide. Behav Res Ther 8:203–206, 1970

Schottenfeld RS, Cullen MR: Occupation-induced posttraumatic stress disorders. Am J Psychiatry 142:198–202, 1985

Schottenfeld RS, Cullen MR: Recognition of occupation-induced posttraumatic stress disorders. Journal of Occupational Medicine 28:365–369, 1986

Mass Hysteria

Alexander RW, Fedoruk MJ: Epidemic psychogenic illness in a telephone operators' building. Journal of Occupational Medicine 28:42–45, 1986

Araki S, Honma T: Mass psychogenic systemic illness in school children in relation to the Tokyo photochemical smog. Arch Environ Health 41:159–162, 1986

Bartholomew R, Wessely S: Epidemic hysteria in Virginia: the case of the phantom gasser of 1933–1934. South Med J 92:762–769, 1999

Bell A, Jones AT: Fumigation with dichlorethyl ether and chlordane: hysterical sequelae. Med J Aust 2:258–263, 1958

Boxer PA, Singal M, Hartle RW: An epidemic of psychogenic illness in an electronics plant. Journal of Occupational Medicine 26:381–385, 1984

Colligan MJ, Murphy LR: A review of mass psychogenic illness in work settings, in Mass Psychogenic Illness: A Social Psychological Analysis. Edited by Colligan MJ, Pennebaker JW, Murphy LR. Hillsdale, NJ, Lawrence Erlbaum, 1982, pp 33–52

Colligan MJ, Urtes M-A, Wisseman C, et al: An investigation of apparent mass psychogenic illness in an electronics plant. J Behav Med 2:297–309, 1979

Donnell HD, Bagby JR, Harmon RG, et al: Report of an illness outbreak at the Harry S Truman State Office Building. Am J Epidemiol 129:550–558, 1989

Gamino LA, Elkins GR, Hackney KU: Emergency management of mass psychogenic illness. Psychosomatics 30:446–449, 1989

Goh KT: Epidemiological enquiries into a school outbreak of an unusual illness. Int J Epidemiol 16:265–270, 1987

Hall EM, Johnson JV: A case study of stress and mass psychogenic illness in industrial workers. Journal of Occupational Medicine 31:243–250, 1989

Jones TF, Craig AS, Hoy D, et al: Mass psychogenic illness attributed to toxic exposure at a high school. N Engl J Med 342:129–130, 2000

Krug SE: Mass illness at an intermediate school: toxic fumes or epidemic hysteria? Pediatr Emerg Care 8:280–282, 1992

Kurtz PH, Esser TE: A variant of mass (epidemic) psychogenic illness in the agricultural work setting. Journal of Occupational Medicine 31:331–334, 1989

Maguire A: Psychic possession among industrial workers. Lancet 1:376–378, 1978

Modan B, Tirosh M, Weissenberg E, et al: The Arjenyattah epidemic: a mass phenomenon: spread and triggering factors. Lancet 2:1472–1476, 1983

Moffatt MEK: Epidemic hysteria in a Montreal train station. Pediatrics 70:308–310, 1982

Murphy LR, Colligan MJ: Mass psychogenic illness in a shoe factory: a case report. Int Arch Occup Environ Health 44:133–138, 1979

Rockney RM, Lemke T: Casualties from a junior-senior high school during the Persian Gulf War: toxic poisoning or mass hysteria? J Dev Behav Pediatr 13:339–342, 1992

Selden BS: Adolescent epidemic hysteria presenting as a mass casualty, toxic exposure incident. Ann Emerg Med 18:892–895, 1989

Small GW, Borus JF: Outbreak of illness in a school chorus: toxic poisoning or mass hysteria? N Engl J Med 308:632–635, 1983

Small GW, Nicholi AM: Mass hysteria among schoolchildren: early loss as a predisposing factor. Arch Gen Psychiatry 39:721–724, 1982

Small GW, Feinberg DT, Steinberg D, et al: A sudden outbreak of illness suggestive of mass hysteria in schoolchildren. Arch Fam Med 3:711–716, 1994

Sparks PJ, Simon GE, Katon WJ, et al: An outbreak of illness among aerospace workers. West J Med 153:28–33, 1990

Sparks PJ, Ayars GH, Simon GE, et al: Depression and panic attacks related to phenol-formaldehyde composite material exposure in an aerospace manufacturing plant. Allergy Proceedings 12:389–393, 1991

Stahl SM, Lebedun M: Mystery gas: an analysis of mass hysteria. J Health Soc Behav 15:44–50, 1974

3

Ionizing Radiation

Beginning early in the twentieth century, physicians recognized that pelvic irradiation of pregnant women often resulted in the birth of deformed and/or severely mentally retarded children. Irradiated fetuses developed mental retardation and/or microcephaly, especially when exposed between 11 and 20 weeks' gestation (Dekaban 1968). In Japan, the Hiroshima and Nagasaki nuclear explosions confirmed this deleterious effect. Many pregnant women exposed to radiation from the bombs, especially those within 2,000 m of the blasts, gave birth to mentally retarded and/or deformed children. The combined radiation and trauma from the explosions produced other forms of psychiatric casualties, including nonspecific "personality abnormalities" (Konuma 1956; Tsuiki and Iregami 1956). Perhaps "A-bomb neurosis," also known as "burabura" or "do nothing sickness," accounted for the largest number of psychiatric casualties. These victims experienced excessive anxiety over symptoms of exposure and fear of future cancer (Irgens et al. 1991; Yamada et al. 1991).

The effects of direct radiation injury of the brain, including radiation necrosis, were already known by the 1930s from experimental studies and case reports (Mulhern et al. 1991; Pennybacker and Russell 1948; Wachowski and Chenault 1945). Evidence mounted that smaller doses of radiation often resulted in necrotizing leukoencephalopathy, mineralizing microangiopathy with dystrophic calcification, and psychological changes (Bleyer and Griffin 1980). Some studies attributed major mental illnesses to radiation treatment of tinea capitis, or scalp ringworm (Albert and Omran 1968).

The equivalent of "A-bomb neurosis" appeared during the Cold War in some "atomic veterans," or military personnel exposed to military atom bomb tests. Some developed "radiation response syndrome," an elaborate belief that radiation harmed them (Vyner 1983, 1988a, 1988b). Civilian communities also succumbed to the syndrome. So strong and universal was the fear of radiation in the general population that persons receiving radiation therapy for cancer became depressed and anxious, believing the radiation damaged them, even though 60% of them were free of cancer within 18–36 months (Peck and Boland 1977). Mass hysteria developed in Seattle, Washington, when hundreds of citizens believed that radioactive fallout from nuclear testing caused thousands of automobile windshields to develop pitting (Medalia and Larsen 1958). Such reactions also occurred after the Bikini atomic test in the Marshall Islands in 1954, in which nearly 300 individuals were exposed to serious levels of radiation (Conrad 1991). Nonexposed islanders developed severe psychiatric problems based on exaggerated and unfounded fears of the "poisonous powder" or fallout.

An incident in Goiânia, Brazil, in 1987 contributed to understanding the susceptibility of both victims and rescuers in radiation accidents. Scavengers removed cesium from an abandoned radiotherapy institute and gave portions of the "fascinating, glowing, blue material" to friends and relatives (de Carvalho 1991). After the exposures caused many to become ill, a government "rescue team" found the sickest victims alone in the hospital, abandoned by frightened and misinformed medical personnel. The rescuers, mostly technicians and laboratory workers, worked 12–15 hours per day in uncomfortable protective equipment to remove contaminated dwellings. They had no experience in dealing with the aftermath of trauma. Victims physically attacked the rescuers who were tearing down contaminated buildings. Both groups eventually became overwhelmed and traumatized.

Smaller nuclear accidents included the Hanford, California, americium incident in 1976. In an explosion, a laboratory worker was exposed to radiation that required years of treatment (Breitenstein 1991; Brown 1983). Posttraumatic stress symptoms did not develop. Protective characteristics of the person included being a male older than 40 years and having occupational experience, above average intelligence, no history of mental health problems, religious belief, and a high level of disaster training or experience.

More literature exists concerning the psychiatric effects of the Three Mile Island nuclear power plant disaster in Pennsylvania than for any other radiation release. A series of equipment failures, inappropriate procedures, and human error led to a regional threat of radioactive exposure (Kask et al. 1981). The Nuclear Regulatory Commission ordered an evacuation, countermanded by the governor, which caused panic in the population already coping with school closures and police orders to "shoot to kill" looters (Trunk and Trunk 1981). Following the acute danger, residents felt threatened by continued technical problems at the plant, occasional intentional leaks to relieve pressure, plans to reopen the damaged reactor, and constant media attention (Bromet et al. 1982).

The Chernobyl accident in Russia released radioactive iodine, cesium, strontium, and plutonium over major European countries. The disaster disrupted life in the Ukraine, Belorussia, and Russia, causing deaths, disease, environmental damage, lifestyle changes, and physical and psychiatric stress in hundreds of thousands of victims and rescuers (Darby and Reeves 1991; Torubarov 1991). More than 4 million people lived in the contaminated area; 130,000 required immediate evacuation, and 1 million became involved in the cleanup. A 30-km "forbidden area" exists around the site, and 300,000 live in "strict control zones" that require constant monitoring (van den Bout et al. 1995).

SYMPTOMS OF RADIATION EXPOSURE

Table 3–1 lists symptoms of ionizing radiation exposure. Ionizing radiation sources include therapeutic and diagnostic radiation, nuclear fuel, and nuclear fallout (Upton 1998). The symptoms of acute radiation syndrome take four different forms depending on dose and distribution of exposure: cerebral, gastrointestinal, hematopoietic, and pulmonary (Upton 1998). These forms have overlapping symptoms; nausea and vomiting are nearly universal. Symptoms of cerebral and gastrointestinal forms develop early; those of hematopoietic and pulmonary forms usually are delayed.

Psychiatric Symptoms

Psychiatric symptoms occur through several mechanisms (see Table 3–2). The review of therapeutic uses of radiation, atom bomb expo-

TABLE 3–1. Signs and symptoms of ionizing radiation exposure

Acute (hours to days)	Nausea, diarrhea, anorexia, vomiting, headache, disorientation, ataxia, loss of consciousness, seizures, death
Delayed (days to months)	Abdominal pain, fever, dehydration from diarrhea, toxemia, leukopenia, thrombocytopenia, bone marrow failure, epilation, respiratory failure, pulmonary fibrosis, death
Delayed (months to years)	Pulmonary fibrosis, cor pulmonale, leukemia,[a] breast cancer,[a] thyroid cancer,[a] mental retardation of irradiated fetus

[a]Inferred from epidemiological data.

Source. Adapted from Upton AC: "Ionizing Radiation," in *Public Health and Preventive Medicine.* New York, Appleton and Lange, 1998. Used with permission of The McGraw-Hill Companies.

sures, and hypothesized radiation reactions during space missions (Bogo 1988) indicates that children and adults experience radiation-induced cognitive and emotional changes through physiological changes. Prenatal exposure causes mental retardation; its severity is dependent on gestational age. Cranial radiation therapy (CRT) for brain cancer and acute lymphoblastic leukemia often causes mild, acute reactions with nausea, vomiting, headache, and anorexia (Pizzo et al. 1979). These may progress over a period of weeks to early delayed reactions consisting of tingling, paresthesias, fever, irritability, and somnolence, often referred to as *postirradiation syndrome* (Pizzo et al. 1979; Sheline et al. 1980). The literature reflects disagreement concerning the long-term intellectual effects of CRT for brain tumors and acute lymphocytic leukemia in treated children. Some studies indicate an increased risk of delayed intellectual decline in children who develop postirradiation syndrome (Ch'ien et al. 1980). Most studies indicate that mental retardation or intellectual decline following CRT affects a significant number of treated children (Copeland et al. 1999; Fletcher and Copeland 1988; Grill et al. 1999; Leung et al. 2000; Nahum et al. 2001; Palmer et al. 2001; Walter et al. 1999). Severity of the decline often correlates with young age at the time of CRT. Radiation necrosis, a more severe reaction to CRT, results from direct physical injury to the brain. The typical case begins 4–12 months after CRT; progressive neurological problems and dementia develop (Bleyer and Griffin 1980). Some cases may appear years later (Pizzo et al. 1979).

TABLE 3–2. Psychiatric signs and symptoms attributed to direct and traumatic effects of radiation

Therapeutic radiation	
Fetus at 11–20 weeks' gestation	Mental retardation and microcephaly
Children	Greater risk of future psychoses, personality disorders, and neuroses; decrease in cognitive and intellectual performance; mental retardation; fatigue; somnolence (postirradiation syndrome)
Adults	Radiation necrosis: decreased appetite, weakness, depression, nightmares, paranoia, psychosis, labile mood, personality changes, cognitive decline, dementia
Nuclear bombs or accidents	
Exposed fetuses	Mental retardation and microcephaly
Children and adults	Acute stress symptoms, posttraumatic stress symptoms
Children	Personality disorders
Adults	"A-bomb neurosis" or "radiation response syndrome": excessive anxiety over symptoms of exposure, fear of cancer, subclinical stress symptoms

Chemotherapy with methotrexate, and to a lesser degree with nitrosoureas and cytosine arabinoside, enhances the neurotoxicity of CRT (DeAngelis and Shapiro 1991). Other factors that increase the neurotoxicity of CRT include young age, leptomeningeal neoplasms, prolonged CRT exposure, and high doses of intrathecal or intravenous methotrexate (DeAngelis and Shapiro 1991). Structural damage to the brain, a history of seizures, young age at the time of treatment, and more than one course of CRT increase the risk for neuropsychological abnormalities (Mulhern et al. 1991). Brain imaging usually detects leukoencephalopathy with white matter hypodensity in both cerebral hemispheres, preserved gray matter, multiple necrotic areas, and vascular changes (DeAngelis and Shapiro 1991). Intracerebral calcification from mineralizing microangiopathy correlates with greater neuropsychological dysfunction than cortical atrophy on computed tomography (Brouwers et al. 1985). Children receiving CRT should have formal psychometric testing before or during treatment followed by yearly testing for 5 years (Mulhern et al. 1991). Some authors recommend 1,800 cGy rather than the previous standard of 2,400 cGy for CRT (Mulhern et al. 1991). Use of hyperfractionated doses may also minimize cognitive decline (Murray et al. 2000; Riva and Giorgi 2000; Wenz et al. 2000).

Experiences at Hiroshima, Three Mile Island, and Chernobyl suggested that stress responses to radiation events are similar regardless of culture. Hiroshima survivors developed "burabura" or "do nothing sickness" in response to trauma (Hocking 1970). At Three Mile Island, residents closest to the facility developed stress symptoms, but women with preschool children developed more severe problems (Dohrenwend et al. 1981). Women around Three Mile Island perceived a greater health threat than did men, wanted to move away, developed worse attitudes toward nuclear power, and had less trust in authorities than did the men (Dohrenwend et al. 1981). Several studies reported that symptoms in mothers persisted for 10 years (Bromet 1991; Bromet et al. 1982; Davidson et al. 1986). Women near Chernobyl also reported more psychiatric symptoms, had greater risk for psychiatric symptoms if they were mothers, and developed greater opposition to nuclear power (Havenaar et al. 1997; Sjoberg and Drottz 1987). Unlike Three Mile Island, where mental health patients in the region did not experience exacerbation of their illnesses, patients with chronic psychiatric illnesses near Chernobyl had worse symptoms for up to 1 year (Spivak 1992). Similar to Hiroshima survivors, Chernobyl victims had acute stress reactions followed by fears about future health, anxiety, and depression (Spivak 1992).

Accounts from Chernobyl (van den Bout et al. 1995) provide a concise description of the expected psychosocial reactions in radiation disasters. Victims attributed every physical ailment to radiation exposure, evacuees experienced hostile receptions, no one could define safe radiation levels, physicians moved away from the disaster area, changes in lifestyle and insecurity over the food supply occurred, universal distrust in official information developed, and anxiety, depression, acute stress, and posttraumatic stress disorder appeared. The invisibility of radiation, the difficulty of measuring exposure, and the unpredictability of prognosis contributed to stress (Vyner 1988a, 1988b). Many victims at Chernobyl developed acute radiation illness accompanied by depression and neurovegetative complaints. Those persons with mild to moderate exposures had especially difficult reactions to the deaths of the severely irradiated persons (Torubarov 1991). At the onset of their symptoms, survivors required medical restrictions and aseptic regimens. They identified with those who died and became fearful of similar outcomes. Their recoveries over 5 years became complicated by uncertainty about the future, loss of home and property, fear of future health consequences, and changes in lifestyles (Torubarov 1991). In the 10 years following the disaster, one study found a significant increase in the incidence of schizophrenia in workers from the contaminated zone around Chernobyl; the increase was attributed to radiation-induced left frontotemporal limbic dysfunction (Loganovsky and Loganovskaya 2000).

Following the acute phase of the Chernobyl disaster, local physicians diagnosed an epidemic of "vegetative dystonia" in children, manifested by fatigue, pallor, inattention, headache, abdominal pain, poor school performance, clammy extremities, and other nonspecific findings. Russian physicians used non-Western techniques of diagnosis, followed by long and ineffective inpatient treatments (Stiehm 1992). Inexperience and ignorance concerning radiation exposures allowed these inappropriate diagnostic and treatment interventions. Stiehm (1992) used Western medical methods and found no abnormalities in the children; they were given diagnoses of "chronic fatigue syndrome by proxy." Recent studies of children exposed in utero to age 15 months at the time of the disaster found no neuropsychological or school performance differences between exposed and control children (Igumnov and Drozdovitch 2000; Litcher et al. 2000).

DIAGNOSIS AND TREATMENT OF RADIATION EXPOSURE

Diagnosis of radiation exposure relies on history and physical symptoms. DSM-IV-TR (American Psychiatric Association 2000) specifies the diagnosis of dementia due to other general medical conditions for instances of dementia secondary to intracranial radiation. Brain imaging assists the diagnosis of radiation necrosis. Neuropsychological testing may help assess cognitive changes after therapeutic or accidental exposures.

Treatment of acute symptoms remains supportive, whereas long-term developments require more specific interventions. Psychiatric treatment of acute exposures requires initial management of acute stress reactions, often in a mass casualty environment, followed by individual treatment for posttraumatic stress disorder or other mood disorders in certain survivors. As seen in nuclear disasters, the lack of training and awareness of dangers in rescuers contributes to the disaster (Torubarov 1991). Ross (1952) emphasized the pertinence of reading John Hersey's (1946) *Hiroshima* in preparing for psychiatric response to nuclear accidents and attacks.

REFERENCES

Albert RE, Omran AR: Follow-up study of patients treated by x-ray epilation for tinea capitis. Arch Environ Health 17:899–918, 1968

American Psychiatric Association: Diagnostic and Statistical Manual of Mental Disorders, 4th Edition, Text Revision. Washington, DC, American Psychiatric Association, 2000

Bleyer WA, Griffin TW: White matter necrosis, mineralizing microangiopathy, and intellectual abilities in survivors of childhood leukemia: associations with central nervous system irradiation and methotrexate therapy, in Radiation Damage to the Nervous System: A Delayed Therapeutic Hazard. Edited by Gilbert HA, Kagan AR. New York, Raven, 1980, pp 155–174

Bogo V: Radiation: behavioral implications in space. Toxicology 49:299–307, 1988

Breitenstein BD Jr: The 1976 Hanford americium accident: psychological effects on the patient, his family, and caregivers, in The Medical Basis for Radiation-Accident Preparedness, III: The Psychological Perspective. Edited by Ricks RC, Berger ME, O'Hara FM Jr. New York, Elsevier, 1991, pp 193–198

Bromet EJ: Psychologic effects of the radiation accident at TMI, in The Medical Basis for Radiation-Accident Preparedness, III: The Psychological Perspective. Edited by Ricks RC, Berger ME, O'Hara FM Jr. New York, Elsevier, 1991, pp 61–70

Bromet E, Parkinson D, Schulberg HC, et al: Mental health of residents near the Three Mile Island reactor: a comparative study of selected groups. Journal of Preventative Psychiatry 1:225–276, 1982

Brouwers P, Riccardi R, Fedio P, et al: Long-term neuropsychologic sequelae of childhood leukemia: correlation with CT brain scan abnormalities. J Pediatr 106:723–728, 1985

Brown WR: 1976 Hanford americium exposure incident: phychological [sic] aspects. Health Phys 45:867–871, 1983

Ch'ien LT, Aur RJ, Stagner S, et al: Long-term neurological implications of somnolence syndrome in children with acute lymphocytic leukemia. Ann Neurol 8:273–277, 1980

Conrad RA: Direct and outside influences on the psychological health of a Marshall Island population exposed to radioactive fallout, in The Medical Basis for Radiation-Accident Preparedness, III: The Psychological Perspective. Edited by Ricks RC, Berger ME, O'Hara FM Jr. New York, Elsevier, 1991, pp 165–171

Copeland DR, deMoor C, Moore BD 3rd, et al: Neurocognitive development of children after a cerebellar tumor in infancy: a longitudinal study. J Clin Oncol 17:3476–3486, 1999

Darby S, Reeves GK: Lessons of Chernobyl: psychological problems seem to be the major health effect at present. BMJ 303:1347–1348, 1991

Davidson LM, Baum A, Fleming R, et al: Toxic exposure and chronic stress at Three Mile Island, in Advances in Environmental Psychology. Edited by Lebovits AH, Baum A, Singer JE. Hillsdale, NJ, Lawrence Erlbaum, 1986, pp 35–46

DeAngelis LM, Shapiro WR: Drug/radiation interactions and central nervous system injury, in Radiation to the Nervous System. Edited by Gutin PH, Leibel SA, Sheline GE. New York, Raven, 1991, pp 361–382

de Carvalho AB: The psychological effects of the Goiania radiological accident on the emergency responders, in The Medical Basis for Radiation-Accident Preparedness, III: The Psychological Perspective. Edited by Ricks RC, Berger ME, O'Hara FM Jr. New York, Elsevier, 1991, pp 131–141

Dekaban AS: Abnormalities in children exposed to x-radiation during various stages of gestation: tentative timetable of radiation injury to the human fetus, part 1. J Nucl Med 9:471–477, 1968

Dohrenwend BP, Dohrenwend BS, Warheit GJ, et al: Stress in the community: a report to the president's commission on the accident at Three Mile Island. Ann N Y Acad Sci 365:159–174, 1981

Fletcher JM, Copeland DR: Neurobehavioral effects of central nervous system prophylactic treatment of cancer in children. J Clin Exp Neuropsychol 10:495–538, 1988

Grill J, Renaux VK, Bulteau C, et al: Long-term intellectual outcome in children with posterior fossa tumors according to radiation doses and volumes. Int J Radiat Oncol Biol Phys 45:137–145, 1999

Havenaar JM, Rumyantzeva GM, van den Brink W, et al: Long-term mental health effects of the Chernobyl disaster: an epidemiologic survey in two former Soviet regions. Am J Psychiatry 154:1605–1607, 1997

Hersey J: Hiroshima. New York, Knopf, 1946

Hocking F: Psychiatric aspects of extreme environmental stress. Diseases of the Nervous System 31:542–545, 1970

Igumnov S, Drozdovitch V: The intellectual development, mental and behavioural disorders in children from Belarus exposed in utero following the Chernobyl accident. Eur Psychiatry 15:244–253, 2000

Irgens LM, Lie RT, Ulstein M, et al: Pregnancy outcome in Norway after Chernobyl. Biomed Pharmacother 45:233–241, 1991

Kask SV, Chisholm RF, Eskenazi B: The impact of the accident at the Three Mile Island on the behavior and well-being of nuclear workers, part 1: perceptions and evaluations, behavioral responses, and work-related attitudes and feelings. Am J Public Health 71:472–483, 1981

Konuma M: Neuropsychiatric case-studies on the atomic bomb casualties at Hiroshima, in Research in the Effects and Influences of the Nuclear Bomb Test Explosions II. Tokyo, Japan Society for the Promotion of Science, 1956, pp 1715–1720

Leung W, Hudson MM, Strickland DK, et al: Late effects of treatment in survivors of childhood acute myeloid leukemia. J Clin Oncol 18:3273–3279, 2000

Litcher L, Bromet EJ, Carlson G, et al: School and neuropsychological performance of evacuated children in Kyiv 11 years after the Chernobyl disaster. J Child Psychol Psychiatry 41:291–299, 2000

Loganovskya KN, Loganovskaya TK: Schizophrenia spectrum disorders in persons exposed to ionizing radiation as a result of the Chernobyl accident. Schizophr Bull 26:751–773, 2000

Medalia NZ, Larsen ON: Diffusion and belief in a collective delusion: the Seattle windshield pitting epidemic. American Sociological Review 23:180–186, 1958

Mulhern RK, Ochs J, Kun LE: Changes in intellect associated with cranial radiation therapy, in Radiation Injury to the Nervous System. Edited by Gutin PH, Leibel SA, Sheline GE. New York, Raven, 1991, pp 325–340

Murray KJ, Scott C, Zachariah B, et al: Importance of the Mini-Mental Status Examination in the treatment of patients with brain metastases: a report from the Radiation Therapy Oncology Group protocol 91-04. Int J Radiat Oncol Biol Phys 48: 59–64, 2000

Nahum MP, Gdal-On M, Kuten A, et al: Long-term follow-up of children with retinoblastoma. Pediatr Hematol Oncol 18:173–179, 2001

Palmer SL, Goloubeva O, Reddick WE, et al: Patterns of intellectual development among survivors of pediatric medulloblastoma: a longitudinal analysis. J Clin Oncol 19:2302–2308, 2001

Peck A, Boland J: Emotional reactions to radiation treatment. Cancer 40:180–184, 1977

Pennybacker J, Russell DS: Necrosis of the brain due to radiation therapy: clinical and pathological observations. J Neurol Neurosurg Psychiatry 11:183–198, 1948

Pizzo PA, Poplack DG, Bleyer WA: Neurotoxicities of current leukemia therapy. American Journal of Pediatric Hematology/Oncology 1:127–140, 1979

Riva D, Giorgi C: The neurodevelopmental price of survival in children with malignant brain tumours. Childs Nerv Syst 16:751–754, 2000

Ross WD: The emotional effects of an atomic incident. Cincinnati Journal of Medicine 33:38–41, 1952

Sheline GE, Wara WM, Smith V: Therapeutic irradiation and brain injury. Int J Radiat Oncol Biol Phys 6:1215–1228, 1980

Sjoberg L, Drottz B-M: Psychological reactions to cancer risks after the Chernobyl accident. Medical Oncology and Tumor Pharmacotherapy 4:259–271, 1987

Spivak LI: Psychiatric aspects of the accident at Chernobyl nuclear power station. European Journal of Psychiatry 6:207–212, 1992

Stiehm ER: The psychologic fallout from Chernobyl. American Journal of Diseases of Children 146:761–762, 1992

Torubarov FS: Psychological consequences of the Chernobyl accident from the radiation neurology point of view, in The Medical Basis for Radiation-Accident Preparedness, III: The Psychological Perspective. Edited by Ricks RC, Berger ME, O'Hara FM Jr. New York, Elsevier, 1991, pp 81–91

Trunk AD, Trunk EV: Three Mile Island: a resident's perspective. Ann N Y Acad Sci 365:175–185, 1981

Tsuiki S, Iregami A: Personality tests on the atomic bomb exposed children, in Research in the Effects and Influences of the Nuclear Bomb Test Explosions II. Tokyo, Japan Society for the Promotion of Science, 1956, pp 1709–1714

Upton AC: Ionizing radiation, in Public Health and Preventive Medicine. Edited by Wallace RB, Doebbeling BN, Last JM. Stamford, CT, Appleton & Lange, 1998, pp 619–626

van den Bout J, Havenaar JM, Meijler-Iljina LI: Health problems in areas contaminated by the Chernobyl disaster, in Beyond Trauma: Cultural and Societal Dynamics. Edited by Kleber RJ, Figley CR, Gersons BPR. New York, Plenum, 1995, pp 213–231

Vyner HM: The psychological effects of ionizing radiation. Cult Med Psychiatry 7: 241–261, 1983

Vyner HM: Invisible Trauma: The Psychosocial Effects of Invisible Environmental Contaminants. Lexington, MA, Lexington Books, 1988a

Vyner HM: The psychological dimensions of health care for patients exposed to radiation and the other invisible contaminants. Soc Sci Med 27:1097–1103, 1988b

Wachowski TJ, Chenault H: Degenerative effects of large doses of roentgen rays on the human brain. Radiology 45:227–246, 1945

Walter AW, Mulhern RK, Gajjar A, et al: Survival and neurodevelopmental outcome of young children with medulloblastoma at St Jude Children's Research Hospital. J Clin Oncol 17:3720–3728, 1999

Wenz F, Steinvorth S, Lohr F, et al: Prospective evaluation of delayed central nervous system (CNS) toxicity of hyperfractionated total body irradiation (TBI). Int J Radiat Oncol Biol Phys 48:1497–1501, 2000

Yamada M, Kodama K, Wong FL: The long-term psychological sequelae of atomic-bomb survivors in Hiroshima and Nagasaki, in The Medical Basis for Radiation-Accident Preparedness, III: The Psychological Perspective. Edited by Ricks RC, Berger ME, O'Hara FM Jr. New York, Elsevier, 1991, pp 155–163

ADDITIONAL READINGS

Irradiation of Tinea Capitis

Albert RE, Omran AR, Brauer EW, et al: Follow-up study of patients treated by x-ray for tinea capitis. Am J Public Health 56:2114–2120, 1966

Omran AR, Shore RE, Markoff RA, et al: Follow-up study of patients treated by x-ray epilation for tinea capitis: psychiatric and psychometric evaluation. Am J Public Health 68:561–567, 1978

Ron E, Modan B, Floro S, et al: Mental function following scalp irradiation during childhood. Am J Epidemiol 116:149–160, 1982

Shore RE, Albert RE, Pasternack BS: Follow-up study of patients treated by x-ray epilation for tinea capitis. Arch Environ Health 31:17–24, 1976

Yaar I, Ron E, Modan M, et al: Long-term cerebral effects of small doses of x-irradiation in childhood as manifested in adult visual evoked responses. Ann Neurol 8:261–268, 1980

Yaar I, Ron E, Modan B, et al: Long-lasting cerebral functional changes following moderate dose x-radiation treatment to the scalp in childhood: an electroencephalographic power spectral study. J Neurol Neurosurg Psychiatry 45:166–169, 1982

Yaar I, Ron E, Modan B, et al: Long term electroencephalographic changes caused by low therapeutic x-radiation doses to the scalp in childhood: a power spectral study (abstract). Electroencephalogr Clin Neurophysiol 43:494, 1977

Irradiation of Pregnant Women

Goldstein L, Murphy DP: Etiology of the ill-health in children born after maternal pelvic irradiation. American Journal of Roentgenology and Radium Therapy 22:322–331, 1929a

Goldstein L, Murphy DP: Microcephalic idiocy following radium therapy for uterine cancer during pregnancy. Am J Obstet Gynecol 18:189–195, 1929b

Maxfield FN: A case of microcephaly following prenatal roentgen irradiation. American Journal of Mental Deficiency 45:358–365, 1941

Murphy DP: The outcome of 625 pregnancies in women subjected to pelvic radium or roentgen irradiation. Am J Obstet Gynecol 18:179–187, 1929a

Murphy DP: Ovarian irradiation and the health of the subsequent child: a review of more than two hundred previously unreported pregnancies in women subjected to pelvic irradiation. Surgery, Gynecology, and Obstetrics 48:766–779, 1929b

Murphy DP, Shirlock ME, Doll EA: Microcephaly following maternal pelvic irradiation for the interruption of pregnancy: report of a case. American Journal of Roentgenology and Radium Therapy 48:356–359, 1942

Irradiation of Brain Tumors and Acute Lymphocytic Leukemia

Armstrong CL, Corn BW, Ruffer JE, et al: Radiotherapeutic effects on brain function: double dissociation of memory systems. Neuropsychiatry Neuropsychol Behav Neurol 13:101–111, 2000

Aron BS: Medulloblastoma in children twenty-two years' experience with radiation therapy. American Journal of Diseases of Children 121:314–317, 1971

Aronson S, Elmquist D, Garwicz S: Somnolence in children with acute leukaemia (letter). BMJ 3:344, 1974

Bamford FN, Jones PM, Pearson D, et al: Residual disabilities in children treated for intracranial space-occupying lesions. Cancer 37:1149–1151, 1976

Berg RA, Ch'ien LT, Bowman WP, et al: The neuropsychological effects of acute lymphocytic leukemia and its treatment—a three year report: intellectual functioning and academic achievement. Clinical Neuropsychology 5:9–13, 1983a

Berg RA, Ch'ien LT, Lancaster W, et al: Neuropsychological sequelae of postradiation somnolence syndrome. J Dev Behav Pediatr 4:103–107, 1983b

Blonder LX, Hodes JE, Ranseen JD, et al: Short-term neuropsychological outcome following gamma knife radiosurgery for arteriovenous malformations: a preliminary report. Applied Neuropsychology 6:181–186, 1999

Bloom HJG, Wallace ENK, Henk JM: The treatment and prognosis of medulloblastoma in children. American Journal of Roentgenology, Radium Therapy and Nuclear Medicine 105:43–62, 1969

Bouchard J, Peirce CB: Radiation therapy in the management of neoplasms of the central nervous system, with a special note in regard to children: twenty years' experience, 1939–1958. American Journal of Roentgenology, Radium Therapy and Nuclear Medicine 84:610–628, 1960

Broadbent VA, Barnes ND, Wheeler TK: Medulloblastoma in childhood: long-term results of treatment. Cancer 48:26–30, 1981

Catane R, Schwade JG, Yarr I, et al: Follow-up neurological evaluation in patients with small cell lung carcinoma treated with prophylactic cranial irradiation and chemotherapy. Int J Radiat Oncol Biol Phys 7:105–109, 1981

Cetingul N, Aydinok Y, Kantar M, et al: Neuropsychologic sequelae in the long-term survivors of childhood acute lymphoblastic leukemia. Pediatr Hematol Oncol 16:213–220, 1999

Chak LY, Zatz LM, Wasserstein P, et al: Neurologic dysfunction in patients treated for small cell carcinoma of the lung: a clinical and radiological study. Int J Radiat Oncol Biol Phys 12:385–389, 1986

Cheung M, Chan AS, Law SC, et al: Cognitive function of patients with nasopharyngeal carcinoma with and without temporal lobe radionecrosis. Arch Neurol 57: 1347–1352, 2000

Chin HW, Maruyama Y: Age at treatment and long-term performance results in medulloblastoma. Cancer 53:1952–1958, 1984

Copeland DR, Fletcher JM, Pfefferbaum-Levine B, et al: Neuropsychological sequelae of childhood cancer in long-term survivors. Pediatrics 75:745–753, 1985

Craig JB, Jackson DV, Moody D, et al: Prospective evaluation of changes in computed cranial tomography in patients with small cell lung carcinoma treated with chemotherapy and prophylactic cranial irradiation. J Clin Oncol 2:1151–1156, 1984

Danoff BF, Cowchock FS, Marquette C, et al: Assessment of the long-term effects of primary radiation therapy for brain tumors in children. Cancer 49:1580–1586, 1982

Davidson A, Tait DM, Payne GS, et al: Magnetic resonance spectroscopy in the evaluation of neurotoxicity following cranial irradiation for childhood cancer. Br J Radiol 73:421–424, 2000

De Winter AE, Moore BD III, et al: Brain tumors in children with neurofibromatosis: additional neuropsychological morbidity? Neuro-oncology 1:275–281, 1999

Eiser C: Intellectual abilities among survivors of childhood leukaemia as a function of CNS irradiation. Arch Dis Child 53:391–395, 1978

Eiser C, Lansdown R: Retrospective study of intellectual development in children treated for acute lymphoblastic leukaemia. Arch Dis Child 52:525–529, 1977

Ellenberg L, McComb G, Siegel SE, et al: Factors affecting intellectual outcome in pediatric brain tumor patients. Neurology 21:638–644, 1987

Fonseca R, O'Neill BP, Foote RL, et al: Cerebral toxicity in patients treated for small cell carcinoma of the lung. Mayo Clin Proc 74:461–465, 1999

Freeman JE, Johnston PGB, Voke JM: Somnolence after prophylactic cranial irradiation in children with acute lymphoblastic leukaemia. BMJ 4:523–525, 1973

Fuss M, Poljanc K, Hug EB: Full-scale IQ (FSIQ) changes in children treated with whole brain and partial brain irradiation: a review and analysis. Strahlenther Onkol 176:573–581, 2000

Hakansson CH, Lindgren M, Sulg IA: EEG effects of postoperative irradiation treatment of brain tumours. Acta Radiologica Therapy, Physics and Biology 8:301–310, 1969

Hirsch JF, Renier D, Czernichow P, et al: Medulloblastoma in childhood: survival and functional results. Acta Neurochir (Wien) 48:1–15, 1979

Hochberg FH, Slotnick B: Neuropsychologic impairment in astrocytoma survivors. Neurology 30:172–177, 1980

Ivnik RJ, Colligan RC, Obetz SW, et al: Neuropsychologic performance among children in remission from acute lymphocytic leukemia. Dev Behav Pediatr 2:29–34, 1981

Jenkins RDT: Medulloblastoma in childhood: radiation therapy. Canadian Medical Association Journal 100:51–53, 1969

Johnson BE, Becker B, Goff WB, et al: Neurologic, neuropsychologic, and computed cranial tomography scan abnormalities in 2- to 10-year survivors of small-cell lung cancer. J Clin Oncol 3:1659–1667, 1985

Kieffer-Renaux V, Bulteau C, Grill J, et al: I. Patterns of neuropsychological deficits in children with medulloblastoma according to craniospatial irradiation doses. Dev Med Child Neurol 42:741–745, 2000

Kun LE, Mulhern RK, Crisco J: Quality of life in children treated for brain tumors: intellectual, emotional, and academic function. J Neurosurg 58:1–6, 1983

Lansky SB, Cairns NU, Lansky LL, et al: Central nervous system prophylaxis. American Journal of Pediatric Hematology/Oncology 6:183–190, 1984

Lee JS, Umsawasdi T, Lee Y-Y, et al: Neurotoxicity in long-term survivors of small cell lung cancer. Int J Radiat Oncol Biol Phys 12:313–321, 1986

Lieberman AN, Foo SH, Ransohoff J, et al: Long term survival among patients with malignant brain tumors. Neurosurgery 10:450–453, 1982

Lilja AM, Portin RI, Hamalainen PI, et al: Short-term effects of radiotherapy on attention and memory performances in patients with brain tumors. Cancer 91:2361–2368, 2001

Longeway K, Mulhern RK, Crisco J, et al: Treatment of meningeal relapse in childhood acute lymphoblastic leukemia, II: a prospective study of intellectual loss specific to CNS relapse and therapy. American Journal of Pediatric Hematology/Oncology 12:45–50, 1990

Martins AN, Johnston JS, Henry JM, et al: Delayed radiation necrosis of the brain. J Neurosurg 47:336–345, 1977

McIntosh S, Klatskin EH, O'Brien RT, et al: Chronic neurologic disturbance in childhood leukemia. Cancer 37:853–857, 1976

Meadows AT, Massari DJ, Fergusson J, et al: Declines in IQ scores and cognitive dysfunctions in children with acute lymphocytic leukaemia treated with cranial irradiation. Lancet 2:1015–1018, 1981

Mealey J Jr, Hall PV: Medulloblastoma in children: survival and treatment. J Neurosurg 46:56–64, 1977

Merchant TE, Sherwood SH, Mulhern RK, et al: CNS germinoma: disease control and long-term functional outcome for 12 children treated with craniospinal irradiation. Int J Radiat Oncol Biol Phys 46:1171–1176, 2000

Meyers CA, Geara F, Wong PF, et al: Neurocognitive effects of therapeutic irradiation for base of skull tumors. Int J Radiat Oncol Biol Phys 46:51–55, 2000

Moss HA, Nannis ED, Poplack DG: The effects of prophylactic treatment of the central nervous system on the intellectual functioning of children with acute lymphocytic leukemia. Am J Med 71:47–52, 1981

Mulhern RK, Ochs J, Fairclough D, et al: Intellectual and academic achievement status after CNS relapse: a retrospective analysis of 40 children treated for acute lymphoblastic leukemia. J Clin Oncol 5:933–940, 1987

Mulhern RK, Kovnar EH, Kun LE, et al: Psychologic and neurologic function following treatment for childhood temporal lobe astrocytoma. J Child Neurol 3:47–52, 1988

Mulhern R, Reddick WE, Palmer SL, et al: Neurocognitive deficits in medulloblastoma survivors and white matter loss. Ann Neurol 46:834–841, 1999

Mulhern RK, Wasserman AL, Fairclough D, et al: Memory function in disease-free survivors of childhood acute lymphocytic leukemia given CNS prophylaxis with or without 1,800 cGy cranial irradiation. J Clin Oncol 6:315–320, 1988

Nakagawa K, Tago M, Terahara A, et al: A single institutional outcome analysis of Gamma Knife radiosurgery for single or multiple brain metastases. Clin Neurol Neurosurg 102:227–232, 2000

Obetz SW, Smithson WA, Groover RV, et al: Neuropsychologic follow-up study of children with acute lymphocytic leukemia. American Journal of Pediatric Hematology/Oncology 1:207–213, 1979

Ochs J, Parvey LS, Mulhern R: Prospective study of central nervous system changes in children with acute lymphoblastic leukemia receiving two different methods of central nervous system prophylaxis. Neurotoxicology 7:217–226, 1986

Ogawa K, Toita T, Kakinohana Y, et al: A patient with improvement in short-term memory disturbance brought about by radiation therapy for germinoma involving Papez circuit. Radiat Med 17:317–322, 1999

Oi S, Raimondi AJ: Ependymoma in children: the tumor location and its clinical significance. Child's Brain 5:550–551, 1979

O'Neill BP, Wang CH, O'Fallon JR, et al: The consequences of treatment and disease in patients with primary CNS non-Hodgkin's lymphoma: cognitive function and performance status. North Central Cancer Treatment Group. Neuro-oncology 1:196–203, 1999

Parageorgiou C, Dardoufas C, Kouloulias V, et al: Psychophysiological evaluation of short-term neurotoxicity after prophylactic brain irradiation in patients with small cell lung cancer: a study of event related potentials. J Neuro-oncol 50:275–285, 2000

Pavlovsky S, Fisman N, Arizaga R, et al: Neuropsychological study in patients with ALL. American Journal of Pediatric Hematology/Oncology 5:79–86, 1983

Peck FC, McGovern ER: Radiation necrosis of the brain in acromegaly. J Neurosurg 25:536–542, 1966

Pennybacker J, Russell DS: Necrosis of the brain due to radiation therapy: clinical and pathological observations. J Neurol Neurosurg Psychiatry 11:183–198, 1948

Peylan-Ramu N, Poplack DG, Pizzo PA, et al: Abnormal CT scans of the brain in asymptomatic children with acute lymphocytic leukemia after prophylactic treatment of the central nervous system with radiation and intrathecal chemotherapy. N Engl J Med 298:815–818, 1978

Pfefferbaum-Levine B, Copeland DR, Fletcher JM, et al: Neuropsychologic assessment of long-term survivors of childhood leukemia. American Journal of Pediatric Hematology/Oncology 6:123–128, 1984

Raimondi AJ, Tomita T: The disadvantages of prophylactic whole CNS postoperative radiation therapy for medulloblastoma, in Multidisciplinary Aspects of Brain Tumor Therapy. Edited by Paoletti P, Walker MD, Butti G, et al: Amsterdam, Elsevier, 1979, pp 209–218

Regine WF, Scott C, Murray K, et al: Neurocognitive outcome in brain metastases patients treated with accelerated-fractionation vs accelerated-hyperfractioned radiotherapy: an analysis from Radiation Therapy Oncology Group Study 91-04. Int J Radiat Oncol Biol Phys 51:711–717, 2001

Ris MD, Packer R, Goldwin J, et al: Intellectual outcome after reduced-dose radiation therapy plus adjuvant chemotherapy for medulloblastoma: a Children's Cancer Group study. J Clin Oncol 19:3470–3476, 2001

Robison LL, Nesbit ME Jr, Sather HN, et al: Factors associated with IQ scores in long-term survivors of childhood acute lymphoblastic leukemia. American Journal of Pediatric Hematology/Oncology 6:115–121, 1984

Rowland JH, Glidewell OJ, Sibley RF, et al: Effects of different forms of central nervous system prophylaxis on neuropsychologic function in childhood leukemia. J Clin Oncol 2:1327–1335, 1984

Sands SA, Kellie SJ, Davidow AL, et al: Long-term quality of life and neuropsychologic functioning for patients with CNS germ-cell tumors: from the First International CNS Germ-Cell Tumor Study. Neuro-oncology 3:174–183, 2001

Schatz J, Kramer JH, Ablin A, et al: Processing speed, working memory, and IQ: a developmental model of cognitive deficits following cranial radiation therapy. Neuropsychology 14:189–200, 2000

Schuler D, Polcz A, Revesz T, et al: Psychological late effects of leukemia in children and their prevention. Med Pediatr Oncol 9:191–194, 1981

Schwartz AL, Nail LM, Chen S, et al: Fatigue patterns observed in patients receiving chemotherapy and radiotherapy. Cancer Invest 18:11–19, 2000

Skowronska-Gardas A: Radiotherapy of central nervous system tumors in young children: benefits and pitfalls. Med Pediatr Oncol 33:572–576, 1999

Smith RA, Lampe I, Kahn EA: The prognosis of medulloblastoma in children. J Neurosurg 18:91–97, 1961

So NK, O'Neill BP, Frytak S, et al: Delayed leukoencephalopathy in survivors with small cell lung cancer. Neurology 37:1198–1201, 1987

Soni SS, Marten GW, Pitner SE, et al: Effects of central nervous system irradiation on neuropsychologic functioning of children with acute lymphocytic leukemia. N Engl J Med 293:113–118, 1975

Spunberg JJ, Chang CH, Goldman M, et al: Quality of long-term survival following irradiation for intracranial tumors in children under the age of two. Int J Radiat Oncol Biol Phys 7:727–736, 1981

Sundaresan N, Galicich JH, Deck MDF, et al: Radiation necrosis after treatment of solitary intracranial metastases. Neurosurgery 8:329–333, 1981

Sutton LN, Radcliffe J, Goldwein JW, et al: Quality of life of adult survivors of germinomas treated with craniospinal irradiation. Neurosurgery 45:1292–1297; discussion 1297–1298, 1999

Verzosa MS, Aur RJA, Simone JV, et al: Five years after central nervous system irradiation of children with leukemia. Int J Radiat Oncol Biol Phys 1:209–215, 1976

Waber DP, Shapiro BL, Carpentieri SC, et al: Excellent therapeutic efficacy and minimal late neurotoxicity in children treated with 18 grays of cranial radiation therapy for high-risk acute lymphoblastic leukemia: a 7-year follow-up study of the Dana-Farber Cancer Institute Consortium Protocol 87-01. Cancer 92:15–22, 2001

Wachowski TJ, Chenault H: Degenerative effects of large doses of roentgen rays on the human brain. Radiology 45:227–246, 1945

Whitt JK, Wells RJ, Lauria MM, et al: Cranial radiation in childhood acute lymphocytic leukemia. American Journal of Diseases of Children 138:730–736, 1984

Other Therapeutic Uses of Radiation

DiLorenzo N, Nolletti A, Palma L: Late cerebral radionecrosis. Surg Neurol 10:281–290, 1978

French LR, Schuman LM, Mortimer JA, et al: A case-control study of dementia of the Alzheimer type. Am J Epidemiol 121:414–421, 1985

Furchtgott E: Behavioral effects of ionizing radiations: 1955–61. Psychol Bull 60:157–199, 1963

Garwicz S, Aronson AS, Elmqvist D, et al: Postirradiation syndrome and EEG findings in children with acute lymphoblastic leukaemia. Acta Paediatrica Scandinavica 64:399–403, 1975

Gottschalk LA, Kunkel R, Wohl TH, et al: Total and half body irradiation. Arch Gen Psychiatry 21:574–580, 1969

Kokmen E, Beard CM, Bergstralh E, et al: Alzheimer's disease and prior therapeutic radiation exposure: a case-control study. Neurology 40:1376–1379, 1990

McMahon T, Vahora S: Radiation damage to the brain: neuropsychiatric aspects. Gen Hosp Psychiatry 8:437–441, 1986

Peck A, Boland J: Emotional reactions to radiation treatment. Cancer 40:180–184, 1977

Roeleveld N, Zielhuis GA, Gabreels F: Mental retardation and parental occupation: a study on the applicability of job exposure matrices. British Journal of Industrial Medicine 50:945–954, 1993

Rottenberg DA, Chernik NL, Deck MDF, et al: Cerebral necrosis following radiotherapy of extracranial neoplasms. Ann Neurol 1:339–357, 1977

Hiroshima and Nagasaki

Blot WJ, Miller RW: Mental retardation following in utero exposure to the atomic bombs of Hiroshima and Nagasaki. Radiology 106:617–619, 1973

Kawaishi K: Delayed effects of A-bomb irradiation in a group exposed to the Hiroshima A-bomb under identical circumstances, in Research in the Effects and Influences of the Nuclear Bomb Test Explosions II. Tokyo, Japan Society for the Promotion of Science, 1956, pp 1481–1491

Konuma M: Neuropsychiatric case-studies on the atomic bomb casualties at Hiroshima, in Research in the Effects and Influences of the Nuclear Bomb Test Explosions II. Tokyo, Japan Society for the Promotion of Science, 1956, pp 1715–1720

Miller RW: Delayed effects occurring within the first decade after exposure of young individuals to the Hiroshima atomic bomb. Pediatrics 18:1–17, 1956

Miyata H: After effects of the atomic bomb injuries in Hiroshima and Nagasaki, in Research in the Effects and Influences of the Nuclear Bomb Test Explosions II. Ueno, Tokyo, Japan Society for the Promotion of Science, 1956, pp 1634–1640

Otake M, Schull WJ: In utero exposure to A-bomb radiation and mental retardation: a reassessment. Br J Radiol 57:409–414, 1984

Plummer G: Anomalies occurring in children exposed in utero to the atomic bomb in Hiroshima. Pediatrics 10:687–693, 1952

Schull WJ: Effects of Atomic Radiation: A Half-Century of Studies From Hiroshima and Nagasaki. New York, Wiley, 1995

Schull WJ, Neel JV: Maternal radiation and mongolism (letter). Lancet 1:537–538, 1962

Tsuiki S, Iregami A: Personality tests on the atomic bomb exposed children, in Research in the Effects and Influences of the Nuclear Bomb Test Explosions II. Ueno, Tokyo, Japan Society for the Promotion of Science, 1956, pp 1709–1714

Wood JW, Johnson KG, Omori Y: In utero exposure to the Hiroshima atomic bomb: an evaluation of head size and mental retardation: twenty years later. Pediatrics 39:385–392, 1967

Wood JW, Johnson KG, Omori Y, et al: Mental retardation in children exposed in utero to the atomic bombs in Hiroshima and Nagasaki. Am J Public Health 57:1381–1389, 1967

Yamazaki JN, Wright SW, Wright PM: Outcome of pregnancy in women exposed to the atomic bomb in Nagasaki. American Journal of Diseases of Children 87:448–463, 1954

"Atomic Veterans"

Berkun MM, Timiras PS, Pace N: Psychological and physiological responses in observers of an atomic test shot. Psychol Rep 4:679–682, 1958

Three Mile Island

Baum A, Fleming R, Singer JE: Coping with victimization by technological disaster. Journal of Social Issues 39:117–138, 1983a

Baum A, Gatchel RJ, Schaeffer MA: Emotional, behavioral, and physiological effects of chronic stress at Three Mile Island. J Consult Clin Psychol 51:565–572, 1983b

Bromet E, Dunn L: Mental health of mothers nine months after the Three Mile Island accident. The Urban and Social Change Review 14:12–15, 1981

Bromet E, Parkinson D, Schulberg HC, et al: Three Mile Island: Mental Health Findings. Pittsburgh, PA, University of Pittsburgh School of Medicine, 1980

Bromet E, Schulberg HC, Dunn L: Reactions of psychiatric patients to the Three Mile Island nuclear accident. Arch Gen Psychiatry 39:725–730, 1982

Bromet E, Hough L, Connell M: Mental health of children near the Three Mile Island reactor. Journal of Preventative Psychiatry 2:275–301, 1984

Chisholm RF, Kask SV, Dohrenwend BP, et al: Behavioral and mental health effects of the Three Mile Island accident on nuclear workers: a preliminary report. Ann N Y Acad Sci 365:134–145, 1981

Cleary PD, Houts PS: The psychological impact of the Three Mile Island incident. J Human Stress 10:28–34, 1984

Collins DL, Baum A, Singer JE: Coping with chronic stress at Three Mile Island: psychological and biochemical evidence. Health Psychol 2:149–166, 1983

Davidson LM, Baum A: Victimization and self-blame following a technological disaster, in Communities at Risk: Collective Responses to Technological Disasters. Edited by Couch SR, Kroll-Smith JS. New York, Peter Lang, 1991, pp 33–52

Davidson LM, Baum A, Collins DL: Stress and control-related problems at Three Mile Island. Journal of Applied Social Psychology 12:349–359, 1982

Dew MA, Bromet EJ, Schulberg HC: A comparative analysis of two community stressors' long-term mental health effects. Am J Community Psychol 15:167–184, 1987a

Dew MA, Bromet EJ, Schulberg HC, et al: Mental health effects of the Three Mile Island nuclear reactor restart. Am J Psychiatry 144:1074–1077, 1987b

Dohrenwend BP: Psychological implications of nuclear accidents: the case of Three Mile Island. Bull N Y Acad Med 59:1060–1076, 1983

Dohrenwend BP, Dohrenwend BS, Fabrikant JI, et al: Staff Reports to the President's Commission on the Accident at Three Mile Island. Washington, DC, U.S. Government Printing Office, 1979

Dohrenwend BP, Dohrenwend BS, Warheit GJ, et al: Stress in the community: a report to the president's commission on the accident at Three Mile Island. Ann N Y Acad Sci 365:159–174, 1981

Fabrikant JI: The effects of the accident at Three Mile Island on the mental health and behavioral responses of the general population and nuclear workers. Health Phys 45:579–586, 1983

Fleming R, Baum A, Gisriel MM, et al: Mediating influences of social support on stress at Three Mile Island. Journal of Human Stress 8:14–22, 1982

Gatchel RJ, Schaeffer MA, Baum A: A psychophysiological field study of stress at Three Mile Island. Psychophysiology 22:175–181, 1985

Goldsteen R, Schorr JK: The long-term impact of a man-made disaster: an examination of a small town in the aftermath of the Three Mile Island nuclear reactor accident. Disasters 6:50–59, 1982

Goldsteen R, Schorr JK, Goldsteen KS: Longitudinal study of appraisal at Three Mile Island: implications for life event research. Soc Sci Med 28:389–398, 1989

Hakansson CH, Lindgren M, Sulg IA: EEG effects of postoperative irradiation treatment of brain tumours. Acta Radiologica Therapy, Physics and Biology 8:301–310, 1969

Houts PS, Miller RW, Tokuhata GK, et al: Health-Related Behavioral Impact of the Three Mile Island Nuclear Incident (Report), Part I: 1980. Pennsylvania Department of Health, 1980

Kask SV, Chisholm RF, Eskenazi B: The impact of the accident at the Three Mile Island on the behavior and well-being of nuclear workers, Part II: perceptions and evaluations, behavioral responses, and work-related attitudes and feelings. Am J Public Health 71:472–483, 1981a

Kask SV, Chisholm RF, Eskenazi B: The impact of the accident at the Three Mile Island on the behavior and well-being of nuclear workers, Part 11: job tension, psychophysiological symptoms, and indices of distress. Am J Public Health 71:484–495, 1981b

McKinnon W, Weisse CS, Reynolds CP, et al: Chronic stress, leukocyte subpopulations, and humoral response to latent viruses. Health Psychol 8:389–402, 1989

Parkinson DK, Bromet EJ: Correlates of mental health in nuclear and coal-fired power plant workers. Scand J Work Environ Health 9:341–345, 1983

Prince-Embury S, Rooney JF: Psychological symptoms of residents in the aftermath of the Three Mile Island nuclear accident and restart. J Soc Psychol 128:779–790, 1988

Schaeffer MA, Baum A: Adrenal cortical response to stress at Three Mile Island. Psychosom Med 46:227–237, 1984

Wert BJ: Stress due to nuclear accident: a survey of an employee population. Occupational Health Nursing 27:16–24, 1979

Chernobyl

Bromet EJ, Goldgaber D, Carlson G, et al: Children's well-being 11 years after the Chernobyl catastrophe. Arch Gen Psychiatry 57:563–571, 2000

Chinkina OV: Psychological characteristics of patients exposed to accidental irradiation at the Chernobyl atomic-power station, in The Medical Basis for Radiation-Accident Preparedness, III: The Psychological Perspective. Edited by Ricks RC, Berger ME, O'Hara FM Jr. New York, Elsevier, 1991, pp 93–103

Chinkina OV, Torubarov FS: Psychological features of patients with acute radiation sickness following the Chernobyl atomic power station disaster. Human Physiology 17:301–307, 1991

Ginzburg HM: The psychological consequences of the Chernobyl accident—findings from the international atomic energy agency study. Public Health Rep 108:184–192, 1993

Havenaar JM, van den Brink W, van den Bout J, et al: Mental health problems in the Gomel region (Belarus): an analysis of risk factors in an area affected by the Chernobyl disaster. Psychol Med 26:845–855, 1996

Kolominsky Y, Igumnov S, Drozdovitch V: The psychological development of children from Belarus exposed in the prenatal period to radiation from the Chernobyl atomic power plant. J Child Psychol Psychiatry 40:299–305, 1999

Koscheyev VS, Martens VK, Kosenkov AA, et al: Psychological status of Chernobyl nuclear power plant operators after the nuclear disaster. J Trauma Stress 6:561–568, 1993

Spivak LI: Psychiatric aspects of the accident at Chernobyl nuclear power station. European Journal of Psychiatry 6:207–212, 1992

Viinamaki H, Kumpusalo E, Myllykangas M, et al: The Chernobyl accident and mental well-being—a population study. Acta Psychiatr Scand 91:396–401, 1995

Weisceth L: Reactions in Norway to fallout from the Chernobyl disaster, in Radiation and Cancer Risk. Edited by Brustad T, Langmark F, Reitan JB. New York, Hemisphere Publishing, 1990, pp 149–155

Other Accidental Radiation Exposures

Gilberti MV, Wald N: The Pittsburgh radiation accident: twenty-three-year follow-up of clinical and psychological aspects, in The Medical Basis for Radiation-Accident Preparedness, III: The Psychological Perspective. Edited by Ricks RC, Berger ME, O'Hara FM Jr. New York, Elsevier, 1991, pp 199–206

Hurtado RM, Secin R, Marquez M, et al: The radiological accident in El Salvador: psychological aspects, in The Medical Basis for Radiation-Accident Preparedness, III: The Psychological Perspective. Edited by Ricks RC, Berger ME, O'Hara FM Jr. New York, Elsevier, 1991, pp 187–191

Korol M, Green BL, Gleser GC: Children's responses to a nuclear waste disaster: PTSD symptoms and outcome prediction. J Am Acad Child Adolesc Psychiatry 38:368–375, 1999

II

Pesticides

4

Insecticides

EPIDEMIOLOGY

Of the several classes of synthetic insecticides, the chlorinated hydrocarbon (CH) and organophosphate (OP) insecticides have the greatest psychiatric significance (*Pesticides and Neurological Diseases* 1982; Ecobichon 1996). The CH insecticides, also called organochlorine insecticides, include three chemical classes: dichlorodiphenyltrichloroethane (DDT), cyclodienes (aldrin, dieldrin, heptachlor, chlordane, endosulfan), and chlorinated benzene and cyclohexanes (lindane) (Ecobichon 1996). Their ban in the United States and Europe resulted from their high chemical stability and lipid solubility that allowed environmental persistence and magnification in the food chain (Ecobichon 1996; Kaloyanova and El Batawi 1991).

The OP insecticides replaced DDT and other CH insecticides. The first well-known OP insecticide, parathion, appeared on the market in 1944. The severe toxicity of parathion prompted the introduction of the less toxic malathion in 1950, followed by thousands of other formulations, including chlorpyrifos, diazinon, and leptophos (Ecobichon 1982a).

Carbamates, first synthesized in the 1930s and commercialized in the 1960s, constitute the most recently developed class of anticholinesterase insecticides. Developed to replace the more dangerous CH and OP insecticides, their toxic principle derived from the effects on humans of the Calabar bean used in the West African "trial by ordeal" (Ecobichon 1997). Carbamates inhibit nervous tissue cholinesterases, but less irreversibly than OP insecticides, resulting in reduced toxicity (Ecobichon 1997). Common carbamate names include carbaryl, methomyl, and maneb.

Several reviews of the epidemiology of pesticide, including insecticide, poisoning emphasize the increased incidence of poisonings in developing countries compared with the United States (Hall and Rumack 1992; Hodgson and Smith 1992; Jeyaratnam 1990; Kaloyanova and El Batawi 1991; Moses 1992). Open markets in foreign countries still sell dangerous pesticides such as thallium and mercury despite bans on their sales in the United States (Cabrera 1990; Trape 1990). Food contamination by pesticides occurs frequently in some foreign countries (Trape 1990). Developing countries account for 25% of pesticide use, 50% of acute poisonings, and 75%–99% of fatalities (Jeyaratnam 1993; Moses 1992). Estimates of annual poisonings worldwide range from 500,000 to 25 million, most of which are unrecorded (Jeyaratnam 1990; Kaloyanova and El Batawi 1991).

In 1988, United States public health agencies reported 56,674 pesticide poisonings, including 545 deaths (Moses 1992). One regional poison control center in Minnesota logged 2,209 pesticide-related calls in 1988, representing 4.3% of their total for the year (Olson et al. 1991). In California, reported cases possibly represent only 1% or 2% of the actual cases (Kahn 1976). Some poisonings result from violation of state laws or incorrect instructions for the safe application of pesticides (Hall and Rumack 1992). Despite environmental and occupational regulations, the number of poisonings of farm laborers and fieldhands per year in California more than doubled between 1972 and 1982, a trend observed nationwide (Hall and Rumack 1992; Wasserstrom and Wiles 1985). Children represent a large and vulnerable population of poisoning victims (Landrigan 2001). From 1991 to 1993, nearly one-third of hospital admissions for pesticide poisoning in North Carolina and South Carolina were children. In South Carolina, this trend has persisted since at least 1971 (Sumner and Langley 2000). Possible sources of pesticide poisoning evolve with technological advances and cultural changes. Improperly installed automatic insecticide dispensers in restaurants and businesses can pose hazards, and the sale of illegal pesticides, so-called street pesticides, occurs in large cities in the United States ("Illnesses Associated With Use of Automatic Insecticide Dispenser Units" 2000; "Poisonings Associated With Illegal Use of Aldicarbs" 1997). Each year, homeowners in the United States purchase 20 million chlorpyrifos (an OP insecticide) treatments for their lawns, and 82% of U.S. adults have measurable urine levels of 3,5,6-trichloro-2-pyridinol, a chlorpyrifos metabolite (Steenland et al. 2000).

Since World War I, several mass pesticide poisonings have occurred in the United States and elsewhere (Committee on Neurotoxicology and Models for Assessing Risk 1992; Ecobichon 1982b; Farley and McFarland 1999; Ferrer and Cabral 1995; Kaloyanova and El Batawi 1991; Weeks 1967). During Prohibition in the United States, a Jamaican ginger drink adulterated with a compound closely related to OP pesticides, tri-ortho-cresyl phosphate (TOCP), poisoned 20,000 people. Victims developed a paralysis called "Ginger Jake paralysis" or "Jake Leg" (Ecobichon 1982b, 1996). In 1959, olive oil, purposively contaminated with lubricating fluids containing TOCP, poisoned 10,000 Moroccans (Ecobichon 1982b; Gingras and Desmarais 1960). Thousands fell victim to food contaminated with mercury-based insecticides in Middle Eastern countries during the 1950s (Ferrer and Cabral 1995). In the 1960s, endrin killed 26 and hospitalized 874 in Saudi Arabia (Weeks 1967). Thousands more experienced epidemic OP insecticide poisoning in Pakistan during 1976 (Baker et al. 1978). In Guyana during the early 1970s, suicide by malathion poisoning reached epidemic proportions (Nalin 1973). In 1989, Russia allowed a rare announcement of mass intoxications during the potato and onion harvests (Izmerov and Tarasova 1993). In the United States during 1985, watermelons contaminated by a carbamate insecticide poisoned more than 1,000 people, the largest food-borne insecticide poisoning in the United States (Jackson et al. 1986).

Smaller mass poisonings, including community exposures to pesticide waste dumps, also occur (Clark et al. 1982; Farley and McFarland 1999; Ferrer and Cabral 1995; Jackson et al. 1986; Kahn 1976; Kaloyanova and El Batawi 1991; Kreutzer et al. 1994; Sterman and Varma 1983). Exposures of smaller groups, including office workers and schoolchildren, result from inappropriate spraying of insecticides through ventilation systems or in poorly ventilated structures (Hodgson and Parkinson 1985; Hodgson et al. 1986; Sesline et al. 1994).

Table 4–1 lists occupations or other settings at risk for pesticide exposure (Fuortes et al. 1995). Some poisonings result from inappropriate uses of pesticides, unusual environmental sources, "paraoccupational" sources, and children's exploratory behaviors (Glotfelty et al. 1987; Halle and Sloas 1987; Knishkowy and Baker 1997). Some children can be poisoned by insecticides that are nontoxic to adults (Wenzl and Burke 1962). Childhood poisonings result from ingesting improperly stored pesticides, playing on contaminated carpets, entering homes too soon after treatment, or playing with contaminated toys (Kaplan et al. 1993; Markowitz 1992; Zwiener and Ginsburg 1988). Certain pesticides can persist on toys for weeks ("Playing With Pesticides" 1998; Gurunathan et al. 1998). Although no literature exists to support the notion, producers of illegal drug crops probably use illegal or improperly applied pesticides. Illegal drugs in the United States may contain both the drug and the pesticide.

TABLE 4–1. Occupations and environments at increased risk for exposure to pesticides or related compounds

Occupations	Aerial applicators
	Chemical warfare manufacturers
	Emergency workers—road spills, chemical disasters, firefighters, police, emergency department personnel
	Farmers
	Fieldworkers
	Formulators/Manufacturers
	Fumigators
	Gardeners
	Ground applicators
	Livestock workers
	Longshoremen
	Military personnel
	Nurserypersons
	Road construction workers
	Toxic waste workers
	Truckers
	Warehouser
Others/Environments	Children/Infants
	Foreign travel in certain countries
	Residence near toxic waste site

SIGNS AND SYMPTOMS OF INSECTICIDE POISONING

Chlorinated Hydrocarbons

Acute CH poisonings manifest with numerous symptoms (see Table 4–2). Few psychiatric effects appear in the acute stages. Most symptoms, such as irritability and confusion, result from acute physical illness and shock. The cyclodienes, not DDT or its related derivatives, produce the most severe symptoms in Table 4–2. One case report described seizures resulting from the concomitant use of lindane for treatment of head lice with dextroamphetamine for treatment of attention-deficit/hyperactivity disorder (ADHD) (Cox et al. 2000).

Industrial workers producing CH insecticides frequently have electroencephalogram (EEG) changes (Hoogendam et al. 1962, 1965; Mayersdorf et al. 1974; Princi and Spurbeck 1951). Primate studies indicate that EEG changes, from either large or small CH exposures, persist for up to 1 year (Burchfiel et al. 1976). A Poison Control Center study in Nebraska found that 2 of 11 CH-poisoned children had EEG changes (McIntire et al. 1965).

Anticholinesterase Insecticides

Organophosphorus and carbamate insecticides are the two classes of anticholinesterase insecticides. All anticholinesterases inhibit nervous tissue acetylcholinesterase, the enzyme that deactivates the neurotransmitter acetylcholine (Ecobichon 1996). Poisoning causes accumulation of acetylcholine in the synaptic cleft, resulting in continuous electrical stimulation (Chambers 1992; Costa 1988). Described best by Chambers (1992), the mechanism of acute symptoms of poisoning occurs through three pathways:

1. Stimulation of the somatic or voluntary muscles results in twitches, tremors, convulsions, or tetanic paralysis.
2. Stimulation of the parasympathetic and sympathetic branches in the autonomic nervous system results in a wide array of symptoms, depending on which system is more stimulated (Table 4–2). The chemical, route of exposure, and dose determine the symptoms.

Acetylcholine receptors control the primary central nervous system symptoms, including acute and chronic psychiatric symptoms (Costa 1988). The concept that OPs cause psychiatric symptoms developed concurrently with theories that postulated cholinergic involve-

TABLE 4–2. Signs and symptoms of insecticide poisoning

Acute	Chronic
Chlorinated hydrocarbon pesticides	
Acute	**Chronic**
Gastrointestinal	
Vomiting, diarrhea, anorexia, abdominal pain	Weight loss, anorexia, abnormal liver function tests, hepatomegaly
Neurological	
Paresthesias of face and mouth, ataxia, reeling when walking, dizziness, tremor, motor hyperexcitability, hyperreflexia, seizures, coma	Peripheral neuropathy, polyneuritis, ataxia, incoordination, slurred speech, opsoclonus, tremors, twitching, jerking, seizures, electroencephalogram changes, visual changes
Musculoskeletal	
Weakness, fatigue, lethargy, malaise, headache	Weakness, chest pain, arthralgias, headache
Cardiac	
Bradycardia, tachycardia, arrhythmias	Tachycardia, chest pain, dyspnea
Hematological	
None	Anemia, pancytopenia, agranulocytosis, hemolysis, other blood dyscrasias
Other	
Sore throat, metabolic acidosis, fever, rashes, sweating, hematuria, albuminuria, pulmonary edema	Renal failure, impaired spermatogenesis
Organophosphate and carbamate pesticides	
Acute	**Chronic**
Gastrointestinal	
Nausea, vomiting, abdominal pain, diarrhea, fecal incontinence, tenesmus, anorexia, abdominal tightness	Same if chronically exposed
Glands	
Salivation, tearing or lacrimation, perspiration, bronchorrhea, rhinitis, pulmonary edema	Same if chronically exposed
Eyes	
Miosis, ptosis, blurred vision, conjunctival congestion, "bloody tears," eye pain	Same if chronically exposed
Bladder	
Urinary frequency and incontinence	Same if chronically exposed

TABLE 4–2. Signs and symptoms of insecticide poisoning *(continued)*

Acute	Chronic
Organophosphate and carbamate pesticides *(continued)*	
Respiratory	
Bronchorrhea, rhinitis, pulmonary edema, chest tightness, wheezing, bronchoconstriction, cough, dyspnea, bronchospasms	Same if chronically exposed
Cardiovascular	
Bradycardia or tachycardia, dysrhythmias, heart block, hypertension or hypotension	Same if chronically exposed
Musculoskeletal	
Muscle fasciculations, cramps, weakness, loss of reflexes, paralysis, flacid or rigid tone, restlessness, generalized motor activity, tremulousness	Same if chronically exposed
Neurological	
Headache, coma, loss of reflexes, Cheyne-Stokes respiration, seizures, abnormal electroencephalogram findings	Organophosphate-induced delayed polyneuropathy manifested by flaccidity or paralysis of extremities, paresthesias, footdrop, gait ataxia, spasticity; develops 1–2 weeks after exposure Intermediate syndrome manifested by weakness of proximal limb and respirator muscles, loss of knee reflexes, cranial nerve palsy, death; develops 1–4 days after exposure

ment with mood disorders (Janowsky et al. 1972, 1974). Current research focuses on the proposed cholinergic role in learning and memory that correlates with the frequent cognitive complaints following OP poisoning (Fibiger 1991; Muller et al. 1991; Overstreet 2000). Alterations in cholinergic function may mediate the cognitive effects of electroconvulsive therapy (ECT), a notion supported by the reduction of acetylcholine and acetylcholinesterase in the postictal state in rodents (Prudic et al. 1998). Further evidence of a cholinergic role in cognitive function comes from the mechanism of tolerance to OPs. Tolerance that develops through increased density of cholinergic receptors in response to increased acetylcholine levels could compromise higher brain functions (Costa 1996).

After acute effects subside, OPs produce a condition called the "intermediate syndrome" mediated through the enzyme neurotoxic esterase (Annau 1992). Symptoms consist of muscle weakness developing days after initial symptoms. Organophosphate-induced delayed neurotoxicity, a second delayed OP effect, develops weeks after exposure (Davis and Richardson 1980; Ecobichon 1996; Willems et al. 1984). Another condition described as "wasting away" results from toxic by-products generated during synthesis of OP insecticides, especially malathion (Chambers 1992).

Mixed Exposures and Impurities

Certain clinical and chemical circumstances may render an individual more susceptible to insecticides than usual. In animals, concurrent administration of OP agents potentiate CH, OP, and carbamate insecticides (Dubois 1958; Keplinger and Deichmann 1967). Mixed exposures have toxicological and clinical complexities (Genderen 1980). Some insecticides reduce rather than potentiate the effects of other insecticides (Kaloyanova and El Batawi 1991). Some instances of exposure involve many classes of insecticides, which hinders specific conclusions about subjective complaints (Ensberg et al. 1974; Kaloyanova and El Batawi 1991).

Genetic Susceptibility

Many individuals have genetic susceptibility to certain chemicals (Calabrese 1978). The influence of these genetic differences likely produces sub- and supersensitivity to OP insecticides and warfare agents (Russell and Overstreet 1987). Several enzymes with variations or polymorphisms control sensitivity to OPs: red blood cell acetylcholinesterase, serum cholinesterase or pseudocholinesterase, lymphocyte neuropathy target esterase or platelet neuropathy target esterase (NTE), serum paroxonase, butyrylcholinesterase, and serum arylesterase (Costa et al. 1999; LaDu 1988; Li et al. 1993; Mutch et al. 1992). Inhibition of red blood cell acetylcholinesterase, in both the central and the peripheral nervous systems, produces acute symptoms (Mutch et al. 1992). Paroxonase and arylesterase further modify the response (LaDu 1988; Li et al. 1993). Variant, inactive butyrylcholinesterases increase sensitivity to OPs (Lockridge and Masson 2000; Schwarz et al. 1995). OP-induced delayed polyneuropathy results from inhibition of NTE (Schaumburg and Berger 1993). Inhibition of plasma cholinesterase or pseudocholinesterase does not cause acute symptoms but induces sensitivity to the anesthetic agent succinylcholine (Fuortes et al. 1995). Estimates of the frequency of genetic sensitivity to succinylcholine in individuals of European ancestry range from 1 per 1,250 to 1 per 3,500 (Calabrese 1978; Costa 1996). Individuals who attempt suicide with OP insecticides and are later treated with ECT, during which succinylcholine is used for anesthesia, may develop prolonged paralysis (Jaksa and Palahniuk 1995). Long-distance runners, women in early pregnancy or taking oral contraceptives, and cases of liver failure, alcoholism, and dermatomyositis are associated with low plasma cholinesterase (Fuortes et al. 1995). Genetically determined differences in cytochrome P450 and glutathione transferases also may determine OP toxicity (Costa 1996).

Other Potentiating Factors

Phenothiazine derivatives potentiate the acute toxicity of OPs (Arterberry et al. 1962). Individuals treated with phenothiazine derivatives should avoid occupations with high exposure risk to insecticides. Phenothiazines appear contraindicated in treating insecticide-related delirium.

Phenylmethylsulfonyl fluoride prevents delayed neurotoxicity from OPs if administered before exposure but potentiates neurotoxicity if administered after exposure (Pope and Padilla 1990). Alcohol and drug abuse also potentiate insecticide toxicity, but symptoms are not specific (Calabrese 1978). Protein-deficient diets increase susceptibility to OP poisoning (Boyd and Chen 1968; Krijnen and Boyd 1971). Special diets increase risks for infants, “food faddists,” and individuals with protein deficiency, including persons in developing countries with protein-deficient diets. Individuals with vitamin A, vitamin C, or methionine deficiencies may be susceptible to CH insecticides (Calabrese 1978). The environmental temperature and fat solubility of OPs have marked effects on their toxicities (J. E. Davies et al. 1975; Wheeler 1987).

PSYCHIATRIC SIGNS AND SYMPTOMS ATTRIBUTED TO INSECTICIDES

Chlorinated Hydrocarbons

Several psychiatric manifestations result from CH and OP insecticide poisonings (Table 4–3). Assessment of the psychiatric effects of

CH compounds is more difficult than for modern insecticides. Few CH poisoning studies, written during the 1950s and 1960s, used well-conceived control groups or epidemiological methods. Some reflected, and perhaps inflamed, public hysteria over pesticides. An early paper hypothesized a "pandemic" of a highly debilitating syndrome attributed to a hypothetical "virus X" caused by DDT (Biskind and Bieber 1949). In later years, a similar fear developed from OP insecticides in Mississippi, where the public believed that insecticides caused a "cotton poisoning virus" (Quinby et al. 1958). A recent controlled study of malaria-control workers with chronic exposure to DDT found they performed worse on neurobehavioral tests than did controls (van Wendel et al. 2001).

The CH insecticide chlordecone caused a serious neurotoxic epidemic in the United States. Because of poor industrial control at the world's only chlordecone plant in Hopewell, Virginia, a mass industrial poisoning and environmental disaster occurred in the 1970s. An internist and neurologist, working independently, diagnosed the first victims (Cannon et al. 1978; Taylor et al. 1980). Psychiatric symptoms developed in 44% of the 133 workers and 19% of the 158 residents (Cannon et al. 1978). These complaints persisted for several weeks after exposure was terminated and included confusion and auditory and visual hallucinations (Taylor et al. 1978).

An early case report of aldrin poisoning (Spiotta 1951) identified a confounding factor in chemical exposures. Persons may use insecticides in suicide attempts, and a survivor of suicidal poisoning may have a preexisting psychiatric condition. The insecticide may organically modify his or her condition. Most insecticides contain solvents that promote the potential of a combined effect of insecticide and solvent ingestion. Certain symptoms may result from solvent rather than insecticide exposure.

Organophosphate Compounds

Organophosphate pesticides do not cause a significant percentage of major mental illnesses, such as schizophrenia and bipolar disorder, but they do cause severe psychiatric symptoms of both acute and chronic duration. The most prominent psychiatric symptoms include early anxiety and emotional lability, followed by insomnia, excessive dreaming, nightmares, and reduced concentration. Other symptoms listed in Table 4–3 usually develop only after exposures severe enough to cause physical symptoms but may occur at lower doses in individuals with genetic vulnerability. The limited informa-

TABLE 4–3. Psychiatric signs and symptoms attributed to insecticide exposure

Chlorinated hydrocarbons	
Mood	Irritability, nervousness, depression, anxiety, mood lability
Behavior	Agitation, personality change
Cognitive	Memory loss, confusion, academic decline
Perceptual	Hallucinations
Other	Insomnia, poor appetite, loss of libido, nightmares, fatigue, somatic complaints
Organophosphate pesticides	
Mood	Mood lability, anxiety, irritability, depression, giddiness
Behavior	Apathy, restlessness, suicidal ideation, hyperactivity
Cognitive	Confusion, poor concentration, memory loss, academic decline
Perceptual	Hallucinations, paranoia
Other	Dissociation, nightmares, insomnia, excessive dreaming, fatigue, poor appetite, somatic complaints, change in libido
Carbamates	
Mood	Irritability, mood lability
Cognitive	Memory loss, confusion

tion about psychiatric effects of carbamates comes from case reports that suggest that exposures cause aggression, irritability, confusion, and memory loss.

Several reports focused on the risk for suicide from OP exposure. Some studies of suicide in farmers found only a slight excess, but others reported twice the average risk for suicide (Blair et al. 1993; "Suicide Among Farmers Provokes Government Action" 1994). Concern for farmers' mental health comes from several sources. A letter in the *British Medical Journal* warned of the effects of OP sheep dips (Murray et al. 1992). A neuropsychological study of 146 British sheep farmers later found worse performance in sustained attention and speed of information processing compared with control subjects (Beach et al. 1996; Stephens et al. 1995). The sheep farmers also had greater risk for psychiatric disorder, although this finding did not correlate with the insecticide exposure dose. This study was criticized for methodological errors, and its findings remain unclear (Beach et al. 1996; D. R. Davies 1995; Watt 1995).

The role of atropine treatment of OP poisoning in psychiatric, especially psychotic, symptoms remains unclear. Several studies indicated the difficulty of differentiating psychiatric symptoms of OP poisoning from atropine treatment (Penetar et al. 1988). Some investigators reported that atropine alleviates psychiatric symptoms, whereas others concluded that it causes symptoms not attributable to OPs.

Some reports attributed "toxic delirium" with visual hallucinations to atropine (Wadia et al. 1974). Others described hallucinations in chronic poisoning before treatment (Xintaras et al. 1978). The administration of OPs to individuals with schizophrenia exacerbates psychosis in the absence of atropine (Rowntree et al. 1950). One case report described a 17-year-old victim of chronic poisoning with agitation and hallucinations, developing 24 hours after atropine treatment and shortly after pralidoxime administration (Brachfeld and Zavon 1965). Another case report described a female with a history of nonpsychotic depression who ingested fenthion and experienced severe symptoms for 30 days (Merrill and Mihm 1982). She developed delusions and hallucinations but only after atropine was administered. Her psychosis persisted 6 days during which she did not receive atropine, but then the hallucinations cleared when atropine was restarted on the sixth day of psychosis. The authors, aware of atropine's association with psychosis, attributed the symptoms to OP poisoning. It appears that both OPs and atropine cause psychotic reactions, depending on the individual and doses involved.

DIAGNOSIS AND TREATMENT OF INSECTICIDE POISONING

Psychiatric consultation can assist the emergency management of acute insecticide poisonings by evaluating suicidal overdoses with insecticides or by assessing psychiatric symptoms secondary to acute poisoning. Table 4–4 lists tests and consultations helpful in the assessment of insecticide exposure. Chronic exposures require evaluation to rule out somatoform or other psychiatric disorders in the presence of unexplained physical symptoms. Diagnosis may present significant challenges, and misdiagnoses of viral illnesses or mass psychogenic illness arise before later analysis confirms some poisonings (Aldous et al. 1994; Briggs and Levine 1994; Hodgson and Parkinson 1985; Hodgson et al. 1986). Other cases present months or years after exposure or lack a clear history of exposure. *The New Yorker* magazine published a popular account of the difficulty for both patient and physician in this situation (Roueche 1988). Table 4–5 lists the substance-induced disorders attributed by DSM-IV-TR (American Psychiatric Association 2000) to OP insecticides.

TABLE 4–4. Recommended tests for psychiatric evaluation of insecticide exposure

Complete blood count, electrolytes, liver and renal function tests
Red blood cell count and plasma cholinesterase (for organophosphates)
Urinalysis and urine pesticide/metabolite screen—if recent exposure
Lymphocyte and platelet neuropathy target esterase assay
Neurological evaluation
Neuropsychological testing
Electroencephalogram

TABLE 4–5. DSM-IV-TR diagnoses attributed to organophosphate insecticide or nerve gas exposure

Substance-induced delirium
Substance-induced psychotic disorder
Substance-induced mood disorder
Substance-induced persisting amnestic disorder
Substance-induced anxiety disorder

Exposure to insecticides also carries high risk for posttraumatic stress disorder. Insecticides exacerbate preexisting mental conditions, and atropine treatment of OP poisoning may induce psychotic symptoms. Incomplete assessment may overlook organophosphate-induced delayed neuropathy presenting as fatigue or weakness.

Severe symptoms from mild or moderate exposures may indicate a somatoform disorder rather than physiological effects of insecticides. Somatoform disorder can be distinguished from substance-induced disorders by its presentation, which normally includes extreme symptoms involving areas not normally affected by chemical exposure, symptoms worsening in the absence of exposure, and psychological testing indicating a "hysterical" profile (White et al. 1992).

An early case from New Zealand showed the difficulty of differentiating mass hysteria from mass OP poisoning (McLeod 1975). Following the transport of leaking drums of 5,5,5-tributylphosphorotrithioate (DEF) and merphos, the trivalent phosphorus analog of DEF, 643 persons in a New Zealand community sought medical care for various poisoning symptoms. An investigating board ruled that the symptoms were "real" physiological responses to poisoning, but a New Zealand psychiatrist argued that most symptoms resulted from mass panic because both compounds were of low toxicity. Although DEF and merphos do not produce severe acute symptoms, later studies found that both cause delayed toxicity (Lotti et al. 1983). The incident highlighted two important points. First, differential diagnoses of mass hysteria, epidemic chronic fatigue syndrome, and multiple chemical sensitivities should include OP poisoning (Behan and Haniffah 1994; Rosenthal and Cameron 1991). Second, reported toxicities of OPs may change after commercial or experimental use reveals previously unsuspected toxicities.

Treatment of mental disorders secondary to insecticide poisoning should follow certain precautions. Phenothiazine treatment of OP-induced delirium should be avoided. Low-dose succinylcholine can be considered for ECT after OP poisoning (Dillard and Webb 1999). Patients taking phenothiazine medications should avoid jobs with routine or high risk for OP exposure. Treatment should otherwise proceed in accordance with standard practice guidelines for the treatment of mental disorders. Treatment may require additional psychotherapy and pharmacotherapy for posttraumatic stress disorder.

REFERENCES

Aldous JC, Ellam GA, Murray V, et al: An outbreak of illness among schoolchildren in London: toxic poisoning not mass hysteria. J Epidemiol Community Health 48: 41–45, 1994

American Psychiatric Association: Diagnostic and Statistical Manual of Mental Disorders, 4th Edition, Text Revision. Washington, DC, American Psychiatric Association, 2000

Annau Z: Neurobehavioral effects of organophosphorus compounds, in Organophosphates: Chemistry, Fate, and Effects. Edited by Chambers HW, Levi PE. San Diego, CA, Academic Press, 1992, pp 419–432

Arterberry JD, Bonifaci RW, Nash EW, et al: Potentiation of phosphorus insecticides by phenothiazine derivatives. JAMA 182:110–112, 1962

Baker EL, Zack M, Miles JW, et al: Epidemic malathion poisoning in Pakistan malaria workers. Lancet 1:31–34, 1978

Beach JR, Spurgeon A, Stephens R, et al: Abnormalities on neurological examination among sheep farmers exposed to organophosphorous pesticides. Occup Environ Med 53:520–525, 1996

Behan PO, Haniffah BAG: Chronic fatigue syndrome: a possible delayed hazard of pesticide exposure (letter). Clin Infect Dis 18 (suppl 1):S54, 1994

Biskind MS, Bieber I: DDT poisoning—a new syndrome with neuropsychiatric manifestations. Am J Psychother 3:261–270, 1949

Blair A, Dosemeci M, Heineman EF: Cancer and other causes of death among male and female farmers from twenty-three states. Am J Ind Med 23:729–742, 1993

Boyd EM, Chen CP: Lindane toxicity and protein-deficient diet. Arch Environ Health 17:156–163, 1968

Brachfeld J, Zavon MR: Organic phosphate (Phosdrin) intoxication: report of a case and the results of treatment with 2-PAM. Arch Environ Health 11:859–862, 1965

Briggs NC, Levine PH: A comparative review of systemic and neurological symptomatology in 12 outbreaks collectively described as chronic fatigue syndrome, epidemic neuromyasthenia, and myalgic encephalomyelitis. Clin Infect Dis 18 (suppl 1):S32–S42, 1994

Burchfiel JL, Duffy FH, Sim VM: Persistent effects of sarin and dieldrin upon the primate electroencephalogram. Toxicol Appl Pharmacol 35:365–379, 1976

Cabrera MAM: Neurotoxicology in Mexico and its relation to the general and work environment, in Advances in Neurobehavioral Toxicology: Applications in Environmental and Occupational Health. Edited by Johnson BL. Chelsea, MI, Lewis Publishers, 1990, pp 35–57

Calabrese EJ: Pollutants and High-Risk Groups: The Biological Basis of Increased Human Susceptibility to Environmental and Occupational Pollutants. New York, Wiley-Interscience, 1978

Cannon SB, Veazey JM Jr, Jackson RS, et al: Epidemic kepone poisoning in chemical workers. Am J Epidemiol 107:529–537, 1978

Chambers HW: Organophosphorus compounds: an overview, in Organophosphates: Chemistry, Fate and Effects. Edited by Chambers JE, Levi PE. San Diego, CA, Academic Press, 1992, pp 3–17

Clark CS, Meyer CR, Gartside PS, et al: An environmental health survey of drinking water contamination by leachate from a pesticide waste dump in Hardeman County, Tennessee. Arch Environ Health 37:9–18, 1982

Committe on Neurotoxicology and Models for Assessing Risk: Introduction: defining the problem of neurotoxicity, in Environmental Neurotoxicology. Edited by Committe on Neurotoxicology and Models for Assessing Risk. Washington, DC, National Academy Press, 1992, pp 9–19

Costa LG: Organophosphorous compounds, in Recent Advances in Nervous System Toxicology. Edited by Galli CL, Manzo L, Spencer PS. New York, Plenum, 1988, pp 203–245

Costa LG: Biomarker research in neurotoxicity: the role of mechanistic studies to bridge the gap between the laboratory and epidemiological investigations. Environ Health Perspect 104 (suppl 1):55–67, 1996

Costa LG, Li W-F, Richter ED, et al: The role of paraoxonase (PON1) in the detoxication of organophosphates and its human polymorphism. Chem Biol Interact 14:429–438, 1999

Cox R, Krupnick J, Bush N, et al: Seizures caused by concomitant use of lindane and dextroamphetamine in a child with attention deficit hyperactivitiy disorder. J Miss State Med Assoc 41:690–692, 2000

Davies DR: Neuropsychological effects of exposure to sheep dip. Lancet 345:1632–1633, 1995

Davies JE, Barquet A, Freed VH, et al: Human pesticide poisonings by a fat-soluble organophosphate insecticide. Arch Environ Health 30:608–613, 1975

Davis CS, Richardson RJ: Organophosphorus compounds, in Experimental and Clinical Neurotoxicology. Edited by Spencer PS, Schaumburg HH. Baltimore, MD, Williams & Wilkins, 1980, pp 527–544

Dillard M, Webb J: Administration of succinylcholine for electroconvulsive therapy after organophosphate poisoning: a case study. AANA J 67:513–517, 1999

Dubois KP: Potentiation of the toxicity of insecticidal organic phosphates. AMA Archives of Industrial Health 18:488–496, 1958

Ecobichon DJ: Introduction, in Pesticides and Neurological Diseases. Edited by Ecobichon DJ, Joy RM. Boca Raton, FL, CRC Press, 1982a, pp 1–14

Ecobichon DJ: Organophosphorus ester insecticides, in Pesticides and Neurological Diseases. Edited by Ecobichon DJ, Joy RM. Boca Raton, FL, CRC Press, 1982b, pp 151–203

Ecobichon DJ: Toxic effects of pesticides, in Casarett and Doull's Toxicology: The Basic Science of Poisons. Edited by Klaassen CD. New York, McGraw-Hill, 1996, pp 643–689

Ecobichon DJ: Carbamic acid ester pesticides, in Pesticides and Neurological Diseases. Edited by Ecobichon DJ, Joy RM. Boca Raton, FL, CRC Press, 1982, pp 205–233

Ensberg IFG, de Bruin A, Zielhuis RL: Health of workers exposed to a cocktail of pesticides. Internationales Archiv fur Arbeitsmedizin 32:191–201, 1974

Farley TA, McFarland L: Aldicarb as a cause of food poisoning—Louisiana, 1999 (brief report). JAMA 281:1979, 1999

Ferrer A, Cabral R: Recent epidemics of poisoning by pesticides. Toxicol Lett 82/83: 55–63, 1995

Fibiger HC: Cholinergic mechanisms in learning, memory and dementia: a review of recent evidence. Trends Neurosci 14:220–223, 1991

Fuortes LJ, Ayebo A, Kross B: Cholinesterase-inhibiting pesticide toxicity, in Environmental Medicine: Integrating a Missing Element Into Medical Education. Edited by Pope AM, Rall DP. Washington, DC, National Academy Press, 1995, pp 562–584

Genderen HV: Risks from combined exposures to different chemicals, in Field Worker Exposure During Pesticide Application. Edited by Tordoir WF, Heemstra-Lequin EAHV. Amsterdam, Elsevier, 1980, pp 151–156

Gingras G, Desmarais HL: Rehabilitation operation for 10,000 Moroccan paralysis victims. Arch Phys Med Rehabil 41:559–563, 1960

Glotfelty DE, Seiber J, Liljedahl LA: Pesticides in fog. Nature 325:602–605, 1987

Gurunathan S, Robson M, Freeman N, et al: Accumulation of chlorpyrifos on residential surfaces and toys accessible to children. Environ Health Perspect 106:9–16, 1998

Hall AH, Rumack BH: Incidence, presentation and therapeutic attitudes to anticholinesterase poisoning in the USA, in Clinical and Experimental Toxicology of Organophosphates and Carbamates. Edited by Ballantyne B, Marrs TC, Aldridge WN. Oxford, UK, Butterworth Heinemann, 1992, pp 471–512

Halle A, Sloas DD: Percutaneous organophosphate poisoning. South Med J 80:1179–1181, 1987

Hodgson MJ, Parkinson DK: Diagnosis of organophosphate intoxication (letter). N Engl J Med 313:329, 1985

Hodgson MJ, Smith AD: Commercial and residential poisoning with anticholinesterases, in Clinical and Experimental Toxicology of Organophosphates and Carbamates. Edited by Ballantyne B, Marrs TC, Aldridge WN. Oxford, UK, Butterworth Heinemann, 1992, pp 352–363

Hodgson MJ, Block GD, Parkinson DK: Organophosphate poisoning in office workers. J Occup Med 28:434–437, 1986

Hoogendam I, Versteeg JPJ, deVlieger M: Electroencephalograms in insecticide toxicity. Arch Environ Health 4:92–100, 1962

Hoogendam I, Versteeg JPJ, deVlieger M: Nine years' toxicity control in insecticide plants. Arch Environ Health 10:441–448, 1965

Illnesses associated with use of automatic insecticide dispenser units—selected states and United States, 1986–1999. MMWR Morb Mortal Wkly Rep 49:492–495, 2000

Izmerov N, Tarasova L: Occupational diseases developed as a result of severely injured nervous system: acute and chronic neurotic effects. Environ Res 62:172–177, 1993

Jackson RJ, Stratton JW, Goldman LR, et al: Aldicarb food poisoning from contaminated melons—California. JAMA 256:175–176, 1986

Jaksa RJ, Palahniuk RJ: Attempted organophosphate suicide: a unique cause of prolonged paralysis during electroconvulsive therapy. Anesth Analg 80:832–833, 1995

Janowsky DS, El-Yousef MK, Davis JM, et al: A cholinergic-adrenergic hypothesis of mania and depression. Lancet 2:632–635, 1972

Janowsky DS, El-Yousef MK, Davis JM: Acetylcholine and depression. Psychosom Med 36:248–257, 1974

Jeyaratnam J: Acute pesticide poisoning: a major global health problem. World Health Stat Q 43:139–144, 1990

Jeyaratnam J: Occupational health issues in developing countries. Environ Res 60: 207–212, 1993

Kahn E: Pesticide related illness in California farm workers. J Occup Med 18:693–696, 1976

Kaloyanova FP, El Batawi MA: Human Toxicology of Pesticides. Boca Raton, FL, CRC Press, 1991

Kaplan JG, Kessler J, Rosenberg N, et al: Sensory neuropathy associated with Dursban (chlorpyrifos) exposure. Neurology 43:2193–2196, 1993

Keplinger ML, Deichmann WB: Acute toxicity of combinations of pesticides. Toxicol Appl Pharmacol 10:586–595, 1967

Knishkowy B, Baker EL: Transmission of occupational disease to family contacts. Am J Ind Med 9:543–550, 1997

Kreutzer RA, Hewitt DJ, Draper WM: An epidemiological assessment of the Cantara metam sodium spill: acute health effects and methyl isothiocyanate exposure, in Environmental Epidemiology: Effects of Environmental Chemicals on Human Health. Edited by Draper WM. Washington, DC, American Chemical Society, 1994, pp 209–230

Krijnen CJ, Boyd EM: The influence of diets containing from 0 to 81% of protein on tolerated doses of pesticides. Comparative and General Pharmacology 2:373–376, 1971

LaDu BN: Invited editorial: the human serum paraoxonase/arylesterase polymorphism. Am J Hum Genet 43:227–229, 1988

Landrigan PJ: Pesticides and polychlorinated biphenyls (PCBs): an analysis of the evidence that they impair children's neurobehavioral development. Mol Genet Metab 73:11–17, 2001

Li W-F, Costa LG, Furlong CE: Serum paraoxonase status: a major factor in determining resistance to organophosphates. J Toxicol Environ Health 40:337–346, 1993

Lockridge O, Masson P: Pesticides and susceptible populations: people with butyrylcholinesterase genetic variants may be at risk. Neurotoxicology 21:113–126, 2000.

Lotti M, Becker CE, Aminoff MJ, et al: Occupational exposure to the cotton defoliants DEF and Merphos. J Occup Med 25:517–522, 1983

Markowitz SB: Poisoning of an urban family due to misapplication of household organophosphate and carbamate pesticides. Clin Toxicol 30:295–303, 1992

Mayersdorf A, Israeli R, Beer-Sheva I: Toxic effects of chlorinated hydrocarbon insecticides: on the human electroencephalogram. Arch Environ Health 28:159–163, 1974

McIntire MS, Angle CR, Maragos G: Insecticide poisoning of childhood: follow-up evaluation. J Pediatr 67:647–648, 1965

McLeod WR: Merphos poisoning or mass panic? Aust N Z J Psychiatry 9:225–229, 1975

Merrill DG, Mihm FG: Prolonged toxicity of organophosphate poisoning. Crit Care Med 10:550–551, 1982

Moses M: Pesticides, in Public Health and Preventive Medicine. Edited by Last JM, Wallace RB. Norwalk, CT, Appleton & Lange, 1992, pp 479–489

Muller WE, Stoll L, Schubert T, et al: Central cholinergic functioning and aging. Acta Psychiatr Scand Suppl 366:34–39, 1991

Murray VSG, Wiseman HM, Dawling S, et al: Health effects of organophosphate sheep dips (letter). BMJ 305:1090, 1992

Mutch E, Blain PG, Williams FM: Interindividual variations in enzymes controlling organophosphate toxicity in man. Hum Exp Toxicol 11:109–116, 1992

Nalin DR: Epidemic of suicide by malathion poisoning in Guyana. Tropical and Geographical Medicine 25:8–14, 1973

Olson DK, Sax L, Gunderson P, et al: Pesticide poisoning surveillance through regional poison control centers. Am J Public Health 81:750–755, 1991

Overstreet DH: Organophosphate pesticides, cholinergic function and cognitive performance in advanced age. Neurotoxicology 21:75–81, 2000

Penetar DM, Haegerstrom-Portnoy G, Jones RT: Combined atropine and 2-PAM Cl effects on tracking performance and visual, physiological, and psychological functions. Aviat Space Environ Med 59:1125–1132, 1988

Pesticides and Neurological Diseases. Boca Raton, FL, CRC Press, 1982

Playing with pesticides. Environ Health Perspect 106:A10, 1998

Poisonings associated with illegal use of aldicarbs as a rodenticide-New York City, 1994–1997. MMWR Morb Mortal Wkly Rep 46:961–963, 1997

Pope CN, Padilla S: Potentiation of organophosphorus-induced delayed neurotoxicity by phenylmethylsulfonyl fluoride. J Toxicol Environ Health 31:261–273, 1990

Princi F, Spurbeck GH: A study of workers exposed to the insecticides chlordan, aldrin, dieldrin. AMA Archives of Industrial Hygiene and Occupational Medicine 3:64–72, 1951

Prudic J, Sackeim HA, Spricknall K: Potential pharmacologic agents for the cognitive effects of electroconvulsive treatment. Psychiatric Annals 28:40–46, 1998

Quinby G, Walker KC, Durham WF: Public health hazards involved in the use of organic phosphorus insecticides in cotton culture in the delta area of Mississippi. J Econ Entomol 51:831–838, 1958

Rosenthal NE, Cameron CL: Exaggerated sensitivity to an organophosphate pesticide (letter). Am J Psychiatry 148:270, 1991

Roueche B: The fumigation chamber. The New Yorker, January 4, 1988, pp 60–65

Rowntree DW, Nevin S, Wilson A: The effects of diisopropylfluorophosphonate in schizophrenia and manic depressive psychosis. J Neurol Neurosurg Psychiatry 13:47–62, 1950

Russell RW, Overstreet DH: Mechanisms underlying sensitivity to organophosphorus anticholinesterase compounds. Prog Neurobiol 28:97–129, 1987

Schaumburg HH, Berger AR: Human toxic neuropathy due to industrial agents, in Peripheral Neuropathy. Edited by Dyck PJ, Thomas PK, Griffin JW, et al. Philadelphia, PA, WB Saunders, 1993, pp 1533–1548

Schwarz M, Glick D, Loewenstein Y, et al: Engineering of human cholinesterases explains and predicts diverse consequences of administration of various drugs and poisons. Pharmacol Ther 67:283–322, 1995

Sesline D, Ames RG, Howd RA: Irritative and systemic symptoms following exposure to microban disinfectant through a school ventilation system. Arch Environ Health 49:439–444, 1994

Spiotta EJ: Aldrin poisoning in man. AMA Archives of Industrial Hygiene and Occupational Medicine 4:560–566, 1951

Steenland K, Dick RB, Howell RJ, et al: Neurologic function among termiticide applicators exposed to chlorpyrifos. Environ Health Perspect 108:293–300, 2000

Stephens R, Spurgeon A, Calvert IA, et al: Neuropsychological effects of long-term exposure to organophosphates in sheep dip. Lancet 345:1135–1139, 1995

Sterman AB, Varma A: Evaluating human neurotoxicity of the pesticide Aldicarb: when man becomes the experimental animal. Neurobehavioral Toxicology and Teratology 5:493–495, 1983

Suicide among farmers provokes government action. BMJ 308:1001–1001, 1994

Sumner D, Langley R: Pediatric pesticide poisoning in the Carolinas: an evaluation of the trends and proposal to reduce the incidence. Vet Hum Toxicol 42:101–103, 2000

Taylor JR, Selhorst JB, Houff SA, et al: Chlordecone intoxication in man. Neurology 28:626–630, 1978

Taylor JR, Selhorst JB, Calabrese VP: Chlordecone, in Experimental and Clinical Neurotoxicology. Edited by Spencer PS, Schaumburg HH. Baltimore, MD, Williams & Wilkins, 1980, pp 407–421

Trape AZ: Exposure to pesticides—situation in Brazil, in Advances in Neurobehavioral Toxicology: Applications in Environmental and Occupational Health. Edited by Johnson BL. Chelsea, MI, Lewis Publishers, 1990, pp 59–73

van Wendel DJB, Wesseling C, Kromhout H, et al: Chronic nervous-system effects of long-term occupational exposure to DDT. Lancet 357:1014–1016, 2001

Wadia RS, Sadagopan C, Amin RB, et al: Neurological manifestations of organophosphorous insecticide poisoning. J Neurol Neurosurg Psychiatry 37:841–847, 1974

Wasserstrom RF, Wiles R: Field Duty: U.S. Farmworkers and Pesticide Safety. Washington, DC, World Resources Institute, 1985

Watt AH: Neuropsychological effects of exposure to sheep dip. Lancet 345:1631–1632, 1995

Weeks DE: Endrin food-poisoning: a report on four outbreaks caused by two separate shipments of endrin-contaminated flour. Bull World Health Organ 37:499–512, 1967

Wenzl JE, Burke EC: Poisoning from a malathion-aerosol mixture. JAMA 182:495–497, 1962

Wheeler TG: The behavioral effects of anticholinesterase insult following exposure to different environmental temperatures. Aviat Space Environ Med 58:54–59, 1987

White RF, Feldman RG, Proctor SP: Neurobehavioral effects of toxic exposures, in Clinical Syndromes in Adult Neuropsychology: The Practitioner's Handbook. Edited by White RF. Amsterdam, Elsevier, 1992, pp 1–51

Willems JL, Nicaise M, DeBisschop HC: Delayed neuropathy by the organophosphorus nerve agents soman and tabun. Arch Toxicol 55:76–77, 1984

Xintaras C, Burg JR, Tanaka S, et al: NIOSH Health Survey of Velsicol Pesticide Workers: Occupational Exposure to Leptophos and Other Chemicals. Cincinnati, OH, U.S. Department of Health, Education, and Welfare, 1978

Zwiener RJ, Ginsburg CM: Organophosphate and carbamate poisoning in infants and children. Pediatrics 81:121–126, 1988

ADDITIONAL READINGS

Dichlorodiphenyltrichloroethane (DDT)

Case RAM: Toxic effects of 2,2,-bis (p-chlorphenyl) 1,1,1-trichlorethane (D.D.T.) in man. BMJ 2:842–845, 1945

Kaloyanova FP, El Batawi MA: Human Toxicology of Pesticides. Boca Raton, FL, CRC Press, 1991

Misra UK, Nag D, Krishna M: A study of cognitive functions in DDT sprayers. Ind Health 22:199–206, 1984

Stone TT, Gladstone L: DDT (Dichlorodiphenyl-trichloroethane) (clinical note). JAMA 145:1342–1342, 1951

Wigglesworth VB: A case of D.D.T. poisoning in man (medical memorandum). BMJ 1: 517–517, 1945

Aldrin

Avar P, Czegledi-Janko G: Occupational exposure to aldrin: clinical and laboratory findings. British Journal of Industrial Medicine 27:279–282, 1970

Gupta PC: Neurotoxicity of chronic chlorinated hydrocarbon insecticide poisoning—a clinical and electroencephalographic study in man. Indian J Med Res 63:601–606, 1975

Kazantzis G, McLaughlin AIG, Prior PF: Poisoning in industrial workers by the insecticide aldrin. British Journal of Industrial Medicine 21:46–51, 1964

Dieldrin

Jacobs P, Lurie JB: Acute toxicity of the chlorinated hydrocarbon insecticides. S Afr Med J 41:11–47, 1967

Chlordecone

Taylor JR: Neurological manifestations in humans exposed to chlordecone: follow-up results. Neurotoxicology 6:231–236, 1985

Other Insecticides

Angle CR, McIntire MS, Meile RL: Neurologic sequelae of poisoning in children. J Pediatr 73:531–539, 1968

Bell A, Jones AT: Fumigation with dichlorethyl ether and chlordane: hysterical sequelae. Med J Aust 2:258–263, 1958

Brandt VA, Moon S, Ehler J, et al: Exposure to endosulfan in farmers: two case studies. Am J Ind Med 39:643–649, 2001

Czegledi-Janko G, Avar P: Occupational exposure to lindane: clinical and laboratory findings. British Journal of Industrial Medicine 27:283–286, 1970

Espir MLE, Hall JW, Shirreffs JG, et al: Impotence in farm workers using toxic chemicals. BMJ 1:423–425, 1970

Gladen BC, Rogan WJ, Hardy P, et al: Development after exposure to polychlorinated biphenyls and dichlorodiphenyl dichloroethene transplacentally and through human milk. J Pediatr 113:991–995, 1988

Joy RM: Chlorinated hydrocarbon insecticides, in Pesticides and Neurological Diseases. Edited by Ecobichon DJ, Joy RM. Boca Raton, FL, CRC Press, 1982, pp 91–150

Lessenger JE, Riley N: Neurotoxicities and behavioral changes in a 12-year-old male exposed to dicofol, an organochloride pesticide. J Toxicol Environ Health 33: 255–261, 1991

McIntire MS, Angle CR, Maragos G: Insecticide poisoning of childhood: follow-up evaluation. J Pediatr 67:647–648, 1965

McKee JL: Intellectual and behavioral correlates of chronic exposure to toxic chemicals. Unpublished thesis, University of Denver, Denver, CO, 1970

Peper M, Ertl M, Gerhard I: Long-term exposure to wood-preserving chemicals containing pentachlorophenol and lindane is related to neurobehavioral performance in women. Am J Ind Med 35:632–641, 1999

U.S. House of Representatives, Select Committee to Investigate the Use of Chemicals in Foods and Cosmetics: Chemicals in foods and cosmetics (congressional hearing), 82nd Congress, Washington, DC, 1952

Parathion

Arterberry JD, Durham WF, Elliott JW, et al: Exposure to parathion. Arch Environ Health 3:112–121, 1961

Grob D, Garlick WL, Harvey AM: The toxic effects in man of the anticholinesterase insecticide parathion (p-nitrophenyl diethyl thionophosphate). Bulletin of the Johns Hopkins Hospital 87:106–129, 1950

Harmon GE, Reigart JR, Sandifer SH: Long-term follow-up of survivors of acute pesticide poisoning. J S C Med Assoc 71:253–257, 1976

Hayes WJ Jr, Dixon EM, Batchelor GS, et al: Exposure to organic phosphorus sprays and occurrence of selected symptoms. Public Health Rep 72:787–794, 1957

Holmes JH, Kinzer EJ, Hibbert RW: Parathion poisoning case report. Rocky Mountain Medical Journal 54:1022–1031, 1957

Milby TH, Ottoboni F, Mitchell HW: Parathion residue poisoning among orchard workers. JAMA 189:351–356, 1964

Rehner TA, Kolbo JR, Trump R, et al: Depression among victims of south Mississippi's methyl parathion disaster. Health Soc Work 25:33–40, 2000

Rodnitzky RL, Levin HS, Morgan DP: Effects of ingested parathion on neurobehavioral functions. Clin Toxicol 13:347–359, 1978

Sumerford WT, Hayes WJ Jr, Johnston JM, et al: Cholinesterase response and symptomatology from exposure to organic phosphorus insecticides. AMA Archives of Industrial Hygiene and Occupational Medicine 7:383–398, 1953

Miscellaneous Organophosphate Compounds

Agarwal SB: A clinical, biochemical, neurobehavioral, and sociopsychological study of 190 patients admitted to hospital as a result of acute organophosphorus poisoning, in Neurobehavioral Methods and Effects in Occupational and Environmental Health. Edited by Araki S. San Diego, CA, Academic Press, 1994, pp 787–794

Aldous JC, Ellam GA, Murray V, et al: An outbreak of illness among schoolchildren in London: toxic poisoning not mass hysteria. J Epidemiol Community Health 48: 41–45, 1994

Ames RG, Steenland K, Jenkins B, et al: Chronic neurologic sequelae to cholinesterase inhibition among agricultural pesticide applicators. Arch Environ Health 50: 440–444, 1995

Amr M, Allam M, Osmaan AL, et al: Neurobehavioral changes among workers in some chemical industries in Egypt. Environ Res 63:295–300, 1993

Azaroff LS, Neas LM: Acute health effects associated with nonoccupational pesticide exposure in rural El Salvador. Environ Res 80:158–164, 1999

Barr AM: Further experience in the treatment of severe organic phosphate poisoning. Med J Aust 1:490–492, 1966

Bazylewicz-Walczak B, Majczakowa W, Szymczak M: Behavioral effects of occupational exposure to organophosphorous pesticides in female greenhouse planting workers. Neurotoxicology 20:819–826, 1999

Bellin JS, Chow I: Biochemical effects of chronic low-level exposure to pesticides. Research Communications in Chemical Pathology and Pharmacology 9:325–337, 1974

Bertoncin D, Russolo A, Caroldi S, et al: Neuropathy target esterase in human lymphocytes. Arch Environ Health 40:139–144, 1985

Bhatnagar VK, Saigal S, Singh SP, et al: Survey amongst workers in pesticide factories. Toxicol Lett 10:129–132, 1982

Brenner FE, Bond GG, Mclaren EA, et al: Morbidity among employees engaged in the manufacture or formulation of chlorpyrifos. British Journal of Industrial Medicine 46:133–137, 1989

Conyers RAJ, Goldsmith LE: A case of organophosphorus-induced psychosis. Med J Aust 58:27–29, 1971

Coye MJ, Barnett PG, Midtling JE, et al: Clinical confirmation of organophosphate poisoning of agricultural workers. Am J Ind Med 10:399–409, 1986

Daniell W, Barnhart S, Demers PA, et al: Neuropsychological performance among agricultural pesticide applicators. Environ Res 59:217–228, 1992

Davies GM, Lewis I: Outbreak of food-poisoning from bread made of chemically contaminated flour. BMJ 2:393–398, 1956

Dille JR, Smith PW: Central Nervous System Effect of Chronic Exposure to Organophosphate Insecticides. Oklahoma City, OK, Federal Aviation Agency, Civil Aeromedical Research Institute, 1963

Dille JR, Smith PW: Central nervous system effects of chronic exposure to organophosphate insecticides. Aerospace Medicine 35:475–478, 1964

Durham WF, Wolfe BS, Quinby G: Organophosphorus insecticides and mental alertness. Arch Environ Health 10:55–65, 1965

French LR, Schuman LM, Mortimer JA, et al: A case-control study of dementia of the Alzheimer type. Am J Epidemiol 121:414–421, 1985

Gershon S, Angrist BM: Effects of alterations of cholinergic function on behavior, in Psychopathology and Psychopharmacology. Edited by Cole JO, Freedman AM, Friedhoff AJ. Baltimore, MD, The Johns Hopkins University Press, 1973, pp 15–36

Gershon S, Shaw FH: Psychiatric sequelae of chronic exposure to organophosphorus insecticides. Lancet i:1371–1374, 1961

Grob D, Harvey AM, Langworthy OR, et al: The administration of di-isopropyl fluorophosphate (DFP) to man, III. Bulletin of the Johns Hopkins Hospital 81:257–266, 1947a

Grob D, Lilienthal JL, Harvey AM, et al: The administration of di-isopropyl fluorophosphate (DFP) to man, I. Bulletin of the Johns Hopkins Hospital 81:217–244, 1947b

Gupta SK, Jani JP, Saiyed HN, et al: Health hazards in pesticide formulators exposed to a combination of pesticides. Indian J Med Res 79:666–672, 1984

Hirshberg A, Lerman Y: Clinical problems in organophosphate insecticide poisoning: the use of a computerized information system. Fundamental and Applied Toxicology 4:S209–S214, 1984

Hodgson MJ, Parkinson DK: Diagnosis of organophosphate intoxication (letter). N Engl J Med 313:329, 1985

Hollis GJ: Organophosphate poisoning versus brainstem stroke. Med J Aust 170:596–597, 1999

Ilanis S, Goldsmith JR, Israeli R: Neurotoxicity of organo-phosphate insecticides among a Negev population with long-term exposure, in Progress in Occupational Epidemiology. Edited by Hogstedt C, Reuterwall C. Amsterdam, Excerpta Medica, 1988, pp 253–262

Joubert J, Joubert PH: Chorea and psychiatric changes in organophosphate poisoning. S Afr Med J 74:32–34, 1988

Kashyap SK: Health surveillance and biological monitoring of pesticide formulators in India. Toxicol Lett 33:107–114, 1986

Keifer M, Rivas F, Moon JD, et al: Symptoms and cholinesterase activity among rural residents living near cotton fields in Nicaragua. Occup Environ Med 53:726–729, 1996

Lerman Y, Hirshberg A, Shteger Z: Organophosphate and carbamate pesticide poisoning: the usefulness of a computerized clinical information system. Am J Ind Med 6:17–26, 1984

Levin HS: Behavioral effects of occupational exposure to organophosphate pesticides, in Behavioral Toxicology: Early Detection of Occupational Hazards. Edited by Xintaras C, Johnson BL, de Groot I. Washington, DC, U.S. Department of Health, Education and Welfare, 1974, pp 154–164

Levin HS, Rodnitzky RL: Behavioral effects of organophosphate pesticides in man. Clin Toxicol 9:391–405, 1976

Levin HS, Rodnitzky RL, Mick DL: Anxiety associated with exposure to organophosphate compounds. Arch Gen Psychiatry 33:225–228, 1976

Maizlish N, Schenker M, Weisskopf C, et al: Behavioral evaluation of pest control workers with short-term, low-level exposure to the organophosphate diazinon. Am J Ind Med 12:153–172, 1987

Markowitz JS, Gutterman EM, Link BG: Self-reported physical and psychological effects following a malathion pesticide incident. J Occup Med 23:377–383, 1986

McCrank E, Rabheru K: Four cases of progressive supranuclear palsy in patients exposed to organic solvents. Can J Psychiatry 34:934–935, 1989

Metcalf DR, Holmes JH: EEG, psychological, and neurological alterations in humans with organophosphorus exposure. Ann N Y Acad Sci 160:357–365, 1969

Midtling JE, Barnett PG, Coye MJ, et al: Clinical management of field worker organophosphate poisoning. West J Med 142:514–518, 1985

Misra UK, Nag D, Bhushan V, et al: Clinical and biochemical changes in chronically exposed organophosphate workers. Toxicol Lett 24:187–193, 1985

Ohayo-Mitoko GJ, Kromhout H, Simwa, et al: Self reported symptoms and inhibition of acetylcholinesterase activity among Kenyan agricultural workers. Occup Environ Med 57:195–200, 2000

Otto DA, Soliman S, Svendsgaard D, et al: Neurobehavioral assessment of workers exposed to organophosphorus pesticides, in Advances in Neurobehavioral Toxicology: Applications in Environmental and Occupational Health. Edited by Johnson BL. Chelsea, MI, Lewis Publishers, 1990, pp 305–322

Parron T, Hernandez AF, Pla A, et al: Clinical and biochemical changes in greenhouse sprayers chronically exposed to pesticides. Hum Exp Toxicol 15:957–963, 1996a

Parron T, Hernandez AF, Villanueva E: Increased risk of suicide with exposure to pesticides in an intensive agricultural area: a 12-year retrospective study. Forensic Sci Int 79:53–63, 1996b

Peters HA, Levine RL, Matthews CG, et al: Carbon disulfide-induced neuropsychiatric changes in grain storage workers. Am J Ind Med 3:373–391, 1982

Peters HA, Levine RL, Matthews CG, et al: Synergistic neurotoxicity of carbon tetrachloride/carbon disulfide (80/20 fumigants) and other pesticides in grain storage workers. Acta Pharmacologica et Toxicologica 59 (suppl 6–7):535–546, 1986

Petty CS: Organic phosphate insecticide poisoning. Am J Med 24:467–470, 1958

Ratner D, Oren B, Vigder K: Chronic dietary anticholinesterase poisoning. Isr J Med Sci 19:810–814, 1983

Reidy TJ, Bowler RM, Rauch S, et al: Pesticide exposure and neuropsychological impairment in migrant farm workers. Archives of Clinical Neuropsychology 7:85–95, 1992

Richter ED, Chuwers P, Levy Y, et al: Health effects from exposure to organophosphate pesticides in workers and residents in Israel. Isr J Med Sci 28:584–598, 1992

Rodnitzky RL, Levin HS, Mick DL: Occupational exposure to organophosphate pesticides. Arch Environ Health 30:98–103, 1975

Rosenstock L, Daniell W, Barnhart S, et al: Chronic neuropsychological sequelae of occupational exposure to organophosphate insecticides. Am J Ind Med 18:321–325, 1990

Rosenstock L, Keifer M, Daniell W, et al: Chronic central nervous system effects of acute organophosphate pesticide intoxication. Lancet 338:223–227, 1991

Savage EP, Keefe TJ, Mounce LM, et al: Chronic neurological sequelae of acute organophosphate pesticide poisoning. Arch Environ Health 43:38–45, 1988

Singer R: Neurotoxicity Guidebook. New York, Van Nostrand Reinhold, 1990

Srivastava AK, Gupta BN, Bihari V, et al: Clinical, biochemical and neurobehavioral studies of workers engaged in the manufacture of quinalphos. Food Chem Toxicol 38:65–69, 2000

Steenland K, Jenkins B, Ames RG, et al: Chronic neurological sequelae to organophosphate pesticide poisoning. Am J Public Health 84:731–736, 1994

Stoller A, Krupinski J, Christophers AJ, et al: Organophosphorus insecticides and major mental illness: an epidemiological investigation. Lancet i:1387–1388, 1965

Tabershaw IR, Cooper WC: Sequelae of acute organic phosphate poisoning. J Occup Med 8:5–20, 1966

Warnick SL, Carter JE: Some findings in a study of workers occupationally exposed to pesticides. Arch Environ Health 25:265–270, 1972

White RF, Feldman RG, Proctor SP: Neurobehavioral effects of toxic exposures, in Clinical Syndromes in Adult Neuropsychology: The Practitioner's Handbook. Edited by White RF. Amsterdam, Elsevier, 1992, pp 1–51

Whorton MD, Obrinsky DL: Persistence of symptoms after mild to moderate acute organophosphate poisoning among 19 farm field workers. J Toxicol Environ Health 11:347–354, 1983

Wood W, Gabica J, Brown HW, et al: Implication of organophosphate pesticide poisoning in the plane crash of a duster pilot. Aerospace Medicine 42:1111–1113, 1971

Xintaras C, Burg JR, Johnson BL, et al: Neurotoxic effects of exposed chemical workers. Ann N Y Acad Sci 329:30–38, 1979

Unspecified Pesticides

Bosma H, van Boxtel MP, Ponds RW, et al: Pesticide exposure and risk of mild cognitive dysfunction (letter). Lancet 356:912–913, 2000

Furst JB, Cooper A: Failure of systematic desensitization in 2 cases of obsessive-compulsive neurosis marked by fears of insecticide. Behav Res Ther 8:203–206, 1970

Gauthier E, Fortier I, Courchesne F, et al: Environmental pesticide exposure as a risk factor for Alzheimer's disease: a case-control study. Environ Res 86:37–45, 2001

Carbamates

Bear D, Rosenbaum J, Norman R: Aggression in cat and human precipitated by a cholinesterase inhibitor. Psychosomatics 27:535–536, 1986

Branch RA, Jacqz E: Subacute neurotoxicity following long-term exposure to carbaryl. Am J Med 80:741–745, 1986

Dumont MP: Psychotoxicology: the return of the mad hatter. Soc Sci Med 29:1077–1082, 1989

Ecobichon DJ: Carbamic acid ester pesticides, in Pesticides and Neurological Diseases. Edited by Ecobichon DJ, Joy RM. Boca Raton, FL, CRC Press, 1982, pp 205–233

5

Fumigants

EPIDEMIOLOGY OF METHYL BROMIDE POISONING

Methyl bromide's (MB) severe toxicity and psychiatric effects differentiate it from other fumigants. In the 1960s, it caused more fatalities, mostly from fumigation, than all organophosphate insecticides combined (Klaassen 1985). Despite the well-known toxicity of MB, poisonings go unrecognized because of the delayed onset of symptoms that hinder diagnosis. Some unwary consumers become exposed from unexpected sources, including waterbeds or respiratory protection devices that release MB or fail to protect from MB exposure, respectively (Dempsey and Becker 1992; Deschamps and Turpin 1996). Table 5–1 lists occupations and environmental circumstances with the highest risk of exposure.

SYMPTOMS OF METHYL BROMIDE POISONING

Hours may pass before symptoms of MB poisoning appear. The victim may have no knowledge of exposure to the colorless and odorless

TABLE 5–1. Occupations and other environments at risk for methyl bromide exposure

Occupations	
Chemical workers	
Structural and soil fumigators	
Other	
Fumigation of dwellings or workplaces	

gas, and some exposures result in euphoria, which leads to greater exposure from carelessness (Bleecker 1994). Some poisonings mimic influenza, Reye's syndrome, or encephalitis/meningitis (Gosselin et al. 1984). Poisoning occurs after both dermal and inhalational contact, and residual symptoms can persist for years (O'Donoghue 1985). MB is a vesicant, or blistering agent, with a mechanism of injury similar to that of mustard gas (Collins 1965). Table 5–2 lists the general signs and symptoms of MB poisoning. Table 5–3 lists the psychiatric signs and symptoms attributed to MB poisoning.

TABLE 5–2. Signs and symptoms of methyl bromide poisoning

Respiratory	Pulmonary edema, bronchopneumonia
Gastrointestinal	Gastrointestinal complaints, weight loss, anorexia, jaundice, mild hepatotoxicity
Neurological	Dizziness, headache, giddiness, lassitude, weakness, ataxia, staggering gait, slurred speech, tremor, myoclonus, sensory neuropathy, tinnitus, numbness, paresthesias, seizures, coma, status epilepticus
Other	Hyperthermia, skin blistering, blurred vision, blindness, renal failure

TABLE 5–3. Psychiatric signs and symptoms attributed to methyl bromide poisoning

Mood	Mania, euphoria, "neurosis," "melancholia," depression, anxiety, irritability
Behavior	Apathy, violence, homicidal/suicidal ideation
Cognitive	Mental confusion, poor concentration
Perceptual changes	Hallucinations, delusions, paranoia
Other	Insomnia, hypersomnia, decreased libido, impotence

SUMMARY OF CLINICAL STUDIES OF METHYL BROMIDE POISONING

With the exception of one group study, case reports provide the bulk of information about MB. Case reports leave convincing impressions that serious psychiatric symptoms result from severe poisoning. Significant MB exposure results in mood, thought, and cognitive disorders (Hine 1969; Johnstone 1945; Zatuchni and Hong 1981). The one case-control study suggested that even low-level exposures produce cognitive and mood changes in some individuals (Anger et al. 1986).

OTHER FUMIGANTS

Numerous chemicals are used as fumigants (Fishbein 1976). Flowerbulb workers with low-level exposures to 1,3-dichloropropene, a short-chained chlorinated hydrocarbon, did not have significantly greater psychiatric complaints than did control subjects (Brouwer et al. 1992). Diphenyl, or biphenyl, a fumigant or fungicide for fruits, converts to polychlorinated biphenyl through chlorination. Electrophysiological findings in workers exposed to diphenyl suggest that the chemical has neurotoxic potential (Hakkinen et al. 1973).

DIAGNOSIS AND TREATMENT OF METHYL BROMIDE POISONING

Correlation of a chemical exposure with mild elevations of blood bromide levels suggests MB poisoning. Inorganic bromide poisonings produce much lower blood bromide levels than do poisonings from bromide-containing sleep aids (Bleecker 1994). An abnormal electroencephalogram finding may assist the diagnosis. Standard treatment consists of 2,3-dimercaptopropanol (British Anti-Lewisite) with symptomatic and supportive treatment for mood and thought disorders.

REFERENCES

Anger WK, Moody L, Burg J, et al: Neurobehavioral evaluation of soil and structural fumigators using methyl bromide and sulfuryl fluoride. Neurotoxicology 7:137–156, 1986

Bleecker ML: Clinical presentation of selected neurotoxic compounds, in Occupational Neurology and Clinical Neurotoxicology. Edited by Bleecker ML, Hansen JA. Baltimore, MD, Williams & Wilkins, 1994, pp 207–233

Brouwer EJ, Brouwer DH, Bruynzeel DP, et al: Health in Relation to Occupational Exposure to Pesticides in the Dutch Flower Bulb Culture, Part 1: General Study Design: Results, Conclusions and Recommendations. The Hague, CIP-gegevens Koninklijke Bibliotheek, 1992

Collins RP: Methyl bromide poisoning: a bizarre neurological disorder. California Medicine 103:112–116, 1965

Dempsey DA, Becker CE: Death after entering an apartment building fumigated with methyl bromide and cleared for habitation (abstract). Vet Hum Toxicol 34:356, 1992

Deschamps FJ, Turpin JC: Methyl bromide intoxication during grain store fumigation. Occup Med 46:89–90, 1996

Fishbein L: Potential hazards of fumigant residues. Environ Health Perspect 14:39–45, 1976

Gosselin RE, Smith RP, Hodge HC, et al: Clinical Toxicology of Commercial Products. Baltimore, MD, Williams & Wilkins, 1984

Hakkinen I, Siltanen E, Hernberg S, et al: Diphenyl poisoning in fruit paper production. Arch Environ Health 26:70–74, 1973

Hine CH: Methyl bromide poisoning: a review of ten cases. J Occup Med 11:1–10, 1969

Johnstone RT: Methyl bromide intoxication of a large group of workers. Industrial Medicine 14:495–497, 1945

Klaassen CD: Nonmetallic environmental toxicants: air pollutants, solvents and vapors, and pesticides, in The Pharmacological Basis of Therapeutics. Edited by Gilman AG, Goodman LS, Rall TW, et al. New York, Macmillan, 1985, pp 1628–1650

O'Donoghue JL: Aliphatic halogenated hydrocarbons, alcohols, and acids and thioacids, in Neurotoxicity of Industrial and Commercial Chemicals, Vol II. Edited by O'Donoghue JL. Boca Raton, FL, CRC Press, 1985, pp 99–126

Zatuchni J, Hong K: Methyl bromide poisoning seen initially as psychosis. Arch Neurol 38:529–530, 1981

ADDITIONAL READINGS

Methyl Bromide

Drawneek W, O'Brien MJ, Goldsmith HJ, et al: Industrial methyl-bromide poisoning in fumigators. Lancet 2:855–856, 1964

Goldman LR, Mengle DC, Epstein DM, et al: Acute symptoms in persons residing near a field treated with the soil fumigants methyl bromide and chloropicrin. West J Med 147:95–98, 1987

Greenberg JO: The neurological effects of methyl bromide poisoning. Industrial Medicine 40:27–29, 1971

Herzstein J, Cullen MR: Methyl bromide intoxication in four field-workers during removal of soil fumigation sheets. Am J Ind Med 17:321–326, 1990

Ingram FR: Methyl bromide fumigation and control in the date-packing industry. AMA Archives of Industrial Hygiene and Occupational Medicine 4:193–198, 1951

Irsigler FJ: A case of methyl bromide poisoning: simulating rupture of an intracranial aneurysm. S Afr Med J 25:949–952, 1951

Johnstone RT: Methyl bromide intoxication of a large group of workers. Industrial Medicine 14:495–497, 1945

Longley EO, Jones AT: Methyl bromide poisoning in man. Industrial Medicine and Surgery 34:499–502, 1965

Peters HA, Levine RL, Matthews CG, et al: Carbon disulfide-induced neuropsychiatric changes in grain storage workers. Am J Ind Med 3:373–391, 1982

Peters HA, Levine RL, Matthews CG, et al: Synergistic neurotoxicity of carbon tetrachloride/carbon disulfide (80/20 fumigants) and other pesticides in grain storage workers. Acta Pharmacologica et Toxicologica 59 (suppl 6–7):535–546, 1986
Shield LK, Coleman TL, Markesbery WR: Methyl bromide intoxication: neurologic features, including simulation of Reye syndrome. Neurology 27:959–962, 1977
Verberk MM, Rooyakkers-Beemster T, De Vlieger M, et al: Bromine in blood, EEG and transaminases in methyl bromide workers. British Journal of Industrial Medicine 36:59–62, 1979

Other Fumigants

Flessel P, Goldsmith JR, Kahn E, et al: Acute and possible long-term effects of 1,3-dichloropropene-California. MMWR Morb Mortal Wkly Rep 27:50–55, 1978
Tyas SL, Manfreda J, Strain LA, et al: Risk factors for Alzheimer's disease: a population-based, longitudinal study in Manitoba, Canada. Int J Epidemiol 30:590–597, 2001

III

Metals

6

Aluminum

EPIDEMIOLOGY

In 1937, a study found that aluminum salts caused uniformly fatal, neurotoxic symptoms when injected intracerebrally in animals (Scherp and Church 1937). Experimental work in the 1960s later showed that intracerebral or intrathecal injections of aluminum in rabbits caused neurotoxic reactions and neurofibrillary tangles (NFTs) similar to those observed in Alzheimer's disease (AD) (Klatzo et al. 1965; Terry and Pena 1965). Between 1973 and 1976, three landmark articles reported aluminum in the NFTs of AD patients (Crapper 1974; Crapper et al. 1973, 1976).

In the same decade, five dialysis patients developed dyspraxia and seizures at a dialysis center in Denver, Colorado (Alfrey et al. 1972). Investigators suspected a contaminant in the tap water used for dialysis but did not suspect aluminum until their second study in 1976 found increased aluminum in the gray matter of 12 subjects with "dialysis dementia" (DD) (Alfrey et al. 1976). Two fields of research then merged with additional data from occupational exposures to focus on aluminum's putative role as a cause of dementing illnesses.

Exposures to aluminum can occur at home and work (Table 6–1). The greatest exposures of aluminum result from ingestion of food additives, water treatments, and nonprescription drugs. Significant aluminum ingestion also results from drinking water from aluminum-lined containers, including soda cans, corroded hot water heaters, and coffeepots (Brenner 1989; Duggan et al. 1992; Jackson et al. 1989).

TABLE 6–1. Occupations and other environments at risk for aluminum exposure

Occupations	Household/Medical
Aircraft makers	Antacids
Automobile makers	Antidiarrheal agents
Electrical equipment makers	Cosmetics
Explosives makers	Deodorants
Foundry workers	Dermatological pastes
Grinders	Dialysis fluids
Miners	Food additives
Painters	Formulas
Petroleum refining workers	Intravenous fluids
Rubber makers	Outer skins of many root vegetables
Utensil makers	Tea
Waterwork workers	Utensils
Welders	Water processing/pumping equipment/ boiling/heating appliances

Unlike the clear correlation of aluminum in water with DD, aluminum's role in AD remains unconfirmed. Animal studies confirm that aluminum causes NFTs and damages neuronal structure and function, but other areas of research suggest that aluminum plays no specific role in AD (Goyer 1996; Lukiw 1997). NFTs are seen in more than one neuropsychiatric disorder; they differ chemically and structurally between aluminum encephalopathy and AD, and individuals with increased brain aluminum may not develop dementia (Goyer 1996). Rather than cause injury, aluminum may only accumulate passively in injured neurons, and it increases with normal aging (Gautrin and Gauthier 1989; Katzman 1986). Many geographical studies that correlate high levels of aluminum in drinking water with AD rates have methodological errors and biases (Martyn 1990). Some geographical studies fail to demonstrate an association of AD with aluminum (Emard et al. 1994). Despite these drawbacks, many reviewers argue that aluminum has neuropathological relevance to AD (Flaten 2001;

McLachlan et al. 1991b; Meiri et al. 1993; Yokel 2000). Recent investigations suggest that AD is associated with enhanced bioavailability of certain aluminum species. AD patients have greater gastrointestinal absorption than controls, and specific exposure to organic monomeric aluminum increases risk of AD compared with exposure to other forms of aluminum (Gauthier et al. 2000; Moore et al. 2000).

DD has a stronger association with aluminum than does AD. Symptoms can result from oral aluminum treatment, especially in children (Baluarte et al. 1977; Sedman et al. 1984). Dialysis that uses water with high aluminum levels results in a higher prevalence of DD (Platts et al. 1977; Schreeder et al. 1983). An outbreak of DD occurred after a city added aluminum to the water supply (Rozas et al. 1978a, 1978b). A recent occurrence of DD resulted from an aluminum-containing cement mortar water distribution pipe in a dialysis center (Berend et al. 2001). Prevention of the syndrome is accomplished not only by avoiding aluminum-containing oral phosphate binders in dialysis but also by removing aluminum from water used for dialysis (Goyer 1996; Rozas et al. 1978a, 1978b). Chelation with desferrioxamine arrests the dementia (Goyer 1996).

The literature suggests that children, compared with adults, may have greater sensitivity to aluminum and greater susceptibility to cognitive decline from oral aluminum exposure from food, containers, and utensils. Treatment of children with chronic renal failure with oral aluminum resulted in an encephalopathy similar to DD (Baluarte et al. 1977; Griswold et al. 1983; Nathan and Pedersen 1980; Sedman et al. 1984). One study of aluminum in water consumed by children found no association with psychological test scores (McMillan et al. 1993).

NEUROLOGICAL AND PSYCHIATRIC SYMPTOMS OF ALUMINUM POISONING

Table 6–2 lists the neurological and psychiatric symptoms attributed to aluminum exposure. Most references do not consider aluminum an industrial poison, but chronic inhalation of aluminum dust causes pulmonary irritation leading to lung fibrosis (Shaver's disease) and bronchopneumonia (Katz 1985). An industrial case of pulmonary fibrosis in an aluminum refiner with DD-like symptoms and increased brain aluminum showed the overlap of symptoms between occupational exposures and DD (McLaughlin et al. 1962). Aluminum poisoning from the natural environment is one of several proposed causes of parkinsonism-

TABLE 6–2. Neurological and psychiatric signs, symptoms, and syndromes attributed to aluminum exposure

Alzheimer's disease	Dementia
Dialysis dementia	
Neurological	Dementia, dyspraxia, myoclonus, seizures, grimacing, speech arrest, dysarthria, dysphagia, abnormal electroencephalogram findings, asterixis, tremor
Psychiatric	*Mood:* Mood lability, depression, anxiety *Behavior:* Agitation, violence, personality change, bizarre behavior, suicidal, homicidal *Cognitive:* Memory loss, poor concentration, confusion *Perceptual:* Hallucinations, paranoia *Other:* Insomnia
Other	Pulmonary fibrosis, bronchopneumonia, anemia, osteodystrophy, amyotrophic lateral sclerosis and parkinsonism-dementia of Guam, macrophagic myofasciitis

dementia of Guam (PD). PD occurs frequently with amyotrophic lateral sclerosis on Guam. Aluminum accumulates in tangle-bearing neurons in PD as in AD (Candy and Edwardson 1987; Perl et al. 1985).

Macrophagic myofasciitis (MMF) is a recently identified demyelinating central nervous system disorder attributed to intramuscular injections of aluminum-containing vaccines. Symptoms of 1 of 92 cases included cognitive and behavioral changes (Authier et al. 2001). Another new disorder attributed to an inherited abnormality of aluminum metabolism causes progressive and fatal central nervous system calcification (Meshitsuka et al. 2001).

DD symptoms often develop after 2–3 years of dialysis (Chui and Damasio 1980). In typical cases of DD, the individual presents with speech arrest, dysarthria, or dysphasia, followed by myoclonic jerks, electroencephalogram abnormalities, bizarre behavior, and progressive dementia (Chokroverty et al. 1976; O'Hare et al. 1983). Death often occurs within 6 months of onset (Chui and Damasio 1980).

DIAGNOSIS AND TREATMENT OF ALUMINUM POISONING

Serum and urinary concentrations of aluminum provide good indicators of exposure (Maroni and Catenacci 1994). Diagnosis of dementia relies on criteria specified in DSM-IV-TR (American Psychiatric Association 2000). The diagnosis of DD may be aided by finding bilateral spike and wave complexes on the electroencephalogram (Hughes and Schreeder 1980). Neuropathological studies of brains from patients with DD usually find mild and nonspecific changes (Chokroverty et al. 1976; Lederman and Henry 1978). Chelation of aluminum with desferrioxamine may arrest or slow the dementia (Goyer 1996). Desferrioxamine also might slow the clinical progression of AD (McLachlan et al. 1991a).

REFERENCES

Alfrey AC, Mishell JM, Burks J, et al: Syndrome of dyspraxia and multifocal seizures associated with chronic hemodialysis. Transactions—American Society for Artificial Internal Organs 18:257–261, 1972

Alfrey AC, LeGendre GR, Kaehny WD: The dialysis encephalopathy syndrome: possible aluminum intoxication. N Engl J Med 294:184–188, 1976

American Psychiatric Association: Diagnostic and Statistical Manual of Mental Disorders, 4th Edition, Text Revision. Washington, DC, American Psychiatric Association, 2000

Authier FJ, Cherin P, Creange A, et al: Central nervous system disease in patients with macrophagic myofasciitis. Brain 124 (pt 5):983, 2001

Baluarte HJ, Gruskin AB, Hiner LB, et al: Encephalopathy in children with chronic renal failure. Proceedings of the Clinical Dialysis and Transplant Forum 7:95–98, 1977

Berend K, van der Voet G, Boer WH: Acute aluminum encephalopathy in a dialysis center caused by a cement mortar water distribution pipe. Kidney Int 59:746–753, 2001

Brenner S: Aluminium, hot water tanks, and neurobiology (letter) Lancet 1:781, 1989

Chokroverty S, Bruetman ME, Berger V, et al: Progressive dialytic encephalopathy. J Neurol Neurosurg Psychiatry 39:411–419, 1976

Chui HC, Damasio AR: Progressive dialysis encephalopathy ("dialysis dementia"). J Neurol 222:145–157, 1980

Crapper DR: Dementia: recent observations on Alzheimer's disease and experimental aluminum encephalopathy, in Frontiers in Neurology and Neuroscience Research 1974. Edited by Seeman P, Brown GM. Toronto, ON, University of Toronto Press, 1974, pp 97–111

Crapper DR, Krishnan B, Dalton AJ: Brain aluminium distribution in Alzheimer's disease and experimental neurofibrillary degeneration. Science 180:511–513, 1973

Crapper DR, Krishnan SS, Quittkat S: Aluminium, neurofibrillary degeneration and Alzheimer's disease. Brain 99:67–80, 1976

Duggan JM, Dickeson JE, Tynan PF, et al: Aluminium beverage cans as a dietary source of aluminium. Med J Aust 156:604–605, 1992

Candy JM, Edwardson JA: Aluminum and the pathogenesis of Alzheimer's disease. Trace Elements in Medicine 4:178–178, 1987

Emard JF, Andre P, Thouez J-P, et al: Geographical distribution of Alzheimer's disease cases at birth and the geochemical profile of Saguenay-Lac-Saint-Jean/Quebec, Canada (image project). Water, Air, and Soil Pollution 72:251–264, 1994

Flaten TP: Aluminium as a risk factor in Alzheimer's disease, with emphasis on drinking water. Brain Res Bull 55:187–196, 2001

Gauthier E, Fortier I., Courchesne F, et al: Aluminum forms in drinking water and risk of Alzheimer's disease. Environ Res 84:234–246, 2000

Gautrin D, Gauthier S: Alzheimer's disease: environmental factors and etiologic hypotheses. Can J Neurol Sci 16:375–387, 1989

Goyer RA: Toxic effects of metals, in Casarett and Doull's Toxicology: The Basic Science of Poisons. Edited by Klaassen CD, Amdur MO. New York, McGraw-Hill, 1996, pp 691–736

Griswold WR, Reznik V, Mendoza SA, et al: Accumulation of aluminum in a nondialyzed uremic child receiving aluminum hydroxide. Pediatrics 71:56–58, 1983

Hughes JR, Schreeder MT: EEG in dialysis encephalopathy. Neurology 30:1148–1154, 1980

Jackson JA, Riordan HD, Poling CM: Aluminium from a coffee pot (letter). Lancet 1:781–782, 1989

Katz GV: Metals and metalloids other than mercury and lead, in Neurotoxicity of Industrial and Commercial Chemicals, Vol 1. Edited by O'Donoghue JL. Boca Raton, FL, CRC Press, 1985, pp 171–191

Katzman R: Alzheimer's disease. N Engl J Med 314:964–973, 1986

Klatzo I, Wisniewski H, Streicher E: Experimental production of neurofibrillary degeneration. J Neuropathol Exp Neurol 24:187–199, 1965

Lederman RJ, Henry CE: Progressive dialysis encephalopathy. Ann Neurol 4:199–204, 1978

Lukiw WJ: Alzheimer's disease and aluminum, in Mineral and Metal Neurotoxicology. Edited by Yasui M, Strong MJ, Ota K, et al. Boca Raton, FL, CRC Press, 1997, pp 113–126

Maroni M, Catenacci G: Biological monitoring of neurotoxic compounds, in Occupational Neurology and Clinical Neurotoxicology. Edited by Bleecker ML, Hansen JA. Baltimore, MD, Williams & Wilkins, 1994, pp 43–83

Martyn CN: Aluminium and Alzheimer's disease: an epidemiological approach. Environmental Geochemistry and Health 12:169–171, 1990

McLachlan DRC, Dalton AJ, Kruck TPA, et al: Intramuscular desferrioxamine in patients with Alzheimer's disease. Lancet 337:1304–1308, 1991a

McLachlan DRC, Kruck TP, Lukiw WJ, et al: Would decreased aluminum ingestion reduce the incidence of Alzheimer's disease? CMAJ 145:793–804, 1991b

McLaughlin AIG, Kazantzis G, King E, et al: Pulmonary fibrosis and encephalopathy associated with the inhalation of aluminium dust. British Journal of Industrial Medicine 19:253–263, 1962

McMillan TM, Dunn G, Colwill SJ: Psychological testing on schoolchildren before and after pollution of drinking water in North Cornwall. J Child Psychol Psychiatry 34:1449–1459, 1993

Meiri H, Banin E, Roll M, et al: Toxic effects of aluminium on nerve cells and synaptic transmission. Prog Neurobiol 40:89–121, 1993

Meshitsuka S, Loeda T, Hara T, et al: Abnormal aluminium metabolism in two siblings with progressive CNS calcification (letter). Dev Med Child Neurol 43:287–288, 2001

Moore PB, Day JP, Taylor GA, et al: Absorption of aluminium-26 in Alzheimer's disease, measured using accelerator mass spectrometry. Dement Geriatr Cogn Disord 11:66–69, 2000

Nathan E, Pedersen SE: Dialysis encephalopathy in a non-dialysed uraemic boy treated with aluminium hydroxide orally. Acta Paediatrica Scandinavica 69:793–796, 1980

O'Hare JA, Callaghan NM, Murnaghan DJ: Dialysis encephalopathy: clinical, electroencephalographic and interventional aspects. Medicine 62:129–141, 1983

Perl DP, Munoz-Garcia D, Good PF, et al: Intracytoplasmic aluminum accumulation in neurofibrillary tangle-bearing neurons: detection by laser microprobe mass analyzer (abstract). Ann Neurol 18:143, 1985

Platts MM, Goode GC, Hislop JS: Composition of the domestic water supply and the incidence of fractures and encephalopathy in patients on home dialysis. BMJ 2:657–660, 1977

Rozas VV, Port FK, Easterling RE: An outbreak of dialysis dementia due to aluminum in the dialysate. Journal of Dialysis 2:459–470, 1978a

Rozas VV, Port FK, Rutt WM: Progressive dialysis encephalopathy from dialysate aluminum. Arch Intern Med 138:1375–1377, 1978b

Scherp HW, Church CF: Neurotoxic action of aluminum salts. Proc Soc Exp Biol Med 36:851–853, 1937

Schreeder MT, Favero MS, Hughes JR, et al: Dialysis encephalopathy and aluminum exposure: an epidemiologic analysis. Journal of Chronic Diseases 36:581–593, 1983

Sedman AB, Wilkening GN, Warady BA, et al: Encephalopathy in childhood secondary to aluminum toxicity. J Pediatr 105:836–838, 1984

Terry RD, Pena C: Experimental production of neurofibrillary degeneration. J Neuropathol Exp Neurol 24:200–210, 1965

Yokel RA: The toxicology of aluminum in the brain: a review. Neurotoxicology 21: 813–828, 2000

ADDITIONAL READINGS

Positive Correlation of Aluminum With Alzheimer's Disease

Altmann P, Cunningham J, Dhanesha U, et al: Disturbance of cerebral function in people exposed to drinking water contaminated with aluminium sulphate: retrospective study of the Camelford water incident. BMJ 319:807–811, 1999

Basun H, Forssell L, Wetterberg L, et al: Metals and trace elements in blood and cerebrospinal fluid in normal aging an [sic] Alzheimer's disease (abstract). Neurobiol Aging 13:S96, 1992

Bowdler NC, Beasley DS, Fritze EC, et al: Behavioral effects of aluminum ingestion on animal and human subjects. Pharmacol Biochem Behav 10:505–512, 1979

Candy JM, Klinowski J, Perry RH, et al: Aluminosilicates and senile plaque formation in Alzheimer's disease. Lancet 1:354–356, 1986

Flaten TP: Geographical associations between aluminum in drinking water and dementia, Parkinson's disease and amyotrophic lateral sclerosis in Norway. Trace Elements in Medicine 4:179–180, 1987

Flaten TP: Geographical associations between aluminium in drinking water and death rates with dementia (including Alzheimer's disease), Parkinson's disease and amyotrophic lateral sclerosis in Norway. Environmental Geochemistry and Health 12:152–168, 1990

Forbes WF, McAiney CA: Aluminium and dementia (letter). Lancet 340:668–669, 1992

Good PF, Perl DP, Bierer LM, et al: Selective accumulation of aluminum and iron in the neurofibrillary tangles of Alzheimer's disease: a laser microprobe (LAMMA) study. Ann Neurol 31:286–292, 1992

Heyman A, Wilkinson WE, Stafford JA, et al: Alzheimer's disease a study of epidemiological aspects. Ann Neurol 15:335–341, 1984

Lapresle J, Duckett S, Galle P, et al: [Clinical, anatomical and biophysical data on a case of encephalopathy with aluminum deposits]. C R Seances Soc Biol Fil 169: 282–285, 1975

Lukiw WJ, Kruck TPA, Krishnan B, et al: Aluminum and the genetic apparatus in Alzheimer's disease (abstract). Neurobiol Aging 13:S95, 1992

Martyn CN, Barker DJP, Osmond C, et al: Geographical relation between Alzheimer's disease and aluminium in drinking water. Lancet 1:59–62, 1989

Martyn C, Houeland T, Osmond C: Population based studies of aluminium in Alzheimer's disease (abstract). Neurobiol Aging 11:290, 1990

Mattiello G, Gerotto M, Favarato M, et al: Microelemental analysis of plasma from Alzheimer's and multiinfarctual dementia patients (abstract). Neurobiol Aging 13: S97, 1992

McLachlan DRC, Bergeron C, Smith JE, et al: Risk for neuropathologically confirmed Alzheimer's disease and residual aluminum in municipal drinking water employing weighted residential histories. Neurology 46:401–405, 1996

McMillan TM, Freemont AJ, Herxheimer A, et al: Camelford water poisoning accident: serial neuropsychological assessments and further observations on bone aluminium. Hum Exp Toxicol 12:37–42, 1993

Michel P, Commenges D, Dartigues JF, et al: Study of the relationship between aluminium concentration in drinking water and risk of Alzheimer's disease, in Alzheimer's Disease: Basic Mechanisms, Diagnosis and Therapeutic Strategies. Edited by Iqbal K, McLachlan DRC, Winblad B, et al. New York, Wiley-Interscience, 1991, pp 387–391

Miller TP, Davies HD, Yesavage JA, et al: Presenile dementia associated with elevated aluminum and zinc levels: a case report. Clinical Gerontologist 2:55–59, 1984

Neri LC, Hewitt D: Aluminium, Alzheimer's disease, and drinking water (letter). Lancet 338:390, 1991

Neri LC, Hewitt D, Rifat SL: Aluminium in drinking water and risk for diagnoses of presenile Alzheimer's type dementia (abstract). Neurobiol Aging 13:S115, 1992

Perl DP, Brody AR: Alzheimer's disease: x-ray spectrometric evidence of aluminum accumulation in neurofibrillary tangle-bearing neurons. Science 208:297–299, 1980

Rogers MA, Simon DG: A preliminary study of dietary aluminium intake and risk of Alzheimer's disease. Age Ageing 28:205–209, 1999

Rondeau V, Commenges D, Jacqmin-Gadda H, et al: Relation between aluminum concentrations in drinking water and Alzheimer's disease: an 8-year follow-up study. Am J Epidemiol 152:59–66, 2000

Rowland A, Grainger R, Smith RS, et al: Water contamination in North Cornwall: a retrospective cohort study into the acute and short-term effects of the aluminium sulphate incident in July 1988. J R Soc Health 110:166–172, 1990

Sjogren B, Ljunggren KG, Almkvist O, et al: Aluminosis and dementia (letter). Lancet 344:1154, 1994

Solomon B, Koppel R, Jossiphov J: Immunostaining of calmodulin and aluminium in Alzheimer's disese-affected brains. Brain Res Bull 55:253–256, 2001

Stern AJ, Perl DP, Munoz-Garcia D, et al: Investigation of silicon and aluminum content in isolated senile plaque cores by laser microprobe mass analysis (LAMMA) (abstract). J Neuropathol Exp Neurol 45:361, 1986

Trapp GA, Miner GD, Zimmerman RL, et al: Aluminum levels in brain in Alzheimer's disease. Biol Psychiatry 13:709–718, 1978

No Correlation of Aluminum With Alzheimer's Disease

Amaducci LA, Fratiglioni L, Rocca WA, et al: Risk factors for clinically diagnosed Alzheimer's disease: a case-control study of an Italian population. Neurology 36:922–931, 1986

Broe GA, Henderson AS, Creasey H, et al: A case-control study of Alzheimer's disease in Australia. Neurology 40:1698–1707, 1990

Chafi AH, Hauw J-J, Rancurel G, et al: Absence of aluminium in Alzheimer's disease brain tissue: electron microprobe and ion microprobe studies. Neurosci Lett 123:61–64, 1991

Chandra V, Philipose V, Bell PA, et al: Case-control study of late onset "probable Alzheimer's disease." Neurology 37:1295–1300, 1987

David A: Cerebral dysfunction after water pollution incident in Camelford: results were biased by self selection of cases (letter). BMJ 320:1337–1337, 2000

Delaney JF: Spinal fluid aluminum levels in patients with Alzheimer disease. Ann Neurol 5:580–581, 1979

Esmonde TF: Cerebral dysfunction after water pollution incident in Camelford: study has several methodological errors (letter). BMJ 320:1337–1338, 2000

Forster DP, Newens AJ, Kay DWK, et al: Risk factors in clinically diagnosed presenile dementia of the Alzheimer type: a case-control study in northern England. J Epidemiol Community Health 49:253–258, 1995

French LR, Schuman LM, Mortimer JA, et al: A case-control study of dementia of the Alzheimer type. Am J Epidemiol 121:414–421, 1985

Graves AB, White E, Koepsell TD, et al: The association between aluminum-containing products and Alzheimer's disease. J Clin Epidemiol 43:35–44, 1990

Henderson AS, Jorm AF, Korten AE, et al: Environmental risk factors for Alzheimer's disease: their relationship to age of onset and to familial or sporadic types. Psychol Med 22:429–436, 1992

Hershey CO, Hershey LA, Varnes AW, et al: Cerebrospinal fluid trace element content in dementia: clinical, radiologic, and pathologic correlations. Neurology 33: 1350–1353, 1983

Ijomah G, Corrigan FM, Holliday J, et al: Aluminum, cadmium, lipids and prevalence of dementia in people living near an aluminum smelter. Trace Elements in Medicine 10:6–12, 1993

Jacobs RW, Duong T, Jones RE, et al: A reexamination of aluminum in Alzheimer's disease: analysis by energy dispersive x-ray microprobe and flameless atomic absorption spectrophotometry. Can J Neurol Sci 16:498–503, 1989

Jacqmin H, Commenges D, Letenneur L, et al: Study of exposure to aluminium in drinking water and cognitive impairment (abstract). Neurobiol Aging 13:S116–S117, 1992

Jacqmin H, Commenges D, Letenneur L, et al: Components of drinking water and risk of cognitive impairment in the elderly. Am J Epidemiol 139:48–57, 1994

Kapaki EN, Zournas CP, Segdistsa IT, et al: Cerebrospinal fluid aluminum levels in Alzheimer's disease. Biol Psychiatry 33:679–681, 1993

Landsberg JP, McDonald B, Watt F: Absence of aluminium in neuritic plaque cores in Alzheimer's disease. Nature 360:65–68, 1992

Markesbery WR, Ehmann WD, Hossain TIM, et al: Instrumental neutron activation analysis of brain aluminum in Alzheimer disease and aging. Ann Neurol 10:511–516, 1981

Martyn CN, Coggon DN, Inskip H, et al: Aluminum concentrations in drinking water and risk of Alzheimer's disease. Epidemiology 8:281–286, 1997

McDermott JR, Smith AI, Iqbal K, et al: Aluminium and Alzheimer's disease (letter). Lancet 2:710–711, 1977

McDermott JR, Smith AI, Iqbal K, et al: Brain aluminum in aging and Alzheimer disease. Neurology 29:809–814, 1979

McMillan TM, Dunn G, Colwill SJ: Psychological testing on schoolchildren before and after pollution of drinking water in North Cornwall. J Child Psychol Psychiatry 34:1449–1459, 1993a

McMillan TM, Freemont AJ, Herxheimer A, et al: Camelford water poisoning accident: serial neuropsychological assessments and further observations on bone aluminium. Hum Exp Toxicol 12:37–42, 1993b

Reusche E, Koch V, Lindner B, et al: Alzheimer morphology is not increased in dialysis-associated encephalopathy and long-term hemodialysis. Acta Neuropathol (Berl) 101:211–216, 2001

Salib E, Hillier V: A case-control study of Alzheimer's disease and aluminium occupation. Br J Psychiatry 168:244–249, 1996

Shore D, King SW, Kaye W, et al: Serum and cerebrospinal fluid aluminum and circulating parathyroid hormone in primary degenerative (senile) dementia, in Aluminum Toxicity. Edited by Liss L. Park Forest South, IL, Pathotox, 1980a, pp 55–63

Shore D, Millson M, Holtz JL, et al: Serum aluminum in primary degenerative dementia. Biol Psychiatry 15:971–977, 1980b

Wettstein A, Aeppli J, Gautschi K, et al: Failure to find a relationship between amnestic skills in octogenarians and aluminum in drinking water. Int Arch Occup Environ Health 63:97–103, 1991

Wood DJ, Cooper C, Stevens J, et al: Bone mass and dementia in hip fracture patients from areas with different aluminium concentrations in water supplies. Age Ageing 17:415–419, 1988

Dialysis Dementia

Ackrill P, Ralston AJ, Day JP, et al: Successful removal of aluminium from patient with dialysis encephalopathy (letter). Lancet 2:692–693, 1980

Altmann P, Hamon C, Blair JA, et al: Disturbance of cerebral function by aluminium in haemodialysis patients without overt aluminium toxicity. Lancet 2:7–12, 1989

Arieff AI, Cooper JD, Armstrong D, et al: Dementia, renal failure, and brain aluminum. Ann Intern Med 90:741–747, 1979

Ball JH, Butkus DE, Madison DS: Effect of subtotal parathyriodectomy on dialysis dementia. Nephron 18:151–155, 1977

Barratt LJ, Lawrence JR: Dialysis-associated dementia. Aust N Z J Med 5:62–65, 1975

Branaccio D, Damasso R, Spinnler H, et al: Does chronic kidney failure lead to mental failure? A neuropsychologic survey of self-sufficient outpatients. Arch Neurol 38:757–758, 1981

Burks JS, Huddlestone J, Alfrey AC, et al: A fatal encephalopathy in chronic haemodialysis patients. Lancet 1:764–768, 1976

Davison AM, Walker GS, Oli H, et al: Water supply aluminium concentration, dialysis dementia, and effect of reverse-osmosis water treatment. Lancet 2:785–787, 1982

Dettori P, LaGreca G, Biasioli S, et al: Changes of cerebral density in dialyzed patients. Neuroradiology 23:95–99, 1982

Dunea G, Mahurkar SD, Mamdani B, et al: Role of aluminum in dialysis dementia. Ann Intern Med 88:502–504, 1978

Elliott HL, Dryburgh F, Fell GS, et al: Aluminium toxicity during regular haemodialysis. BMJ 1:1101–1103, 1978

Etheridge WB, O'Neill WM: The "dialysis encephalopathy syndrome" without dialysis. Clin Nephrol 10:250–252, 1978

Geary DF, Fennell RS, Andriola M, et al: Encephalopathy in children with chronic renal failure. J Pediatr 96:41–44, 1980

Gilli P, De Bastiani P: Cognitive function and regular dialysis treatment. Clin Nephrol 19:188–192, 1983

Glick ID, Goldfield MD, Kovnat PJ: Recognition and management of psychosis associated with hemodialysis. California Medicine 119:56–59, 1973

Hart RP, Pederson JA, Czerwinski AW, et al: Chronic renal failure, dialysis, and neuropsychological function (abstract). J Clin Neuropsychol 5:301–312, 1983

Ladurner G, Wawschinek O, Poggliysch H, et al: Neurophysiological findings and serum aluminium in dialysis encephalopathy. Eur Neurol 21:335–339, 1982

Madison DP, Baehr ET, Bazell M, et al: Communicative and cognitive deterioration in dialysis dementia: two case studies. Journal of Speech and Hearing Disorders 42:238–246, 1977

Mahurkar SD, Salta R, Smith EC, et al: Dialysis dementia. Lancet 1:1412–1415, 1973

Masramon J, Ricart MJ, Caralps A, et al: Dialysis encephalopathy (letter). Lancet 1:1370, 1978

Masselot JP, Adhemar JP, Jaudon MC, et al: Reversible dialysis encephalopathy: role for aluminium-containing gels (letter). Lancet 2:1386–1387, 1978

McDermott JR, Smith AI, Ward MK, et al: Brain-aluminium concentration in dialysis encephalopathy. Lancet 1:901–904, 1978

McKinney TD, Basinger M, Dawson E, et al: Serum aluminum levels in dialysis dementia. Nephron 32:53–56, 1982

Merrill RH, Collins JL: Acute psychosis in chronic renal failure: case reports. Mil Med 139:622–624, 1974

Nadel AM, Wilson WP: Dialysis encephalopathy: a possible seizure disorder. Neurology 26:1130–1134, 1976

Parkinson IS, Ward MK, Feest TG, et al: Fracturing dialysis osteodystrophy and dialysis encephalopathy. Lancet 1:406–409, 1979

Pascoe MD: Clonazepam in dialysis encephalopathy (letter). Ann Neurol 9:200, 1981

Phelps KR, Naylor K, Brien TP, et al: Encephalopathy after bladder irrigation with alum: case report and literature review. Am J Med Sci 318:181–185, 1999

Platts MM, Anastassiades E: Dialysis encephalopathy: precipitating factors and improvement in prognosis. Clin Nephrol 15:223–228, 1981

Poisson M, Mashaly R: Dialysis encephalopathy: recovery after interruption of aluminium intake (case report). BMJ 2:1610–1611, 1978

Poisson M, Mashaly R, Lafforgue B: Progressive dialysis encephalopathy (letter). Ann Neurol 6:88, 1979

Rosati G, De Bastiani P, Gilli P, et al: Oral aluminum and neuropsychological functioning: a study of dialysis patients receiving aluminum hydroxide gels. J Neurol 223: 251–257, 1980

Rovelli E, Luciani L, Pagani C, et al: Correlation between serum aluminum concentration and signs of encephalopathy in a large population of patients dialyzed with aluminum-free fluids. Clin Nephrol 29:294–298, 1988

Savazzi GM, Cusmano F, Degasperi T: Cerebral atrophy in patients on long-term regular hemodialysis treatment. Clin Nephrol 23:89–95, 1985

Scheiber SC, Ziesat H Jr: Clinical and psychological test findings in cerebral dyspraxia associated with hemodialysis. J Nerv Ment Dis 162:212–214, 1976a

Scheiber SC, Ziesat H Jr: Dementia dialytica: a new psychotic organic brain syndrome. Compr Psychiatry 17:781–785, 1976b

Smith DB, Lewis JA, Burks JS, et al: Dialysis encephalopathy in peritoneal dialysis. JAMA 244:365–366, 1980

Sprague SM, Corwin HL, Tanner CM, et al: Relationship of aluminum to neurocognitive dysfunction in chronic dialysis patients. Arch Intern Med 148:2169–2172, 1988

Trauner DA, Clayman M: Dialysis encephalopathy treated with clonazepam. Ann Neurol 6:555–556, 1979

Warady BA, Belden B, Kohaut E: Neurodevelopmental outcome of children initiating peritoneal dialysis in early infancy. Pediatr Nephrol 13:759–765, 1999

Infant Formulas

Bishop NJ, Robinson MJ, Lendon M, et al: Increased concentration of aluminium in the brain of a parenterally fed preterm infant. Arch Dis Child 64:1316–1317, 1989

Bishop NJ, Morley R, Day JP, et al: Aluminum neurotoxicity in preterm infants receiving intravenous-feeding solutions. N Engl J Med 336:1557–1561, 1997

Freundlich M, Abitbol C, Zilleruelo G, et al: Infant formula as a cause of aluminium toxicity in neonatal uraemia. Lancet 2:527–529, 1985

Occupational Exposures

Akila R, Stollery BT, Riihimaki V: Decrements in cognitive performance in metal inert gas welders exposed to aluminium. Occup Environ Med 56:632–639, 1999

Bast-Pettersen R, Drablos PA, Goffeng LO, et al: Neuropsychological deficit among elderly workers in aluminum production. Am J Ind Med 25:649–662, 1994

Bast-Pettersen R, Skaug V, Ellingsen D, et al: Neurobehavioral performance in aluminum welders. Am J Ind Med 37:184–192, 2000

Hanninen H, Matikainen E, Kovala T, et al: Internal load of aluminum and the central nervous system function of aluminum welders. Scand J Work Environ Health 20: 279–285, 1994

Iregren A, Sjogren B, Gustafsson K, et al: Effects on the nervous system in different groups of workers exposed to aluminium. Occup Environ Med 58:453–460, 2001

Kilburn KH: Neurobehavioural impairment and symptoms associated with aluminum remelting. Arch Environ Health 53:329–335, 1998

Kilburn KH, Warshaw RH: Neurobehavioral testing of subjects exposed residentially to groundwater contaminated from an aluminum die-casting plant and local referents. J Toxicol Environ Health 39:483–496, 1993

Kobayashi S, Hirota N, Saito K, et al: Aluminum accumulation in tangle-bearing neurons of Alzheimer's disease with Balint's syndrome in a long-term aluminum refiner. Acta Neuropathol (Berl) 74:47–52, 1987

Letzel S, Lang CJ, Schaller KH, et al: Longitudinal study of neurotoxicity with occupational exposure to aluminum dust. Neurology 54:997–1000, 2000

Longstreth WT Jr, Rosenstock L, Heyer NJ: Potroom palsy? Neurologic disorder in three aluminum smelter workers. Arch Intern Med 145:1972–1975, 1985

Moulin JJ, Clavel T, Buclez B, et al: A mortality study among workers in a French aluminium reduction plant. Int Arch Occup Environ Health 73:323–330, 2000

Rifat S, Eastwood MR, McLachlan DR, et al: Evidence regarding the effect of prolonged aluminum exposure on cognitive behavior (abstract). Neurobiol Aging 11:295, 1990a

Rifat SL, Eastwood MR, McLachlan DRC, et al: Effect of exposure of miners to aluminium powder. Lancet 336:1162–1165, 1990b

Riihimaki V, Hanninen H, Akila R, et al: Body burden of aluminum in relation to central nervous system function among metal inert-gas welders. Scand J Work Environ Health 26:118–130, 2000

Sim M, Dick R, Russo J, et al: Are aluminium potroom workers at increased risk of neurological disorders? Occup Environ Med 54:229–235, 1997

Sjogren B, Gustavsson P, Hogstedt C: Neuropsychiatric symptoms among welders exposed to neurotoxic metals. British Journal of Industrial Medicine 47:704–707, 1990

Spofforth J: Case of aluminum poisoning (letter). Lancet 1:1301, 1921

White DM, Longstreth WT, Rosenstock L, et al: Neurologic syndrome in 25 workers from an aluminum smelting plant. Arch Intern Med 152:1443–1448, 1992

Other

van Rensburg SJ, Potocnik FC, Kiss T, et al: Serum concentrations of some metals and steroids in patients with chronic fatigue syndrome with reference to neurological and cognitive abnormalities. Brain Res Bull 55:319–325, 2001

7

Arsenic

EPIDEMIOLOGY

Industrial and environmental sources cause most modern cases of arsenic poisoning. A National Institute for Occupational Safety and Health study in 1975 estimated that 1.5 million workers had potential exposure to arsenic (Hartman 1988). Poisonings have resulted from veterinary compounds, paints, herbicides, pesticides, rodenticides, treated lumber, and Chinese herbal products (Garvey et al. 2001; Gosselin et al. 1984; Peters et al. 1983). Table 7–1 lists occupations with the greatest risk of exposure to arsenic.

Arsenic poisoning occurs infrequently in the United States, but other countries have a higher incidence. Since 1900, massive epidemics of arsenic poisoning involving thousands of persons occurred in France and Japan (Katz 1985; Pershagen 1983). The poisoning of 200,000 Indians in West Bengal as recently as 1996 from village wells caused a serious health crisis ("Getting a Grip on Arsenic" 1998; Bagla and Kaiser 1996). A hostage held by foreign terrorists returned with various psychiatric manifestations and elevated serum arsenic levels (Holloway and Benedek 1999).

TABLE 7–1. Occupations and other environmental factors at risk for arsenic exposure

	Occupational	
Antifouling paint users Artificial flower makers Artificial leather workers Bookbinders Brass workers Bronzers Cosmetics workers Disinfectant users/makers Electroplating workers Enamel makers Etching workers Feather users Fertilizer makers/users Fungicide makers/users Glassblowers Herbicide makers/users	Insecticide makers/users Insulator makers Jewelers Linoleum makers Metallurgy workers Miners Pigment/dye makers/users Rubber makers Salt-impregnated materials for fires with multicolored flames—workers/users Semiconductor makers Sheep dippers Silicon microfilm makers Smelter workers	Soap/detergent makers Solderers Storage battery makers Taxidermists Textile workers Treated wood makers/burners Velvet makers Veterinary drug makers/users Watch diode makers Wax makers Welders
	Environmental	
Antique copper kettles Drug abuse (adulteration of the substance)	Illegal alcohol ("moonshine" liquor) Residence near smelter	Seafood Water from rock formations high in arsenic

SYMPTOMS OF ARSENIC POISONING

Arsenic poisoning results from exposure to one of three major groups of arsenic compounds: inorganic compounds, organic compounds, and arsine gas (Maroni and Catenacci 1994). Arsine gas, the most toxic form of arsenic, hemolyzes red blood cells and causes renal failure (Squibb and Fowler 1983). The inorganic salts of arsenic generally have greater toxicity than do organic forms (Squibb and Fowler 1983).

Susceptibility to arsenic poisoning varies genetically and according to nutritional status (Bagla and Kaiser 1996; Brouwer et al. 1992; Calabrese 1978). Table 7–2 lists signs and symptoms of arsenic poisoning. The presence of skin pigmentation, exfoliation, and Mees' lines indicates arsenic poisoning (Goetz 1985).

Summary of Psychiatric Symptoms

Table 7–3 lists the psychiatric signs and symptoms attributed to arsenic poisoning. Acute arsenic poisoning may induce an encepha-

TABLE 7–2. Signs and symptoms of arsenic poisoning

Acute	
Pulmonary	Pulmonary edema (arsine)
Gastrointestinal	Anorexia, severe gastritis, gastroenteritis, nausea, vomiting
Cardiovascular	Arrhythmia, shock, cardiac arrest
Renal	Renal failure from hemolysis (arsine)
Neurological	Headache, vertigo, convulsions, delirium, coma
Skin	Melanosis, bronzed skin (arsine)
Other	Muscle pain, fever
Subacute and chronic	
Respiratory	Inflamed upper respiratory tract
Gastrointestinal	Anorexia, liver damage
Cardiovascular	Peripheral vascular disease
Neurological	Sensory loss 1–2 weeks postexposure, paresthesias, painful peripheral neuropathy, headache, weakness, encephalopathy
Skin	Numercus skin disorders, white bands in nails (Mees' lines), exfoliation, pigmentation
Other	Anemia, leukopenia, muscle tenderness, gangrene of lower extremities

TABLE 7–3. Psychiatric signs and symptoms attributed to arsenic poisoning

Mood	Anxiety, irritability
Behavior	Agitation, singing, muttering, personality change, suicidal
Cognitive	Confabulation, poor memory and concentration
Perceptual	Visual hallucinations, disordered thinking, psychosis, Korsakoff's psychcsis, paranoia

lopathy leading to death. The resulting delirium manifests as confabulation, confusion, memory loss, agitation, and hallucinations. In less severe or chronic poisonings, psychotic symptoms or neuropsychological impairments appear in the victims. Some poisonings mimic major depressive or psychotic disorders. In some cases, arsenic poisoning is associated with a form of Korsakoff's psychosis that has a peripheral neuropathy unlike the neuropathy in Korsakoff's psychosis secondary to alcohol.

DIAGNOSIS AND TREATMENT OF ARSENIC POISONING

Detection of arsenic in urine indicates recent exposure (Maroni and Catenacci 1994). Diet, especially seafood, influences organic arsenic levels, and a dietary history must be obtained to interpret inorganic arsenic levels (Goetz 1985; Maroni and Catenacci 1994). Hair and nail content of arsenic indicates inorganic arsenic exposure, but levels vary with the type of arsenic and route of exposure (Maroni and Catenacci 1994). Physicians should consider suicide, homicide, and alcohol and drug abuse in circumstances of arsenic poisoning in the absence of occupational or environmental risk factors. Some illicit drug dealers may adulterate drugs with arsenic. The illegal production of alcohol also may produce arsenic contaminants.

Chemical warfare during World War I spurred the development of British Anti-Lewisite (2,3-dimercaptopropanol) for the treatment of arsenic poisoning from the warfare gas Lewisite. British Anti-Lewisite may improve the dermal, pulmonary, and neuropsychological symptoms but not the neuropathy from arsenic (Bolla-Wilson and Bleecker 1987; Goetz 1985; Goyer 1996). Arsine intoxication responds better to hemodialysis (Gosselin et al. 1984). Some authors suggest treating with D-penicillamine, although some life-threatening reactions result from its use (Gosselin et al. 1984).

REFERENCES

Bagla P, Kaiser J: India's spreading health crisis draws global arsenic experts (news). Science 274:174–175, 1996

Bolla-Wilson K, Bleecker ML: Neuropsychological impairment following inorganic arsenic exposure. J Occup Med 29:500–503, 1987

Brouwer OF, Onkenhout W, Edelbroek PM, et al: Increased neurotoxicity of arsenic in methylenetetrahydrofolate reductase deficiency. Clin Neurol Neurosurg 94:307–310, 1992

Calabrese EJ: Pollutants and High-Risk Groups: The Biological Basis of Increased Human Susceptibility to Environmental and Occupational Pollutants. New York, Wiley-Interscience, 1978

Garvey GJ, Hahn G, Lee RV, et al: Heavy metal hazards of Asian traditional remedies. Int J Environ Health Res 11:63–71, 2001

Getting a grip on arsenic (news). Science 281:1261, 1998

Goetz CG: Arsenic, in Neurotoxins in Clinical Practice. New York, Medical & Scientific Books, 1985, pp 36–44

Gosselin RE, Smith RP, Hodge HC, et al: Clinical Toxicology of Commercial Products. Baltimore, MD, Williams & Wilkins, 1984

Goyer RA: Toxic effects of metals, in Casarett and Doull's Toxicology: The Basic Science of Poisons. Edited by Klaassen CD, Amdur MO. New York, McGraw-Hill, 1996, pp 691–736

Hartman DE: Neuropsychological toxicology of metals, in Neuropsychological Toxicology: Identification and Assessment of Human Neurotoxic Syndromes. New York, Pergamon, 1988, pp 55–107

Holloway HC, Benedek DM: The changing face of terrorism and military psychiatry. Psychiatric Annals 29:363–375, 1999

Katz GV: Metals and metalloids other than mercury and lead, in Neurotoxicity of Industrial and Commercial Chemicals, Vol 1. Edited by O'Donoghue JL. Boca Raton, FL, CRC Press, 1985, pp 171–191

Maroni M, Catenacci G: Biological monitoring of neurotoxic compounds, in Occupational Neurology and Clinical Neurotoxicology. Edited by Bleecker ML, Hansen JA. Baltimore, MD, Williams & Wilkins, 1994, pp 43–83

Pershagen G: The epidemiology of human arsenic exposure, in Biological and Environmental Effects of Arsenic. Edited by Fowler BA. Amsterdam, Elsevier, 1983, pp 199–232

Peters HA, Croft WA, Woolson EA, et al: Arsenic, chromium, and copper poisoning from burning treated wood (letter). N Engl J Med 308:1360–1361, 1983

Squibb KS, Fowler BA: The toxicity of arsenic and its compounds, in Biological and Environmental Effects of Arsenic. Edited by Fowler BA. Amsterdam, Elsevier, 1983, pp 233–269

ADDITIONAL READINGS

Beckett WS, Moore JL, Keogh JP, et al: Acute encephalopathy due to occupational exposure to arsenic. British Journal of Industrial Medicine 43:66–67, 1986

Calderon J, Navarro ME, Jimenz-Capdeville ME, et al: Exposure to arsenic and neuropsychological development in Mexican children. Environ Res 85:69–76, 2001

DePalma AE: Arsine intoxication in a chemical plant. J Occup Med 11:582–587, 1969

Eagle H, Magnuson HJ: The systemic treatment of 227 cases of arsenic poisoning (encephalitis, dermatitis, blood dyscrasias, jaundice, fever) with 2,3-dimercaptopropanol (BAL). American Journal of Syphilis, Gonorrhea, and Venereal Diseases 30:420–441, 1946

Frank G: Neurologische und psychiatrische folgesymptome bei akuter arsen-wasserstoff-vergiftung (English abstract). J Neurol 213:59–70, 1976

Freeman JW, Couch JR: Prolonged encephalopathy with arsenic poisoning. Neurology 28:853–855, 1978

Heyman A, Pfeiffer JB, Willett RW, et al: Peripheral neuropathy caused by arsenical intoxication. N Engl J Med 254:401–409, 1956

Jenkins RB: Inorganic arsenic and the nervous system. Brain 89:479–498, 1966

Krainer L, Black DAK, McGill RJ, et al: Arsenical encephalopathy in Indian troops. J Neurol Neurosurg Psychiatry 10:171–182, 1947

Levinsky WJ, Smalley RV, Hillyer PN, et al: Arsine hemolysis. Arch Environ Health 20:436–440, 1970

Minogue SJ: Korsakoff's disease due to lead and arsenic poisoning. Med J Aust 2:16–17, 1956

Morton WE, Caron GA: Encephalopathy: an uncommon manifestation of workplace arsenic poisoning? Am J Ind Med 15:1–5, 1989

Peters HA, Croft WA, Woolson EA, et al: Seasonal arsenic exposure from burning chromium-copper-arsenate-treated wood. JAMA 251:2393–2396, 1984

Peters HA, Croft WA, Woolson EA, et al: Hematological, dermal and neuropsychological disease from burning and power sawing chromium-copper-arsenic (CCA)-treated wood. Acta Pharmacologica et Toxicologica 59 (suppl 7):39–43, 1986

Prickman LE, Millikan CH: Hemorrhagic encephalopathy during arsenic therapy for asthma. JAMA 152:1710–1713, 1953

Reynolds ES: An account of the epidemic outbreak of arsenical poisoning occurring in beer-drinkers in the north of England and the mid-land counties in 1900. Lancet 1:166–170, 1901

Schenk VWD, Stolk PJ: Psychosis following arsenic (possibly thallium) poisoning. Psychiatria, Neurologia, Neurochirurgia 70:31–37, 1967

Tay C-H, Seah C-S: Arsenic poisoning from anti-asthmatic herbal preparations. Med J Aust 2:424–428, 1975

8

Lead

EPIDEMIOLOGY

Of the neurotoxic elements, lead is the most controversial, has the greatest atomic weight, has the largest quantity of literature, and has the most extensive history. Numerous reviews document the controversial history of lead poisoning in this century (Lin-fu 1992), the history of lead poisoning prevention (Fee 1990; Rice 1990; Silbergeld 1997), and the politics and policymaking concerning lead (Hays 1992; Wedeen 1993).

Adult Poisonings

In the twentieth century, epidemics in the United States resulted from contaminated "moonshine" or illegal whiskey, burning battery cases, improperly glazed earthenware, and contaminated food or water (Committee on Biologic Effects of Atmospheric Pollutants 1972; Eskew et al. 1961; Lin-fu 1992). Moonshine consumption still occurs and carries the risk of lead poisoning (Montgomery and Finkenbine 1999; Moore and Adler 2000). Until the phasing out of leaded gasoline in the 1970s, many cases of combined lead and solvent poisoning resulted from the intentional inhalation, sniffing, or "huffing" of gasoline. Leaded gasoline remains available in other parts of the world (Carson et al. 1987; Grandjean 1983). In Australia, lead poisoning still complicates "petrol sniffer's encephalopathy" (Brady and Torzillo 1994; Burns et al. 1994; Currie et al. 1994).

Lead poisoning continues to occur (Centers for Disease Control 1990; Markowitz et al. 1994). Table 8–1 lists past and present occupations at risk for lead exposure. Professions with unexpected risks for lead poisoning include stained glass workers and renovators of old structures (Landrigan et al. 1980, 1982; Marino et al. 1990). Family members living with lead workers can develop lead poisoning from dust carried home (Knishkowy and Baker 1997). Intravenous methamphetamine abuse carries the risk of lead poisoning (Centers for Disease Control 1990). Modern hair coloring products contain lead levels that could contaminate the home if proper procedures are not followed (Mielke et al. 1997). In Mexico, lead tetroxide is marketed over the counter for indigestion. "Clandestine" lead foundries melt lead battery casings in Mexican family kitchens, often causing epidemic poisonings (Lakatos 1993). One case report described lead poisoning resulting from ingestion of an imported "pure medicinal herb" intended to "strengthen the brain" of the user (Moore and Adler 2000).

Many cases of lead poisoning result from unusual sources of lead, including indoor firing ranges; cosmetics from outside the United States; homemade wine; artist's paint; Hispanic, Asian, and Middle Eastern folk and herbal remedies; and aphrodisiacs (Ackerman et al. 1982; Chiba et al. 1980; Gosselin et al. 1984; Graham et al. 1981; Lane and Lawrence 1961; Levitt et al. 1983; Nriagu 1992; Royce and Needleman 1995).

Childhood Poisonings

Childhood lead poisoning, first described in Australia in 1904, frequently results from pica, or the ingestion of nonfood items. Federal law banned household leaded paints in the 1970s, but in 1987, the Public Health Service estimated that 3–4 million children lived in dilapidated homes with high-risk lead concentrations (Agency for Toxic Substances and Disease Registry 1987). Even if children do not eat paint, the exposure of a crawling infant to lead paint dust increases the risk for poisoning (Charney et al. 1983; Riess and Needleman 1992). Inner-city, low-income inhabitants of pre-1970 housing have the greatest risk (Royce and Needleman 1995).

The acknowledgment of a public health problem concerning childhood lead poisoning occurred in the 1960s when the United

TABLE 8–1. Past and present occupations at risk for lead exposure

Antique ceramic doll painters	Electronic devices	Lacquer makers
Ammunition/lead shot makers	Electroplaters	Lead burners
Automobile/boat repairperson	Electrotypers	Lead flooring makers
Battery makers	Emery wheel users	Lead foil/sheeting makers
Bookbinders	Enamel burners/makers	Lead millers
Bottle cap makers	Etchers	Lead miners
Brass founders/polishers	Farmers	Lead pipe makers
Bearing alloy makers	Fertilizer (sludge) makers	Lead salt makers/users
Brick burners/makers	File cutters	Lead shield (nuclear) makers
Bridge reconstructors	Firing range employees	Lead stearate makers
Bronzers	Fishing sinker makers	Lead weight makers
Brush makers	Florists (artificial flowers)	Linoleum makers
Cable makers/splicers	Foundry moulders	Linotypers
Canners	Galvanizers	Lithographers
Cartridge makers	Glassmakers	Match makers
Cement workers	Gold refiners	Metal burners/cutters
Ceramics makers	Gun barrel browners	Metal grinders
Chemical equipment workers	Herbal remedy users	Metal miners/refiners
Construction workers	Home remodelers	Metal polishers
Cutlery makers	Incandescent lamp makers	Mirror silverers
Demolition workers	Ink (color) makers	"Moonshine" whiskey makers
Dental technicians	Insecticide workers	Motor fuel blenders
Diamond polishers	Jewelers	Musical instrument makers
Dye makers	Junk dealers	Newsprint makers

TABLE 8–1. Past and present occupations at risk for lead exposure *(continued)*

Painters	Riveters	Tannery workers
Paint/pigment makers	Roofers	Taxi drivers
Papermakers	Rubber workers	Tetraethyl lead workers
Patent leather workers	Scrap metal workers	Tetramethyl lead workers
Pearl (imitation) makers	Sheet metal workers	Textile workers
Petroleum industry workers	Shellac makers	Tile workers
Photography equipment makers	Ship builders/repairpersons	Tin foil
Pipe makers/fitters	Ship dismantlers	Traffic police officers
Plastics workers	Shoe stainers/makers/repairpersons	Type founders
Plumbers	Smelter workers	Typesetters
Potters	Solderers	Varnish
Printers	Stained glass workers	Wallpaper printers
Putty makers	Steel cutters	Welders
Radiator repairpersons	Steel engravers, welders	Zinc mill/smelter workers
Recycling plant workers	Stereotypers	

States surgeon general recommended screening for lead poisoning. The recommendation established 40 µg of lead per 100 mL of blood as the maximum acceptable blood level in children (Lin-fu 1982). Numerous mass screenings and studies in the 1970s and 1980s allowed large critical reviews and meta-analyses of the findings.

Conclusions from meta-analyses and major reviews of childhood exposures fall into three general categories of opinion. The first category of opinion supports a strong, unquestionable association between lead and intelligence (Needleman and Gatsonis 1990; Schwartz 1994). The second category supports an unequivocal association between low-dose lead and intellectual deficits in children, but errors in methodological methods limit extrapolation to large populations (Ehle and McKee 1990; Gatsonis and Needleman 1992; Thacker et al. 1992; Yule and Rutter 1985). For certain small groups of individuals, especially disadvantaged populations, the effects of low lead levels seem greater (Yule and Rutter 1985). The third category disputes an association of low-level lead with lower children's intelligence. These critics state that most studies do not control for social factors in a person's life that modulate toxic effects of exposures (Ernhart 1995; Pocock et al. 1994). Inconsistencies or contradictory findings support this opinion (Bornschein et al. 1980; Ernhart 1992). Other critics claim that children's reduced intelligence, in the presence of low lead levels, results from inadequate parenting, not lead (Hunt et al. 1982; Milar et al. 1980). Blood lead levels in children in need of foster care are more likely to be elevated compared with the general population and with children already in foster care (Chung et al. 2001). Lack of adequate parenting also enhances the opportunity for a child to engage in pica. Pica then causes an increased lead burden mistakenly identified as the cause rather than the result of low intelligence.

SIGNS AND SYMPTOMS OF LEAD POISONING

Inorganic lead poisoning results from inhalation and ingestion; organic lead poisoning results from oral, dermal, and inhalation exposure (Hamilton and Hardy 1974). Symptoms of inorganic lead poisoning develop after a period of hours. Organic lead poisoning may evolve over days, weeks, or months (Gosselin et al. 1984). Toxic lead levels from chronic exposure may take months to accumulate but can present acutely or even after removal from exposure (Gosselin et al. 1984). Table 8–2 summarizes the most frequently reported signs and symptoms of inorganic and organic lead poisoning.

TABLE 8–2. Signs and symptoms of lead poisoning

Inorganic lead	
Gastrointestinal	Anorexia, abdominal pain, constipation, vomiting, mild jaundice, gingival lead line
Neurological	Ataxia, coma, convulsions, papilledema, headache, peripheral neuritis, wristdrop or footdrop, weakness, paralysis, mild facial or ocular motor nerve paresis, aphonia, laryngeal paralysis, fasciculations, encephalopathy, death
Renal	Albuminuria, cylindruria, porphyrinuria, nephrotic syndrome, renal insufficiency
Special senses	Metallic taste, visual disturbances, optic atrophy, hearing deficits
Other	Facial pallor, anemia, basophilic stippling of red blood cells, muscular wasting, arthralgia, myalgia, hypertension, sterility, gout, miscarriage, stillbirth, inhibition of vitamin D levels, psychiatric symptoms (see Table 8–4)
Organic lead	
Neurological	Tremor, myoclonus, chorea, spasticity, ataxia, convulsions, neuropathy, exaggerated tendon reflexes, headache, vertigo, incoordination, cerebellar signs, delirium, seizures, coma, psychiatric symptoms (see Table 8–4)
Other	Nausea, anorexia, vomiting, weakness, fatigue, body pains, pallor, hypotension, hypothermia, weight loss, metallic taste

Neurological and psychiatric impairments dominate the picture in both acute and chronic intoxications by organic lead. Chorea, myoclonus, and seizures develop after 5–7 days (Edminster and Bayer 1985). The effects of organic lead, when poisoning results from leaded gasoline exposure, mimic or enhance gasoline's solvent properties (Edminster and Bayer 1985).

Ataxia, coma, and convulsions with gastrointestinal symptoms constitute the classical triad of acute inorganic lead poisoning (Marsh 1985). Chronic inorganic poisoning presents with gastrointestinal, neurological, hematological, renal, and psychiatric symptoms. The well-known signs of basophilic stippling of red blood cells and gingival lead lines do not always appear in either organic or inorganic lead poisoning.

Certain genetic, medical, or nutritional conditions render a person susceptible to lead poisoning (Table 8–3). A genetic indicator of susceptibility may be polymorphism of the enzyme δ-aminolevulinic acid de-

TABLE 8–3. Genetic, medical, and nutritional predispositions to lead poisoning

Genetic	Glucose-6-phosphate dehydrogenase deficiency, glutathione deficiency, glutathione reductase deficiency, thalassemia, tyrosinemia, Wilson's disease, δ-aminolevulinic acid dehydratase deficiency
Nutritional deficiencies	Vitamins C, E; calcium, iron, phosphorus, riboflavin
Other conditions	Porphyrias, pregnancy, cystinosis, cystinuria, kidney disease, smoking, alcohol consumption, gout

hydratase (Todd et al. 1996). High serum levels of ascorbic acid correlate with decreased prevalence of elevated blood lead levels and may have implications for prevention of lead toxicity (Simon and Hudes 1999).

PSYCHIATRIC SIGNS AND SYMPTOMS ATTRIBUTED TO LEAD POISONING

Children—Inorganic Lead

For many years, most physicians believed that children's psychiatric symptoms from inorganic lead poisoning resolved without sequelae (Needleman 1993). Byers and Lord (1943) and others challenged this idea with reports of children who developed mental retardation, behavior problems, and developmental delays after poisoning (Levinson and Zeldes 1939; McKhann and Vogt 1933; McKhann et al. 1932; Rodgers et al. 1934).

The dangerous, long-term effects of lead poisoning of children now have wide acceptance with the exception of to what degree low-level lead exposure affects childhood IQ and development (Mushak et al. 1989). Despite methodological errors in many studies, major reviews and meta-analyses agree that the lowest observable effect level of 10–15 μg of lead per deciliter of blood correlates with deficits of neurobehavioral development and lowered IQ in children (Mushak et al. 1989). Higher levels correlate with severe problems. One study found decrements in cognitive abilities in children having blood lead levels less than 5 μg/dL (Lanphear et al. 2000). Table 8–4 summarizes the most commonly reported psychiatric sequelae from lead poisoning at or above the lowest observable effect level.

TABLE 8–4. Psychiatric signs and symptoms attributed to lead poisoning

Inorganic	
Mood	Depression, mood lability, anger, tension
Behavior	Agitation, personality change *Children:* antisocial, impulsivity, crying, distractibility, hyperactivity
Cognitive	Dementia, poor memory, confusion *Children:* Lack of attention
Perceptual	Hallucinations, delusions, paranoia
Other	Decreased libido, insomnia *Children:* Mental retardation, developmental delays, learning disorders, insomnia, academic problems
Organic	
Mood	Nervousness, irritability, anxiety, depression, mood swings
Behavior	Aggression, mania, agitation, suicidality, impulsivity
Cognitive	Poor concentration, memory loss, confusion
Perceptual	Auditory/visual hallucinations, delusions, paranoia
Other	Academic problems/behavior changes, hyperactivity, loss of libido, insomnia

Current opinion comes from the intellectual functioning observed in case reports or large groups of children with varying levels of exposure measured with blood or dentine lead levels. Several reports link mental retardation or autism to higher blood lead levels, but few can determine whether higher lead levels cause the impairment or result from increased pica often observed in mentally impaired children.

Hair lead levels do not accurately reflect blood lead levels and only help make the diagnosis in extreme cases of symptomatic poisoning (Roper et al. 1993). Research continues in the field of hair lead, but the bulk of work appeared in the 1970s and 1980s (Rimland and Larson 1983).

Adults—Inorganic Lead

The earliest American reports of psychiatric symptoms from adult exposures to inorganic lead described symptoms of "insanity." With the institution of better working conditions and environmental controls, the frequency of severe poisonings declined in recent decades. Modern studies describe symptoms of depression, other mood complaints, or cognitive decline as primary effects of exposure. One meta-analysis of four studies comparing the risk of Alzheimer's disease from occupational lead exposure found no increased risk (Graves et al. 1991).

Organic Lead

The presentations of child and adult organic lead poisoning are similar to the solvent-induced toxic properties of gasoline. Some cases resolved with chelation, supporting the notion that organic lead caused the psychiatric symptoms. Early reports of tetraethyl lead poisoning and later group studies of organic lead workers found that organic lead in the absence of gasoline causes psychosis and other severe psychiatric symptoms. One recent study of organolead manufacturing workers suggests that their cognitive function declined as a result of their occupational exposure to lead (Schwartz et al. 2000). The end of leaded gasoline in the United States spelled the end of combined lead and solvent poisoning from gasoline "huffing" or intentional inhalation or sniffing. The one case of tetramethyl lead poisoning found no psychiatric symptoms from that formulation (Gething 1975).

Both children and adults become aggressive when exposed to either organic lead or solvents. Some reviews suggest that antisocial personality predisposes a person to solvent abuse, not that solvents cause antisocial behavior. This may be true for some solvent abusers, but consistent findings of aggression occurring after exposure to organic lead suggest that it directly causes aggression.

DIAGNOSIS AND TREATMENT OF LEAD POISONING

Blood lead levels provide the best indicators of lead poisoning but do not reflect total body burden (Lee and Moore 1990). The inhibition of erythrocyte δ-aminolevulinic acid indicates lead exposure, but most centers still use blood lead levels for screening (Lee and Moore 1990; Roper et al. 1993; Schaffer and Campbell 1994). Zinc protoporphyrin indicates neurotoxicity from lead but does not have the sensitivity for assessing low levels of exposure (Anger and Johnson 1985; Royce and Needleman 1995). Radiological examination of the abdomen and long bones does not reliably portray exposure. The same holds true for the examination of red blood cells for basophilic stippling and the assay of hair and nail levels for lead (Roper et al. 1993). The Centers for Disease Control and Prevention (CDC) does not recommend use of scarification of the forearm with 25% sodium sulfate solution to assess for black discoloration of skin, a procedure recommended in some sources. Medical centers perform an edetate disodium calcium provocative chelation test with urinalysis and complete blood cell counts to determine exposure and overall medical status, respectively (Roper et al. 1993; Royce and Needleman 1995). Blood iron levels can rule out iron deficiency, which enhances lead toxicity (Roper et al. 1993). Lead toxicity results in several nonspecific electroencephalogram findings (Burchfiel et al. 1980).

In 1991, the CDC recommended nearly universal screening of 1- to 2-year-old children, a recommendation that remains controversial (Chisholm et al. 1994; Harvey 1994). The CDC further reduced the level of blood lead requiring intervention from 25 μg/dL in 1985 to 10 μg/dL in 1991 (Roper et al. 1993). Table 8–5 lists the CDC-recommended actions for varying blood levels (Taylor 1992).

DSM-IV-TR (American Psychiatric Association 2000) recognizes four disorders resulting from lead poisoning (Table 8–6). The lack of consistency between DSM-IV-TR disorders and the literature probably reflects a developing psychiatric nosology, not an absence of association. The literature supports inclusion of substance-induced psychotic and mood disorders and delirium in addition to the four already listed in DSM-IV-TR.

TABLE 8–5. Centers for Disease Control and Prevention–recommended actions for blood levels in children

Blood lead (μg/dL)	Action
10–14	Recheck in 3 months Community lead-poisoning prevention
15–19	Individual case management Nutritional/educational intervention
20–44	Medical evaluation/treatment Environmental remediation
45–69	Medical/environmental intervention Chelation
≥70	Acute medical emergency Treatment by physician experienced in treatment of lead poisoning

TABLE 8–6. DSM-IV-TR diagnoses associated with lead poisoning

Mental retardation
Substance-induced anxiety disorder[a]
Substance-induced persisting amnestic disorder
Symptoms of dementia

[a]DSM-IV-TR lists heavy metals as cause.

Medical treatment with chelation uses four different agents: British Anti-Lewisite (2,3-dimercaptopropanol), edetate calcium disodium, D-penicillamine, and succimer or *meso*-2,3-dimercaptosuccinic acid (Roper et al. 1993). British Anti-Lewisite is contraindicated in children allergic to peanuts and in glucose-6-phosphate dehydrogenase deficiency; D-penicillamine is contraindicated in penicillin allergy (Roper et al. 1993).

Special psychiatric considerations include the necessity of evaluating mentally retarded and autistic children for lead poisoning. Lead poisoning may not necessarily be an etiological agent of their primary psychiatric disorder but a possible result from the increased risk for pica in these individuals (Cohen et al. 1976).

REFERENCES

Ackerman A, Cronin E, Rodman D, et al: Lead poisoning from lead tetroxide used as a folk remedy—Colorado. MMWR Morb Mortal Wkly Rep 30:647–648, 1982

Agency for Toxic Substances and Disease Registry: The Nature and Extent of Lead Poisoning in Children in the United States: A Report to Congress. Atlanta, GA, U.S. Department of Health and Human Services, 1987

American Psychiatric Association: Diagnostic and Statistical Manual of Mental Disorders, 4th Edition, Text Revision. Washington, DC, American Psychiatric Association, 2000

Anger WK, Johnson BL: Chemicals affecting behavior, in Neurotoxicity of Industrial and Commercial Chemicals, Vol 1. Edited by O'Donoghue JL. Boca Raton, FL, CRC Press, 1985, pp 51–148

Bornschein R, Pearson D, Reiter L: Behavioral effects of moderate lead exposure in children and animal models, part 1: clinical studies. Crit Rev Toxicol 8:43–99, 1980

Brady M, Torzillo P: Petrol sniffing down the track. Med J Aust 160:176–177, 1994

Burchfiel JL, Duffy FH, Bartels PH, et al: The combined discriminating power of quantitative electroencephalography and neuropsychologic measures in evaluating central nervous system effects of lead at low levels, in Low Level Lead Exposure: The Clinical Implications of Current Research. Edited by Needleman HL. New York, Raven, 1980, pp 75–89

Burns CB, Burt T, Currie BJ: Petrol sniffer's encephalopathy and lead exposure. Med J Aust 161:452, 1994

Byers RK, Lord EE: Late effects of lead poisoning on mental development. American Journal of Diseases of Children 5:471–494, 1943

Carson BL, Stockton RA, Wilkinson RR: Organomercury, -lead, and -tin compounds in the environment and the potential for human exposure, in Neurotoxicants and Neurobiological Function: Effects of Organoheavy Metals. Edited by Tilson HA, Sparber SB. New York, Wiley, 1987, pp 1–79

Centers for Disease Control: Lead poisoning associated with intravenous-methamphetamine use—Oregon, 1988. JAMA 263:797–798, 1990

Charney E, Kessler B, Farfel M, et al: Childhood lead poisoning: a controlled trial of the effect of dust-control measures on blood lead levels. N Engl J Med 309:1089–1093, 1983

Chiba M, Toyoda T, Inaba Y, et al: Acute lead poisoning in an adult from ingestion of paint (letter). N Engl J Med 303:459, 1980

Chisholm J, Goldstein G, Cory-Slechta D, et al: Lead debate goes on (letter). Pediatrics 94:408–409, 1994

Chung EK, Webb D, Clampet-Lundquist S, et al: A comparison of elevated blood lead levels among children living in foster care, their siblings, and the general population. Pediatrics 107:e81, 2001

Cohen DJ, Johnson WT, Caparulo BK: Pica and elevated blood lead level in autistic and atypical children. American Journal of Diseases of Children 130:47–48, 1976

Committee on Biologic Effects of Atmospheric Pollutants: Biologic effects of lead in man, in Lead: Airborne Lead in Perspective. Edited by Committee on Biologic Effects of Atmospheric Pollutants. Washington, DC, National Academy of Sciences, 1972, pp 71–313

Currie B, Burrow J, Fisher D, et al: Petrol sniffer's encephalopathy. Med J Aust 160: 800–801, 1994

Edminster SC, Bayer MJ: Recreational gasoline sniffing: acute gasoline intoxication and latent organolead poisoning: case reports and literature review. J Emerg Med 3:365–370, 1985

Ehle AL, McKee DC: Neuropsychological effect of lead in occupationally exposed workers: a critical review. Crit Rev Toxicol 20:237–255, 1990

Ernhart CB: A critical review of low-level prenatal lead exposure in the human, 2: effects on the developing child. Reprod Toxicol 6:21–40, 1992

Ernhart CB: Inconsistencies in the lead-effects literature exists and cannot be explained by "effect modification." Neurotoxicol Teratol 17:227–233, 1995

Eskew AE, Crutcher JC, Zimmerman SL, et al: Lead poisoning resulting from illicit alcohol consumption. J Forensic Sci 6:337–350, 1961

Fee E: Public health in practice: an early confrontation with the 'silent epidemic' of childhood lead paint poisoning. J Hist Med Allied Sci 45:570–606, 1990

Gatsonis CA, Needleman HL: Recent epidemiologic studies of low-level lead exposure and the IQ of children: a meta-analytic review, in Human Lead Exposure. Edited by Needleman HL. Boca Raton, FL, CRC Press, 1992, pp 243–255

Gething J: Tetramethyl lead absorption: a report of human exposure to a high level of tetramethyl lead. British Journal of Industrial Medicine 32:329–333, 1975

Gosselin RE, Smith RP, Hodge HC, et al: Clinical Toxicology of Commercial Products. Baltimore, MD, Williams & Wilkins, 1984

Graham JAG, Maxton DG, Twort CHC: Painter's palsy: a difficult case of lead poisoning. Lancet 2:1159–1160, 1981

Grandjean P: Health significance of organolead compounds, in Lead Versus Health: Sources and Effects of Low Level Lead Exposure. Edited by Rutter M, Jones RR. Chichester, UK, Wiley, 1983, pp 179–189

Graves AB, van Duijn CM, Chandra V, et al: Occupational exposures to solvents and lead as risk factors for Alzheimer's disease: a collaborative re-analysis of case-control studies. Int J Epidemiol 20:S58–S61, 1991

Hamilton A, Hardy HL: Lead, in Industrial Toxicology. Acton, MA, Publishing Sciences Group, 1974, pp 85–121

Harvey B: Should blood lead screening recommendations be revised? Pediatrics 93: 201–204, 1994

Hays SP: The role of values in science and policy: the case of lead, in Human Lead Exposure. Edited by Needleman HL. Boca Raton, FL, CRC Press, 1992, pp 267–283

Hunt TJ, Hepner R, Seaton KW: Childhood lead poisoning and inadequate child care. American Journal of Diseases of Children 136:538–542, 1982

Knishkowy B, Baker EL: Transmission of occupational disease to family contacts. Am J Ind Med 9:543–550, 1997

Lakatos L: Mythology of lead poisoning (letter). Pediatrics 91:160–161, 1993

Landrigan P, Tamblyn PB, Nelson M, et al: Lead exposure in stained glass workers. Am J Ind Med 1:177–180, 1980

Landrigan PJ, Baker EL Jr, Himmelstein JS, et al: Exposure to lead from the Mystic River Bridge: the dilemma of deleading. N Engl J Med 306:673–676, 1982

Lane CR, Lawrence A: Home-made wine as a cause of lead-poisoning: report of a case. BMJ 2:939–940, 1961

Lanphear BP, Dietrich K, Auinger P, et al: Cognitive deficits associated with blood lead concentrations <10 μg/dL in US children and adolescents. Public Health Rep 15:521ñ529, 2000

Lee WR, Moore MR: Low level exposure to lead: the evidence for harm accumulates. BMJ 301:504–506, 1990

Levinson A, Zeldes M: Lead intoxication in children: a study of 26 cases. Arch Pediatr 56:738–748, 1939

Levitt C, Paulson D, Duvall K, et al: Folk remedy-associated lead poisoning in Hmong children—Minnesota. MMWR Morb Mortal Wkly Rep 32:555–556, 1983

Lin-fu JS: The evolution of childhood lead poisoning as a public health problem, in Lead Absorption in Children: Management, Clinical, and Environmental Aspects. Edited by Chisolm JJ Jr, O'Hara DM. Baltimore, MD, Urban & Schwarzenberg, 1982, pp 1–10

Lin-fu JS: Modern history of lead poisoning: a century of discovery and rediscovery, in Human Lead Exposure. Edited by Needleman HL. Boca Raton, FL, CRC Press, 1992, pp 23–43

Marino PE, Landrigan PJ, Graef J, et al: A case report of lead paint poisoning during renovation of a Victorian farmhouse. Am J Public Health 80:1183–1185, 1990

Markowitz SB, Nunez CM, Klitzman S, et al: Lead poisoning due to Hai Ge Fen: the porphyrin content of individual erythrocytes. JAMA 271:932–934, 1994

Marsh DO: The neurotoxicity of mercury and lead, in Neurotoxicity of Industrial and Commercial Chemicals, Vol 1. Edited by O'Donoghue JL. Boca Raton, FL, CRC Press, 1985, pp 159–169

McKhann CF: Lead poisoning in children: the cerebral manifestations. Archives of Neurology and Psychiatry 27:294–304, 1932

McKhann CF, Vogt EC: Lead poisoning in children. JAMA 101:1131–1135, 1933

Mielke HW, Taylor MD, Gonzales CR, et al: Lead-based hair coloring products: too hazardous for household use. J Am Pharm Assoc (Wash) NS37:85–89, 1997

Milar CR, Schroeder SR, Mushak P, et al: Contributions of the caregiving environment to increased lead burden of children. American Journal of Mental Deficiency 84:339–344, 1980

Montgomery R, Finkenbine R: A brief review of moonshine use (brief review). Psychiatr Serv 50:1088, 1999

Moore C, Adler R: Herbal vitamins: lead toxicity and developmental delay. Pediatrics 106:600–602, 2000

Mushak P, Davis JM, Crocetti AF, et al: Prenatal and postnatal effects of low-level lead exposure: integrated summary of a report to the U.S. Congress on childhood lead poisoning. Environ Res 50:11–36, 1989

Needleman HL: The current status of childhood lead toxicity. Adv Pediatr 40:125–139, 1993

Needleman HL, Gatsonis CA: Low-level lead exposure and the IQ of children. JAMA 263:673–678, 1990

Nriagu JO: Saturnine drugs and medicinal exposure to lead: an historical outline, in Human Lead Exposure. Edited by Needleman HL. Boca Raton, FL, CRC Press, 1992, pp 3–21

Pocock SJ, Smith M, Baghurst P: Environmental lead and children's intelligence: a systematic review of the epidemiological evidence. BMJ 309:1189–1197, 1994

Rice DC: The health effects of environmental lead exposure: closing Pandora's box, in Behavioral Measures of Neurotoxicity. Edited by Russell RW, Flattau PE, Pope AM. Washington, DC, National Academy Press, 1990, pp 243–267

Riess JA, Needleman HL: Cognitive, neural, and behavioral effects of low-level lead exposure, in The Vulnerable Brain and Environmental Risks. Edited by Isaacson RL, Jensen KF. New York, Plenum, 1992, pp 111–126

Rimland B, Larson GE: Hair mineral analysis and behavior: an analysis of 51 studies. J Learn Disabil 16:279–285, 1983

Rodgers TS, Peck JRS, Jupe MH: Lead poisoning in children with a case record. Lancet 2:129–133, 1934

Roper WL, Houk VN, Falk H, et al: Preventing Lead Poisoning in Young Children: A Statement by the Centers for Disease Control—October 1991. Washington, DC, U.S. Government Printing Office, 1993

Royce SE, Needleman HL: Lead toxicity, in Environmental Medicine: Integrating a Missing Element Into Medical Education. Edited by Pope AM, Rall DP. Washington, DC, National Academy Press, 1995, pp 410–435

Schaffer SJ, Campbell JR: The new CDC and AAP lead poisoning prevention recommendations: consensus versus controversy. Pediatr Ann 23:592–599, 1994

Schwartz BS, Stewart WF, Bolla KI., et al: Past adult lead exposure is associated with longitudinal decline in cognitive function. Neurology 55:1144–1150, 2000

Schwartz J: Low-level lead exposure and children's IQ: a meta-analysis and search for a threshold. Environ Res 65:42–55, 1994

Silbergeld EK: Preventing lead poisoning in children. Annu Rev Public Health 18:187–210, 1997

Simon JA, Hudes ES: Relationship of ascorbic acid to blood lead levels. JAMA 281:2289–2293, 1999

Taylor JR: Disorders of the nervous system, in Principles and Practice of Environmental Medicine. Edited by Tarcher AB. New York, Plenum, 1992, pp 217–240

Thacker SB, Hoffman DA, Smith J, et al: Effect of low-level body burdens of lead on the mental development of children: limitations of meta-analysis in a review of longitudinal data. Arch Environ Health 47:336–346, 1992

Todd AC, Wetmur JG, Moline JM, et al: Unraveling the chronic toxicity of lead: an essential priority for environmental health. Environ Health Perspect 104 (suppl 1): 141–146, 1996

Wedeen RP: The politics of lead, in Toxic Circles: Environmental Hazards From the Workplace Into the Community. Edited by Sheehan HS, Wedeen RP. New Brunswick, NJ, Rutgers University Press, 1993, pp 168–200

Yule W, Rutter M: Effect of lead on children's behavior and cognitive performance: a critical review, in Dietary and Environmental Lead: Human Health Effects. Edited by Mahaffey KR. Amsterdam, Elsevier, 1985, pp 211–259

ADDITIONAL READINGS

Inorganic Lead—Adults

A Awad El Karim M, Hamed AAS, Elhaimi YAA, et al: Effects of exposure to lead among lead-acid battery factory workers in Sudan. Arch Environ Health 41:261–265, 1986

Amr M, Allam M, Osmaan AL, et al: Neurobehavioral changes among workers in some chemical industries in Egypt. Environ Res 63:295–300, 1993

Araki S, Yokoyama K, Aono H, et al: Psychological performance in relation to central and peripheral nerve conduction in workers exposed to lead, zinc, and copper. Am J Ind Med 9:535–542, 1986

Arnvig E, Grandjean P, Beckmann J: Neurotoxic effects of heavy lead exposure determined with psychologic tests. Toxicol Lett 5:399–404, 1980

Baker EL, Feldman RG, White R: Neuropsychiatric effects of occupational lead exposure—preliminary findings of a longitudinal study, in Biological Psychiatry 1981: Proceedings of the IIIrd World Congress of Biological Psychiatry Held From June 28th to July 3rd, 1981 in Stockholm, Sweden. Edited by Perris C, Struwe G, Jansson B. Amsterdam, Elsevier, 1981, pp 114–121

Baker EL, Feldman RG, White RF, et al: The role of occupational lead exposure in the genesis of psychiatric and behavioral disturbances. Acta Psychiatr Scand Suppl 303:38–48, 1983

Baker EL, Feldman RG, White RF, et al: Occupational lead neurotoxicity: a behavioural and electrophysiological evaluation: study design and year one results. British Journal of Industrial Medicine 41:352–361, 1984

Baker EL, White RF, Murawski BJ: Clinical evaluation of neurobehavioral effects of occupational exposure to organic solvents and lead. International Journal of Mental Health 14:135–158, 1985a

Baker EL, White RF, Pothier LJ, et al: Occupational lead neurotoxicity: improvement in behavioural effects after reduction of exposure. British Journal of Industrial Medicine 42:507–516, 1985b

Baker EL Jr, Landrigan PJ, Barbour AG, et al: Occupational lead poisoning in the United States: clinical and biochemical findings related to blood lead levels. British Journal of Industrial Medicine 36:314–322, 1979

Balestra DJ: Adult chronic lead intoxication: a clinical review. Arch Intern Med 151:1718–1720, 1991

Bleecker ML, Agnew J, Keogh JP, et al: Neurobehavioral evaluation in workers following a brief exposure to lead, in Neurobehavioral Methods in Occupational Health. Edited by Gilioli R, Cassitto MG, Foa V. Oxford, UK, Pergamon, 1983, pp 255–262

Bromet EJ, Ryan CM, Parkinson DK: Psychosocial correlates of occupational lead exposure, in Advances in Environmental Psychology, Vol 6: Exposure to Hazardous Substances: Psychological Parameters. Edited by Lebovits AH, Baum A, Singer JE. Hillsdale, NJ, Lawrence Erlbaum Associates, 1986, pp 19–31

Campara P, Andrea FD, Micciolo R, et al: Psychological performance of workers with blood-lead concentration below the current threshold limit value. Int Arch Occup Environ Health 53:233–246, 1984

Cirksena WJ, Deller JJ, Marcarelli JL: Adult chronic lead intoxication. Arch Environ Health 4:65–72, 1962

Cullen MR, Robins JM, Eskenazi B: Adult inorganic lead intoxication: presentation of 31 new cases and a review of recent advances in the literature. Medicine 62:221–247, 1983

Dumont MP: Psychotoxicology: the return of the mad hatter. Soc Sci Med 29:1077–1082, 1989

Espinosa AS, Canepa CD, Hermosilla PD, et al: Study of neurobehavioral disturbances from lead exposure using neuropsychological indicators, in Advances in Neurobehavioral Toxicology: Applications in Environmental and Occupational Health. Edited by Johnson BL. Chelsea, MI, Lewis Publishers, 1990, pp 339–352

Fischbein A, Thornton JC, Lilis R, et al: Zinc protoporphyrin, blood lead and clinical symptoms in two occupational groups with low-level exposure to lead. Am J Ind Med 1:391–399, 1980

Goldman RH, Baker EL, Hannan M, et al: Lead poisoning in automobile radiator mechanics. N Engl J Med 317:214–218, 1987

Grandjean P, Arnvig E, Beckmann J: Psychological dysfunctions in lead-exposed workers: relation to biological parameters of exposure. Scand J Work Environ Health 4:295–303, 1978

Grandjean P, Beckmann J, Ditlev G: Relation between subjective symptoms and psychometric test results, in Neurobehavioral Methods in Occupational Health. Edited by Gilioli R, Cassitto MG, Foa V. Oxford, UK, Pergamon, 1983, pp 301–308

Haenninen H, Hernberg S, Mantere P, et al: Psychological performance of subjects with low exposure to lead. J Occup Med 20:683–689, 1978

Hai-Wang T, You-Xin L, Xiao-Hong H, et al: Alterations of monoamine metabolites and neurobehavioral function in lead-exposed workers. Biomed Environ Sci 8:23–29, 1995

Hanninen H, Mantere P, Hernberg S, et al: Subjective symptoms in low-level exposure to lead. Neurotoxicology 1:333–347, 1979

Hartman DE: Neuropsychological toxicology of metals, in Neuropsychological Toxicology: Identification and Assessment of Human Neurotoxic Syndromes. New York, Pergamon, 1988, pp 55–107

Hay W: Lead encephalopathy in a cooperage. British Journal of Industrial Medicine 7:177–186, 1950

Hogstedt C, Hane M, Agrell A, et al: Neuropsychological test results and symptoms among workers with well-defined long-term exposure to lead. British Journal of Industrial Medicine 40:99–105, 1983

Jeyaratnam J, Boey KW, Ong CN, et al: Neuropsychological studies on lead workers in Singapore. British Journal of Industrial Medicine 43:626–629, 1986

Johnson BL, Burg JR, Xintaras C, et al: A neurobehavioral examination of workers from a primary nonferrous smelter. Neurotoxicology 1:561–581, 1980

Johnson G, Mullan B, Rich G: A case of factitious disorder presenting as plumbism. Med J Aust 146:264–266, 1987

Jones R: Insanity in lead workers. BMJ 2:794–804, 1900

Kiernan JG: Contributions to psychiatry, VI: psychoses from traumatism. J Nerv Ment Dis 8:445–463, 1881

Kirkby H, Nielsen CJ, Nielsen VK, et al: Subjective symptoms after long term lead exposure in secondary lead smelting workers. British Journal of Industrial Medicine 40:314–317, 1983

Lancranjan I, Popescu HI, Gavanescu O, et al: Reproductive ability of workmen occupationally exposed to lead. Arch Environ Health 30:396–401, 1975

Landrigan P, Straub WE: Occupational lead exposure aboard a tall ship. Am J Ind Med 8:233–239, 1985

Lilis R, Fischbein A, Diamond S, et al: Lead effects among secondary lead smelter workers with blood lead levels below 80ug/100mg. Arch Environ Health 32:256–266, 1977a

Lilis R, Fischbein A, Eisinger J, et al: Prevalence of lead disease among secondary lead smelter workers and biological indicators of lead exposure. Environ Res 14:225–285, 1977b

Lilis R, Valciukas JA, Kon S, et al: Assessment of lead health hazards in a body shop of an automobile assembly plant. Am J Ind Med 3:33–51, 1982

Lilis R, Valciukas JA, Malkin J, et al: Effects of low-level lead and arsenic exposure on copper smelter workers. Arch Environ Health 40:38–47, 1985

Lockhart PB: Gingival pigmentation as the sole presenting sign of chronic lead poisoning in a mentally retarded adult. Oral Surgery, Oral Medicine, and Oral Pathology 52:143–149, 1981

Lucchini R, Albini E, Cortesi I, et al: Assessment of neurobehavioral performance as a function of current and cumulative occupational lead exposure. Neurotoxicology 21:805–811, 2000

Maizlish NA, Parra G, Feo O: Neurobehavioural evaluation of Venezuelan workers exposed to inorganic lead. Occup Environ Med 52:408–414, 1995

Mantere P, Hanninen H, Hernberg S: Subclinical neurotoxic lead effects: two-year follow-up studies with psychological test methods. Neurobehavioral Toxicology and Teratology 4:725–727, 1982

Mantere P, Hanninen H, Hernberg S, et al: A prospective follow-up study on psychological effects in workers exposed to low levels of lead. Scand J Work Environ Health 10:43–50, 1984

Meyer-Baron M, Seeber A: A meta-analysis for neurobehavioural results due to occupational lead exposure with blood lead concentrations <70 μg/100 ml. Arch Toxicol 73:510ñ518, 2000

Minogue SJ: Korsakoff's disease due to lead and arsenic poisoning. Med J Aust 2:16–17, 1956

Morris CE, Heyman A, Pozefsky T: Lead encephalopathy caused by ingestion of illicitly distilled whiskey. Neurology 14:493–499, 1964

Muldoon SB, Cauley JA, Kuller LH, et al: Effects of blood lead levels on cognitive function of older women. Neuroepidemiology 15:62–72, 1996

Murata K, Araki S, Yokoyama K, et al: Autonomic and central nervous system effects of lead in female glass workers in China. Am J Ind Med 28:233–244, 1995

Neri LC, Johansen H, Hewitt D: Health effects of low level occupational exposure to lead: the Trail, British Columbia study. Arch Environ Health 38:180–189, 1983

Nordberg M, Winblad B, Fratiglioni L, et al: Lead concentrations in elderly urban people related to blood pressure and mental performance: results from a population-based study. Am J Ind Med 38:290–294, 2000

Parkinson DK, Ryan C, Bromet EJ, et al: A psychiatric epidemiologic study of occupational lead exposure. Am J Epidemiol 123:261–269, 1986

Pasternak G, Becker CE, Lash A, et al: Cross-sectional neurotoxicology study of lead-exposed cohort. Clin Toxicol 27:37–51, 1989

Repko JD, Morgan BB Jr, Nicholson J: Behavioral Effects of Occupational Exposure to Lead (HSM-99-72-123, 1-90). Cincinnati, OH, U.S. Department of Health, Education, and Welfare, Public Health Service, 1975

Repko JD, Corum CR, Jones PD, et al: The Effects of Inorganic Lead on Behavioral and Neurologic Function (Final Report 210-75-0054, 1-69). Cincinnati, OH, U.S. Department of Health, Education, and Welfare, Public Health Service, 1978

Rodezno RA, Lundberg I, Escalona E: Development of a questionnaire in Spanish on neurotoxic symptoms. Am J Ind Med 28:505–520, 1995

Ryan CM, Morrow L, Parkinson D, et al: Low level lead exposure and neuropsychological functioning in blue collar males. Int J Neurosci 36:29–39, 1987

Schottenfeld RS: Psychiatric manifestations of occupational toxic exposure. Resident and Staff Physician 30:54–62, 1984

Schottenfeld RS, Cullen MR: Organic affective illness associated with lead intoxication. Am J Psychiatry 141:1423–1426, 1984

Schwartz BS, Bolla KI, Stewart W, et al: Decrements in neurobehavioral performance associated with mixed exposure to organic and inorganic lead. Am J Epidemiol 137:1006–1021, 1993

Schwartz BS, Lee BK, Lee GS, et al: Associations of blood lead, dimercaptosuccinic acid–chelatable lead, and tibia lead with neurobehavioral test scores in South Korean lead workers. Am J Epidemiol 153:453–464, 2001

Sherman JD: Case reports based on the review-of-systems approach, in Chemical Exposure and Disease. Edited by Sherman JD. New York, Van Nostrand Reinhold, 1988, pp 97–137

Singer R: Neurotoxicity Guidebook. New York, Van Nostrand Reinhold, 1990

Stephenson TJ, Lewis SW: Factitious plumbism (letter). Lancet 2:335, 1985

Stollery BT, Banks HA, Broadbent DE, et al: Cognitive functioning in lead workers. British Journal of Industrial Medicine 46:698–707, 1989

Stollery BT, Broadbent DE, Banks HA, et al: Short term prospective study of cognitive functioning in lead workers. British Journal of Industrial Medicine 48:739–749, 1991

Tola S, Nordman C-H: Subjective symptoms and exposure to lead. Int Arch Occup Environ Health 40:153–162, 1977

Valciukas JA, Lilis R, Eisinger J, et al: Behavioral indicators of lead neurotoxicity: results of a clinical field survey. Int Arch Occup Environ Health 41:217–236, 1978a

Valciukas JA, Lilis R, Fischbein A, et al: Central nervous system dysfunction due to lead exposure. Science 201:465–467, 1978b

Whitfield CL, Ch'ien LT, Whitehead JD: Lead encephalopathy in adults. Am J Med 52:289–298, 1972

Williamson AM, Teo RKC: Neurobehavioural effects of occupational exposure to lead. British Journal of Industrial Medicine 43:374–380, 1986

Winegar DA, Levy BS, Andrews JS Jr, et al: Chronic occupational exposure to lead: an evaluation of the health of smelter workers. J Occup Med 19:603–606, 1977

Yokoyama K, Araki S, Aono H: Reversibility of psychological performance in subclinical lead absorption. Neurotoxicology 9:405–410, 1988

Zimmermann-Tansella C, Campara P, Andrea FD, et al: Psychological and physical complaints of subjects with low exposure to lead. Human Toxicology 2:615–623, 1983

Inorganic Lead—Children: Blood and Tooth Levels

Accardo P, Whitman B, Caul J, et al: Autism and plumbism: a possible association. Clin Pediatr 27:41–44, 1988

Akelaitis AJ: Lead encephalopathy in children and adults: a clinico-pathological study. J Nerv Ment Dis 93:313–332, 1959

Albert RE, Shore RE, Sayers AJ, et al: Follow-up of children overexposed to lead. Environ Health Perspect 7:33–39, 1974

Atkinson SE, Crocker TD, Needleman HL: The importance of specification uncertainty and intolerance to measurement error in a study of the impact of dentine lead on children's IQs. International Journal of Environmental Studies 29:127–138, 1987

Baghurst PA, Robertson EF, McMichael AJ, et al: The Port Pirie cohort study: lead effects on pregnancy outcome and early childhood development. Neurotoxicology 8:395–402, 1987

Baghurst PA, McMichael AJ, Wigg NR, et al: Environmental exposure to lead and children's intelligence at the age of seven years. N Engl J Med 327:1279–1284, 1992

Baloh R, Sturm R, Green B, et al: Neuropsychological effects of chronic asymptomatic increased lead absorption. Arch Neurol 32:326–330, 1975

Beattie AD, Moore MR, Goldberg A, et al: Role of chronic low-level lead exposure in the aetiology of mental retardation. Lancet 1:589–592, 1975

Bellinger DC, Needleman HL: Lead and the relationship between maternal and child intelligence. J Pediatr 102:523–527, 1983

Bellinger D, Needleman HL, Bromfield R, et al: A followup study of the academic attainment and classroom behavior of children with elevated dentine lead levels. Biol Trace Elem Res 6:207–223, 1984

Bellinger D, Leviton A, Needleman HL, et al: Low-level lead exposure and infant development in the first year. Neurobehavioral Toxicology and Teratology 8:151–161, 1986

Bellinger D, Leviton A, Waternaux C, et al: Longitudinal analyses of prenatal and postnatal lead exposure and early cognitive development. N Engl J Med 316:1037–1043, 1987

Bellinger D, Leviton A, Waternaux C, et al: Low-level lead exposure, social class, and infant development. Neurotoxicol Teratol 10:497–503, 1989

Bellinger D, Leviton A, Sloman J: Antecedents and correlates of improved cognitive performance in children exposed in utero to low levels of lead. Environ Health Perspect 89:5–11, 1990

Bellinger D, Sloman J, Leviton A, et al: Low-level lead exposure and children's cognitive function in the preschool years. Pediatrics 87:219–227, 1991

Bellinger DC, Stiles KM, Needleman HL: Low-level lead exposure, intelligence and academic achievement: a long-term follow-up study. Pediatrics 90:855–861, 1992

Bellinger D, Hu H, Titlebaum L, et al: Attentional correlates of dentin and bone lead levels in adolescents. Arch Environ Health 49:98–105, 1994a

Bellinger D, Leviton A, Allred E, et al: Pre- and postnatal lead exposure and behavior problems in school-aged children. Environ Res 66:12–30, 1994b

Benetou-Marantidou A, Nakou S, Micheloyannis J: Neurobehavioral estimation of children with life-long increased lead exposure. Arch Environ Health 43:392–395, 1988

Benignus VA, Otto DA, Muller KE, et al: Effects of age and body lead burden on CNS function in young children, II: EEG spectra. Electroencephalogr Clin Neurophysiol 52:240–248, 1981

Bergomi M, Borella P, Fantuzzi G, et al: Relationship between lead exposure indicators and neuropsychological performance in children. Dev Med Child Neurol 31:181–190, 1989

Bicknell J: Selective pica and lead poisoning in a severely subnormal child. Journal of Mental Deficiency Research 11:278–281, 1967

Bicknell J, Clayton BE, Delves HT: Lead in mentally retarded children. Journal of Mental Deficiency Research 12:282–293, 1968

Bradley JE, Baumgartner RJ: Subsequent mental development of children with lead encephalopathy, as related to type of treatment. J Pediatr 53:311–315, 1958

Bruhl HH, Foni J, Lee YH, et al: Plasma concentrations of magnesium, lead, lithium, copper, and zinc in mentally retarded persons. American Journal of Mental Deficiency 92:103–111, 1987

Burrows NFE, Rendle-Short J, Hanna D: Lead-poisoning in children: report of five cases, with special reference to pica. BMJ 1:329–334, 1951

Byers RK: Lead poisoning: review of the literature and report on 45 cases. Pediatrics 23:585–603, 1959

Cabrera MAM: Neurotoxicology in Mexico and its relation to the general and work environment, in Advances in Neurobehavioral Toxicology: Applications in Environmental and Occupational Health. Edited by Johnson BL. Chelsea, MI, Lewis Publishers, 1990, pp 35–57

Calderon J, Navarro ME, Jimenez-Capdeville ME, et al: Exposure to arsenic and lead and neuropsychological development in Mexican children. Environ Res 85:69–76, 2001

Campbell M, Petti TA, Green WH, et al: Some physical parameters of young autistic children. Journal of the American Academy of Child Psychiatry 19:193–212, 1980

Catterjee P: Lead poisoning: subculture as a facilitating agent? Am J Clin Nutr 25:324–330, 1972

Chisolm JJ, Harrison HE: The exposure of children to lead. Pediatrics 18:943–958, 1956

Chisolm JJ, Harrison HE: The treatment of acute lead encephalopathy in children. Pediatrics 19:2–19, 1957

Coffin R, Phillips JL, Staples WI, et al: Treatment of lead encephalopathy in children. J Pediatr 69:198–206, 1966

Cohen GJ, Ahrens WE: Chronic lead poisoning: a review of seven years' experience at the Children's Hospital, District of Columbia. J Pediatr 54:271–284, 1959

Conaway MR, Waternaux C, Allred E, et al: Pre-natal blood lead levels and learning difficulties in children: an analysis of non-randomly missing categorical data. Stat Med 11:799–811, 1992

Cooney GH, Bell A, McBride W, et al: Low-level exposures to lead: the Sydney Lead Study. Dev Med Child Neurol 31:640–649, 1989a

Cooney GH, Bell A, McBride W, et al: Neurobehavioral consequences of prenatal low level exposures to lead. Neurotoxicol Teratol 11:95–104, 1989b

David OJ: Association between lower level lead concentrations and hyperactivity in children. Environ Health Perspect 7:17–25, 1974

David O, Clark J, Voeller K: Lead and hyperactivity. Lancet 2:900–903, 1972

David OJ, Hoffman SP, Sverd J, et al: Lead and hyperactivity: behavioral response to chelation: a pilot study. Am J Psychiatry 133:1155–1158, 1976a

David O, Mcgann B, Clark J, et al: Low lead levels and mental retardation. Lancet 2:1376–1379, 1976b

David OJ, Hoffman SP, Sverd J, et al: Lead and hyperactivity: lead levels among hyperactive children. J Abnorm Child Psychol 5:405–416, 1977

David OJ, Grad G, Mcgann B, et al: Mental retardation and "nontoxic" lead levels. Am J Psychiatry 139:806–809, 1982

David OJ, Hoffman SP, Clark J, et al: The relationship of hyperactivity to moderately elevated lead levels. Arch Environ Health 38:341–346, 1983

David OJ, Katz S, Clark J: Chelation therapy in children as treatment of sequelae in severe lead toxicity. Arch Environ Health 40:109–113, 1985

de la Burde B, Choate MS: Does asymptomatic lead exposure in children have latent sequelae? J Pediatr 81:1088–1091, 1972

de la Burde B, Choate MS: Early asymptomatic lead exposure and development at school age. J Pediatr 87:638–642, 1975

Dietrich KN: The neurobehavioural effects of pre-natal and early post-natal lead exposure: an interim report from the Cincinnati Longitudinal Study, in Health Effects of Lead. Edited by Hotz MCB. Ottawa, Ontario, The Royal Society of Canada/The Commission on Lead in the Environment, 1986, pp 269–294

Dietrich KN, Krafft KM, Bornschein RL, et al: Low-level fetal lead exposure effect on neurobehavioral development in early infancy. Pediatrics 80:721–730, 1987a

Dietrich KN, Krafft KM, Shukla R, et al: The neurobehavioral effects of early lead exposure, in Toxic Substances and Mental Retardation: Neurobehavioral Toxicology and Teratology. Edited by Schroeder SR. Washington, DC, American Association on Mental Deficiency, 1987b, pp 71–95

Dietrich KN, Succop PA, Bornschein RL, et al: Lead exposure and neurobehavioral development in later infancy. Environ Health Perspect 89:13–19, 1990

Dietrich KN, Succop PA, Berger OG, et al: Lead exposure and the cognitive development of urban preschool children: the Cincinnati lead study cohort at age 4 years. Neurotoxicol Teratol 13:203–211, 1991

Dietrich KN, Succop PA, Berger OG, et al: Lead exposure and the central auditory processing abilities and cognitive development of urban children: the Cincinnati lead study cohort at age 5 years. Neurotoxicol Teratol 14:51–56, 1992

Dietrich KN, Berger OG, Succop PA, et al: The developmental consequences of low to moderate prenatal and postnatal lead exposure: intellectual attainment in the Cincinnati lead study cohort following school entry. Neurotoxicol Teratol 15:37–44, 1993a

Dietrich KN, Berger OG, Succop PA: Lead exposure and the motor developmental status of urban six-year-old children in the Cincinnati prospective study. Pediatrics 91:301–307, 1993b

Dolcourt JL, Finch C, Coleman GD, et al: Hazard of lead exposure in the home from recycled automobile storage batteries. Pediatrics 68:225–230, 1981

Elwood PC, Morton M, St Leger AS: Lead in water and mental retardation (letter). Lancet 1:590–591, 1976

Emory E, Pattillo R, Archibold E, et al: Neurobehavioral effects of low-level lead exposure in human neonates. Am J Obstet Gynecol 181(suppl):S2–S11, 1999

Ennis JM, Harrison HE: Treatment of lead encephalopathy with BAL (2.3-dimercaptopropanol). Pediatrics 5:853–867, 1950

Ernhart CB, Landa B, Schell NB: Subclinical levels of lead and developmental deficit—a multivariate follow-up reassessment. Pediatrics 67:911–919, 1981

Ernhart CB, Landa B, Wolf AW: Subclinical lead level and developmental deficit: reanalyses of data. J Learn Disabil 18:475–479, 1985

Ernhart CB, Kennard MJ, Erhard P, et al: Intrauterine exposure to low levels of lead: the status of the neonate. Arch Environ Health 41:287–291, 1986
Ernhart CB, Morrow-Tlucak M, Marler MR, et al: Low level lead exposure in the prenatal and early preschool periods: early preschool development. Neurotoxicol Teratol 9:259–270, 1987
Ernhart CB, Morrow-Tlucak M, Wolf AW: Low level lead exposure and intelligence in the preschool years. Sci Total Environ 71:453–459, 1988
Ernhart CB, Morrow-Tlucak M, Wolf AW, et al: Low level lead exposure in the prenatal and early preschool periods: intelligence prior to school entry. Neurotoxicol Teratol 11:161–170, 1989
Evans HL, Daniel SA, Marmor M: Reversal learning tasks may provide rapid determination of cognitive deficits in lead-exposed children. Neurotoxicol Teratol 16: 471–477, 1994
Faust D, Brown J: Moderately elevated blood lead levels: effects on neuropsychologic functioning in children. Pediatrics 80:623–629, 1987
Fejerman N, Gimenez ER, Vallejo NE, et al: Lennox's syndrome and lead intoxication. Pediatrics 52:227–234, 1973
Fergusson DM, Horwood LJ: The effects of lead levels on the growth of word recognition in middle childhood. Int J Epidemiol 22:891–897, 1993
Fergusson DM, Fergusson JE, Horwood LJ, et al: A longitudinal study of dentine lead levels, intelligence, school performance and behaviour, part II: dentine lead and cognitive ability. J Child Psychol Psychiatry 29:793–809, 1988a
Fergusson DM, Fergusson JE, Horwood LJ, et al: A longitudinal study of dentine lead levels, intelligence, school performance and behaviour, part III: dentine lead levels and attention/activity. J Child Psychol Psychiatry 29:811–824, 1988b
Fergusson DM, Horwood LJ, Lynskey MT: Early dentine lead levels and subsequent cognitive and behavioural development. J Child Psychol Psychiatry 34:215–227, 1993
Freeman R: Chronic lead poisoning in children: a review of 90 children diagnosed in Sydney, 1948–1967, 1: epidemiological aspects. Med J Aust 1:640–647, 1970a
Freeman R: Chronic lead poisoning in children: a review of 90 children diagnosed in Sydney, 1948–1967, 2: clinical features and investigations. Med J Aust 1:648–651, 1970b
Fulton M, Thomson G, Hunter R, et al: Influence of blood lead on the ability and attainment of children in Edinburgh. Lancet 1:1221–1225, 1987
Giannattasio RC, Bedo AV, Pirozzi MJ: Lead poisoning: observations in fourteen cases. American Journal of Diseases of Children 84:316–321, 1952
Gibb JWG, MacMahon JF: Arrested mental development induced by lead-poisoning. BMJ 1:320–323, 1955
Gibson SLM, Lam CN, McCrae WM, et al: Blood lead levels in normal and mentally deficient children. Arch Dis Child 42:573–578, 1967
Gillberg C, Noren JG, Wahlstrom J, et al: Heavy metals and neuropsychiatric disorders in six-year-old children: aspects of dental lead and cadmium. Acta Paedopsychiatrica 48:253–263, 1982
Gittelman R, Eskenazi B: Lead and hyperactivity revisited: an investigation of nondisadvantaged children. Arch Gen Psychiatry 40:827–833, 1983
Gordon N, King E, Mackay RI: Lead absorption in children. BMJ 2:480–482, 1967
Greene T, Ernhart CB: Dentine lead and intelligence prior to school entry: a statistical sensitivity analysis. J Clin Epidemiol 46:323–339, 1993
Greene T, Ernhart CB, Boyd TA: Contributions of risk factors to elevated blood and dentine lead levels in preschool children. Sci Total Environ 115:239–260, 1992
Guerit JM, Meulders M, Amand G, et al: Lead neurotoxicity in clinically asymptomatic children living in the vicinity of an ore smelter. Clin Toxicol 18:1257–1267, 1981

Hansen ON, Trillingsgaard A, Beese I, et al: A neuropsychological study of children with elevated dentine lead level: assessment of the effect of lead in different socio-economic groups. Neurotoxicol Teratol 11:205–213, 1989

Haritos NP: Chronic lead intoxication: a report of 21 treated cases at Children's Hospital. Clinical Proceedings of the Children's Hospital 17:110–115, 1961

Harvey PG, Hamlin MW, Kumar R: Blood lead, behaviour and intelligence test performance in preschool children. Sci Total Environ 40:45–60, 1984

Hawk BA, Schroeder SR, Robinson G, et al: Relation of lead and social factors to IQ of low-SES children: a partial replication. American Journal of Mental Deficiency 91:178–183, 1986

Hebel JR, Kinch D, Armstrong E: Mental capability of children exposed to lead pollution. British Journal of Preventive and Social Medicine 30:170–174, 1976

Holt LE: Lead poisoning in infancy. American Journal of Diseases of Children 25:229–233, 1923

Jenkins CD: Lead poisoning in children: a study of forty-six cases. AMA Archives of Neurology and Psychiatry 77:70–78, 1957

Karpinski FE, Rieders F, Girsh LS: Calcium disodium versenate in the therapy of lead encephalopathy. J Pediatr 42:687–699, 1953

Kirkconnell SC, Hicks LE: Residual effects of lead poisoning on Denver Developmental Screening Test scores. J Abnorm Child Psychol 8:257–267, 1980

Kotok D: Development of children with elevated blood lead levels: a controlled study. J Pediatr 80:57–61, 1972

Kotok D, Kotok R, Heriot JT: Cognitive evaluation of children with elevated blood lead levels. American Journal of Diseases of Children 131:791–793, 1977

Krall V, Sachs H, Rayson B, et al: Effects of lead poisoning on cognitive test performance. Percept Mot Skills 50:483–486, 1980

Landrigan PJ, Whitworth RH, Baloh RW, et al: Neuropsychological dysfunction in children with chronic low-level lead absorption. Lancet 1:708–712, 1975

Lansdown RG, Shepherd J, Clayton BE, et al: Blood-lead levels, behaviour, and intelligence: a population study. Lancet 1:538–541, 1974

Lansdown R, Yule W, Urbanowicz M-A, et al: Blood lead, intelligence, attainment and behaviour in school children: overview of a pilot study, in Lead Versus Health. Edited by Rutter M, Jones RR. Chichester, UK, Wiley, 1983, pp 267–296

Lansdown R, Yule W, Urbanowicz M-A, et al: The relationship between blood-lead concentrations, intelligence, attainment and behaviour in a second population: the second London study. Int Arch Occup Environ Health 57:225–235, 1986

Lavigne K, Batzer W: Survey of lead levels in patients presenting to child and adolescent psychiatry. Hawaii Med J 54:671–672, 1995

Leviton A, Bellinger D, Allred EN, et al: Pre- and postnatal low-level lead exposure and children's dysfunction in school. Environ Res 60:30–43, 1993

Lewendon G, Kinra S, Nelder R, et al: Should children with developmental and behavioural problems be routinely screened for lead? Arch Dis Child 85:286–288, 2001

Lewis M, Worobey J, Ramsay DS, et al: Prenatal exposure to heavy metals: Effect on childhood cognitive skills and health status. Pediatrics 89:1010–1015, 1992

Ling W, Su-en X, Guo-Dong Z, et al: Study of lead absorption and its effect on children's development. Biomed Environ Sci 2:325–330, 1989

Lyngbye T, Hansen ON, Grandjean P: Neurological deficits in children: medical risk factors and lead exposure. Neurotoxicol Teratol 10:531–537, 1989

Lyngbye T, Hansen ON, Trillingsgaard A, et al: Learning disabilities in children: significance of low-level lead-exposure and confounding factors. Acta Paediatrica Scandinavica 79:352–360, 1990

Marecek J, Shapiro IM, Burke A, et al: Low-level lead exposure in childhood influences neuropsychological performance. Arch Environ Health 38:355–359, 1983

McBride WG, Black BP, English BJ: Blood lead levels and behaviour of 400 preschool children. Med J Aust 2:26–29, 1982

Mccracken JT: Lead intoxication psychosis in an adolescent. J Am Acad Child Adolesc Psychiatry 26:274–276, 1987

McMichael AJ, Baghurst PA, Wigg NR, et al: Port Pirie cohort study: environmental exposure to lead and children's abilities at the age of four years. N Engl J Med 319:468–475, 1988

McMichael AJ, Baghurst PA, Vimpani GV, et al: Sociodemographic factors modifying the effect of environmental lead on neuropsychological development in early childhood. Neurotoxicol Teratol 14:321–327, 1992

McMichael AJ, Baghurst PA, Vimpani GV, et al: Tooth lead levels and IQ in school-age children: the Port Pirie cohort study. Am J Epidemiol 140 489–499, 1994

Mellins RB, Jenkins CD: Epidemiological and psychological study of lead poisoning in children. JAMA 158:15–20, 1955

Mendelsohn AL, Dreyer BP, Fierman AH, et al: Low-level lead exposure and cognitive development in early childhood. J Dev Behav Pediatr 20:425–431, 1999

Milar CR, Schroeder SR, Mushak P, et al: Failure to find hyperactivity in preschool children with moderately elevated lead burden. J Pediatr Psychol 6:85–95, 1981

Millar JA, Battistini V, Cumming RL, et al: Lead and delta-aminolevulinic acid dehydratase levels in mentally retarded children and in lead-poisoned suckling rats. Lancet 2:695–698, 1970

Millican FK, Lourie RS, Layman EM: Emotional factors in the etiology and treatment of lead poisoning. American Journal of Diseases of Children 91:144–149, 1956

Molina G, Zuniga MA, Cardenas A, et al: Psychological alterations in children exposed to a lead-rich home environment. Bulletin of the Pan American Health Organization 17:186–192, 1983

Moncrieff AA, Koumides OP, Clayton BE, et al: Lead poisoning in children. Arch Dis Child 39:1–13, 1964

Moore MR, Meredith PA, Goldberg A: A retrospective analysis of blood-lead in mentally retarded children. Lancet 1:717–719, 1977

Munoz H, Romieu I, Palazuelos E, et al: Blood lead level and neurobehavioral development among children living in Mexico City. Arch Environ Health 48:132–139, 1993

Needleman HL: Lead at low dose and the behavior of children. Acta Psychiatr Scand Suppl 303:26–37, 1983a

Needleman HL: Low level lead exposure and neuropsychological performance, in Lead Versus Health: Sources and Effects of Low Level Lead Exposure. Edited by Rutter M, Jones RR. Chichester, UK, Wiley, 1983b, pp 229–248

Needleman HL: The persistent threat of lead: medical and sociological issues. Curr Probl Pediatr 18:697–744, 1988

Needleman HL, Gunnoe C, Leviton A, et al: Deficits in psychologic and classroom performance of children with elevated dentine lead levels. N Engl J Med 300:689–695, 1979

Needleman HL, Geiger SK, Frank R: Lead and IQ scores: a reanalysis. Science 227: 701–704, 1985

Needleman HL, Schell A, Bellinger D, et al: The long-term effects of exposure to low doses of lead in childhood: an 11-year follow-up report. N Engl J Med 322:83–88, 1990

Needleman HL, Riess JA, Tobin MJ, et al: Bone lead levels and delinquent behavior. JAMA 275:363–369, 1996

Nevin R: How lead exposure relates to temporal changes in IQ, violent crime, and unwed pregnancy. Environ Res 83:1–22, 2000

Niklowitz WJ, Mandybur TI: Neurofibrillary changes following childhood lead encephalopathy. J Neuropathol Exp Neurol 34:445–455, 1975

Oliver BE, Gorman GO: Pica and blood led in psychotic children. Dev Med Child Neurol 8:704–707, 1966
Otto DA, Benignus VA, Muller KE, et al: Effects of age and body lead burden on CNS function in young children, I: slow cortical potentials. Electroencephalogr Clin Neurophysiol 52:229–239, 1981
Otto D, Benignus V, Muller K, et al: Effects of low to moderate lead exposure on slow cortical potentials in young children: two year follow-up study. Neurobehavioral Toxicology and Teratology 4:733–737, 1982
Otto D, Benignus V, Muller K, et al: Electrophysiological evidence of changes in CNS function at low-to-moderate blood lead levels in children, in Lead Versus Health: Sources and Effects of Low Level Lead Exposure. Edited by Rutter M, Jones RR. Chichester, UK, Wiley, 1983a, pp 319–331
Otto D, Benignus V, Muller K, et al: Event-related slow brain potential changes in asymptomatic children with secondary exposure to lead, in Neurobehavioral Methods in Occupational Health. Edited by Gilioli R, Cassitto MG, Foa V. Oxford, UK, Pergamon, 1983b, pp 295–300
Otto D, Robinson G, Baumann S, et al: 5-Year follow-up of children with low-to-moderate lead absorption: electrophysiological evaluation. Environ Res 38:168–186, 1985
Padich RA, Dietrich KN, Pearson DT: Attention, activity level, and lead exposure at 18 months. Environ Res 38:137–143, 1985
Pedraza MA, Anzinger F: Lead encephalopathy: report of a case associated with industrial exposure. Ohio State Medical Journal 70:319–321, 1974
Perino J, Ernhart CB: The relation of subclinical lead level to cognitive and sensorimotor impairment in black preschoolers. J Learn Disabil 7:616–620, 1974
Perlstein MA, Attala R: Neurologic sequelae of plumbism in children. Clin Pediatr 5:292–298, 1966
Pocock SJ, Ashby D, Smith MA: Lead exposure and children's intellectual performance. Int J Epidemiol 16:57–67, 1987
Prpic-Majic D, Bobicc J, Simicc D, et al: Lead absorption and psychological function in Zagreb (Croatia) school children. Neurotoxicol Teratol 22:347–356, 2000
Pueschel SM: Neurological and psychomotor functions in children with an increased lead burden. Environ Health Perspect 7:13–16, 1974
Pueschel SM, Kopito L, Schwachman H: Children with an increased lead burden: a screening and follow-up study. JAMA 222:462–466, 1972
Rabinowitz MB, Wang J-D, Soong W-T: Dentine lead and child intelligence in Taiwan. Arch Environ Health 46:351–360, 1991
Rabinowitz MB, Wang J-D, Soong W-T: Children's classroom behavior and lead in Taiwan. Bull Environ Contam Toxicol 48:282–288, 1992
Ratcliffe JM: Developmental and behavioural functions in young children with elevated blood lead levels. Br J Prev Soc Med 31:258–264, 1977
Rigby EP: Low lead levels and mental retardation (letter). Lancet 1:421, 1977
Rogan WJ, Dietrich KN, Ware JH, et al: The effect of chelation therapy with succimer on neuropsychological development in children exposed to lead. N Engl J Med 344:1421–1426, 2001
Rothenberg SJ, Schnaas L, Cansino-Ortiz S, et al: Neurobehavioral deficits after low level lead exposure in neonates: the Mexico City pilot study. Neurotoxicol Teratol 11:85–93, 1989
Routh DK, Mushak P, Boone L: A new syndrome of elevated blood lead and microcephaly. J Pediatr Psychol 4:67–76, 1979
Ruff HA, Bijur PE, Markowitz M, et al: Declining blood lead levels and cognitive changes in moderately lead-poisoned children. JAMA 269:1641–1646, 1993
Rummo JH, Routh DK, Rummo NJ, et al: Behavioral and neurological effects of symptomatic and asymptomatic lead exposure in children. Arch Environ Health 34: 120–124, 1979

Sachs HK, Krall V, McCaughran DA, et al: IQ following treatment of lead poisoning: a patient-sibling comparison. J Pediatr 93:428–431, 1978

Sachs HK, McCaughran DA, Krall V, et al: Lead poisoning without encephalopathy: effect of early diagnosis on neurologic and psychologic salvage. American Journal of Diseases of Children 133:786–790, 1979

Sachs HK, Krall V, Drayton MA: Neuropsychological assessment after lead poisoning without encephalopathy. Percept Mot Skills 54:1283–1288, 1982

Schnaas L, Rothernberg SJ, Perroni E, et al: Temporal pattern in the effect of postnatal blood lead level on intellectual development of young children. Neurotoxicol Teratol 22:805–810, 2000

Schroeder SR, Hawk B, Otto DA, et al: Separating the effects of lead and social factors on IQ. Environ Res 38:144–154, 1985

Schwartz J, Otto D: Blood lead, hearing thresholds, and neurobehavioral development in children and youth. Arch Environ Health 42:153–160, 1987

Sciarillo WG, Alexander G, Farrell KP: Lead exposure and child behavior. Am J Public Health 82:1356–1360, 1992

Shaheen SJ: Neuromaturation and behavior development: the case of childhood lead poisoning. Dev Psychol 20:542–550, 1984

Shapiro IM, Marecek J: Dentine lead concentration as a predictor of neuropsychological functioning in inner-city children. Biol Trace Elem Res 6:69–78, 1984

Silva PA, Hughes P, Williams S, et al: Blood lead, intelligence, reading attainment, and behaviour in eleven year old children in Dunedin, New Zealand. J Child Psychol Psychiatry 29:43–52, 1988

Smith M, Delves T, Landown R, et al: The effects of lead exposure on urban children: the Institute of Child Health/Southhampton Study. Dev Med Child Neurol 25 (suppl 47):1–54, 1983

Soong WT, Chao KY, Jang CS, et al: Long-term effect of increased lead absorption on intelligence of children. Arch Environ Health 54:297–301, 1999

Spivey GH, Brown CP, Baloh RW, et al: Subclinical effects of chronic increased lead absorption—a prospective study, I: study design and analysis of symptoms. J Occup Med 21:423–429, 1979

Stiles KM, Bellinger DC: Neuropsychological correlates of low-level lead exposure in school-age children: a prospective study. Neurotoxicol Teratol 15:27–35, 1993

Stretesky PB, Lynch MJ: The relationship between lead exposure and homicide. Arch Pediatr Adolesc Med 155:579–582, 2001

Tang HW, Huel G, Campagna D, et al: Neurodevelopmental evaluation of 9-month-old infants exposed to low levels of lead in utero: involvement of monoamine neurotransmitters. J Appl Toxicol 19:167–172, 1999

Tanis AL: Lead poisoning in children including nine cases treated with edathamil calcium-disodium. American Journal of Diseases of Children 89:325–331, 1955

Telisman S, Prpic-Majic D, Beritic T: PbB and ALAD in mentally retarded and normal children. Int Arch Occup Environ Health 52:361–369, 1983

Thomson GOB, Raab GM, Hepburn WS, et al: Blood-lead levels and children's behaviour—results from the Edinburgh lead study. J Child Psychol Psychiatry 30:515–528, 1989

Thurston DL, Middelkamp JN, Mason E: The late effects of lead poisoning. J Pediatr 47:413–423, 1955

Tillman P, Grot J, Steinke J: Blood lead levels in an institutionalized developmentally disabled population (abstract). Ment Retard 16:265–266, 1978

Tong IS, Lu Y: Identification of confounders in the assessment of the relationship between lead exposure and child development. Ann Epidemiol 11:38–45, 2001

Tong S, McMichael AJ, Baghurst PA: Interactions between environmental lead exposures and sociodemographic factors on cognitive development. Arch Environ Health 55:330–335, 2000

Vivoli G, Bergomi M, Borella P, et al: Study of biological indicators related to early effects of lead on central nervous system of children: preliminary results, in International Conference: Heavy Metals in the Environment, Vol 1, Athens, September 1985. Edited by Lekkas TD. Edinburgh, CEP Consultants, 1985, pp 454–456

Wasserman GA, Graziano JH, Factor-Litvak P, et al: Independent effects of lead exposure and iron deficiency anemia on developmental outcome at age 2 years. J Pediatr 121:695–703, 1992

Wasserman GA, Graziano JH, Factor-Litvak P, et al: Consequences of lead exposure and iron supplementation on childhood development at age 4 years. Neurotoxicol Teratol 16:233–240, 1994

Wasserman GA, Liu X, Popovac D, et al: The Yugoslavia Prospective Lead Study: contributions of prenatal and postnatal lead exposure to early intelligence. Neurotoxicol Teratol 22:811–818, 2000

Wasserman GA, Liu X, Pine DS, et al: Contribution of maternal smoking during pregnancy and lead exposure to early child behavior problems. Neurotoxicol Teratol 23:13–21, 2001

White HH, Fowler FD: Chronic lead encephalopathy: a diagnostic consideration in mental retardation. Pediatrics 25:309–315, 1960

White RF, Diamond R, Proctor S, et al: Residual cognitive deficits 50 years after lead poisoning during childhood. British Journal of Industrial Medicine 50:613–622, 1993

Wigg NR, Vimpani GV, McMichael AJ, et al: Port Pirie cohort study: childhood blood lead and neuropsychological development at age two years. J Epidemiol Community Health 42:213–219, 1988

Winneke G, Kraemer U: Neuropsychological effects of lead in children: interactions with social background variables. Neuropsychobiology 11:195–202, 1984

Winneke G, Hrdina K-G, Brockhaus A: Neuropsychological studies in children with elevated tooth-lead concentrations, I: pilot study. Int Arch Occup Environ Health 51:169–183, 1982

Winneke G, Kramer U, Brockhaus A, et al: Neuropsychological studies in children with elevated tooth-lead concentrations. Int Arch Occup Environ Health 51:231–252, 1983

Winneke G, Beginn J, Ewert T, et al: Comparing the effects of perinatal and later childhood lead exposure on neuropsychological outcome. Environ Res 38:155–167, 1985

Winneke G, Brockhaus A, Collet W, et al: Modulation of lead-induced performance deficit in children by varying signal rate in a serial choice reaction test. Neurotoxicol Teratol 11:587–592, 1989

Winneke G, Brockhaus A, Ewers U, et al: Results from the European multicenter study on lead neurotoxicity in children: implications for risk assessment. Neurotoxicol Teratol 12:553–559, 1990

Winneke G, Altmann L, Kramer U, et al: Neurobehavioral and neurophysiological observations in six year old children with low lead levels in East and West Germany. Neurotoxicology 15:705–714, 1994

Wolf AW, Ernhart CB, White CS: Intrauterine led exposure and early development, in International Conference: Heavy Metals in the Environment, Athens, September 1985, Vol 2. Edited by Lekkas TD. Edinburgh, CEP Consultants, 1985, pp 153–155

Wolf AW, Jimenez E, Lozoff B: No evidence of developmental ill effects of low-level exposure in a developing country. J Dev Behav Pediatr 15:224–231, 1994

Woods GE, Walters RM: Lead poisoning in mentally subnormal children (letter). Lancet 2:592, 1964

Xiao-ming S, Di G, Ji-de X, et al: The adverse effect of marginally higher lead level on intelligence development of children: a Shanghai study. Indian J Pediatr 59:233–238, 1992

Yamins J: The relationship of subclinical lead intoxication to cognitive and language functioning in preschool children. Unpublished thesis, Hofstra University, Hempstead, NY, 1976

Youroukos S, Lyberatos C, Philippidou A, et al: Increased blood lead levels in mentally retarded children in Greece. Arch Environ Health 33:297–300, 1978

Yule W, Lansdown R, Millar IB, et al: The relationship between blood lead concentrations, intelligence and attainment in a school population: a pilot study. Dev Med Child Neurol 23:567–576, 1981

Organic Lead: Industrial and Accidental Sources

Beattie AD, Moore MR, Goldberg A: Tetraethyl-lead poisoning. Lancet 2:12–15, 1972

Bolter JF, Stanczak DE, Long CJ: Neuropsychological consequences of acute, high-level gasoline inhalation. Clinical Neuropsychology 5:4–7, 1983

Boyd PR, Walker G, Henderson IN: The treatment of tetraethyl lead poisoning. Lancet 1:181–185, 1957

Cassells DAK, Dodds EC: Tetra-ethyl lead poisoning. BMJ 2:681–685, 1946

Grandjean P, Nielsen T: Organolead compounds: environmental health aspects. Residue Reviews 72:97–148, 1979

Hamilton A, Reznikoff P, Burnham GM: Tetra-ethyl lead. JAMA 84:1481–1486, 1925

Hardy HL, Maloof CC: Evidence of systemic effect of tetryl: with summary of available literature. AMA Archives of Industrial Hygiene and Occupational Medicine 1:545–549, 1950

Kahan VL: Paranoid states occurring in leaded-petrol handlers. Journal of Mental Science 96:1043–1047, 1950

Kehoe RA: Tetra-ethyl lead poisoning: clinical analysis of a series of nonfatal cases. JAMA 85:108–110, 1925

Machle WF: Tetra-ethyl lead intoxication and poisoning by related compounds of lead. JAMA 105:578–585, 1935

Mitchell CS, Shear MS, Bolla KI, et al: Clinical evaluation of 58 organolead manufacturing workers. J Occup Environ Med 38:372–378, 1996

Norris C, Gettler AO: Poisoning by tetra-ethyl lead: postmortem and chemical findings. JAMA 85:818–820, 1925

Schwartz BS, Bolla KI, Stewart W, et al: Decrements in neurobehavioral performance associated with mixed exposure to organic and inorganic lead. Am J Epidemiol 137:1006–1021, 1993

Seeber A, Kiesswetter E, Neidhart B, et al: Neurobehavioral effects of a long-term exposure to tetraalkyllead. Neurotoxicol Teratol 12:653–655, 1990

Lead Poisoning Associated With Inhalant Abuse

Boeckx RL, Coodin FJ: An epidemic of gasoline sniffing, in Voluntary Inhalation of Industrial Solvents. Edited by Sharp CW, Carroll LT. Rockville, MD, U.S. Government Printing Office, 1978, pp 179–186

Boeckx RL, Postl B, Coodin FJ: Gasoline sniffing and tetraethyl lead poisoning in children. Pediatrics 60:140–145, 1977

Brown A: Petrol sniffing lead encephalopathy. N Z Med J 96:421–422, 1983

Carroll HG, Abel GG: Chronic gasoline inhalation. South Med J 66:1429–1430, 1973

Coulehan JL, Hirsch W, Brillman J, et al: Gasoline sniffing and lead toxicity in Navajo adolescents. Pediatrics 71:113–117, 1983

de Silva P, Christophers AJ: Lead exposure and children's intelligence: do low levels of lead in blood cause mental deficit? J Paediatr Child Health 33:12–17, 1997

Edminster SC, Bayer MJ: Recreational gasoline sniffing: acute gasoline intoxication and latent organolead poisoning: case reports and literature review. J Emerg Med 3:365–370, 1985

Goldings AS, Stewart RM: Organic lead encephalopathy: behavioral change and movement disorder following gasoline inhalation. J Clin Psychiatry 43:70–72, 1982

Hansen KS, Sharp FR: Gasoline sniffing, lead poisoning, and myoclonus. JAMA 240: 1375–1376, 1978

Kaufman A, Wiese W: Gasoline sniffing leading to increased lead absorption in children. Clin Pediatr 17:475–477, 1978

Law WR, Nelson ER: Gasoline-sniffing by an adult: report of a case with the unusual complication of lead encephalopathy. JAMA 204:144–146, 1968

Mccracken JT: Lead intoxication psychosis in an adolescent. J Am Acad Child Adolesc Psychiatry 26:274–276, 1987

Robinson RO: Tetraethyl lead poisoning from gasoline sniffing. JAMA 240:1373–1374, 1978

Seshia SS, Rajani KR, Boeckx RL, et al: The neurological manifestations of chronic inhalation of leaded gasoline. Dev Med Child Neurol 20:323–334, 1978

Valpey R, Sumi M, Copass MK, et al: Acute and chronic progressive encephalopathy due to gasoline sniffing. Neurology 28:507–510, 1978

Young RSK, Grzyb SE, Crismon L: Recurrent cerebellar dysfunction as related to chronic gasoline sniffing in an adolescent girl. Clin Pediatr 16:706–708, 1977

9

Manganese

EPIDEMIOLOGY

The first American report of manganese poisoning appeared in 1913, followed by occupational poisonings in Spain, Morocco, Germany, Cuba, Italy, India, Mexico, Japan, United Arab Republic, and the former Soviet Union (Hamilton and Hardy 1974; Katz 1985). Later investigations in mining villages of Chile identified a previously unknown condition—*locura manganica,* or manganese madness—that developed in manganese miners (Donaldson 1987).

Case reports and group studies of industrial poisonings continue to appear. Several occupations carry greater risk for exposure (Table 9–1). Most modern exposures occur in mining and manufacturing, but some cases of manganese intoxication result from long-term total parenteral nutrition (Alves et al. 1997; Fell et al. 1996; Masumoto et al. 2001). One case report associated the consumption of large doses of vitamins and minerals with manganese poisoning (Banta and Markesbery 1977). In countries without strict pesticide regulations, manganese intoxication from manganese-based pesticides continues (Ferraz et al. 1988). The recent introduction of methylcyclopenta-

TABLE 9–1. Occupational settings at risk for manganese exposure

Animal food additive	Manufacturing chlorine gas
Ceramics	Matches
Cleaning and coloring molten glass	Mining and ore mills
Coloring and graining soap	Oxidizers
Disinfectants	Paints
Dyes	Production of steel, aluminum, magnesium, and cast iron
Electric coils	Pyrotechnics
Enamel	Smelters
Fertilizers	Storage batteries
Gasoline additives	Welding and welding rods
Hydroquinone production	
Linoleum	

dienylmanganese (MMT) as a gasoline additive mandates the continued awareness of manganese toxicity (Frumkin and Solomon 1997).

In 1980, an endemic neurological disorder consisting of cerebellar, upper motor, and psychiatric symptoms developed on Groote Eylandt, a large island off northern Australia (Kiloh et al. 1980). Researchers suspected manganese poisoning based on the presence of a large manganese mining operation on the island. Residents also had a tradition of eating clay cakes for medicinal purposes (Cawte 1984, 1985; Cawte and Florence 1989; Kilburn 1987; Kiloh et al. 1980).

SIGNS AND SYMPTOMS OF MANGANESE POISONING

Manganese poisoning results from oral or inhalation exposure (Goetz 1985; Goyer 1996). Symptoms appear with a gradual onset 1–9 months after exposure (Goetz 1985). Neurotoxic symptoms without multisystemic injury predominate. Table 9–2 lists physical symptoms associated with poisoning. Occasional reports appear of pneumonia from inhalation of manganese dust.

Several conditions increase the risk for manganese poisoning, including iron deficiency, unspecified genetic susceptibility, liver failure, and Alagille syndrome (Calabrese 1978; Cawte and Florence 1989). Alagille syndrome consists of dysmorphic facies, mild icterus, and pulmonary stenosis. Persons with Alagille syndrome have abnormal excretion of manganese in the bile after absorption in the gastrointestinal tract. One case report of Alagille syndrome described an

TABLE 9–2. Physical signs and symptoms of manganese poisoning

Weakness	Profuse sweating, possibly with metallic odor
Fatigue	Muscle cramps
Apathy	Twitching
Sleepiness	Nocturnal leg cramps
Awkward gait	Ankle/patellar clonus
Broad slapping "cock-step"	Headache
Retropulsion	Slow movement
Propulsion	Rigidity
Fine, resting tremor	Hyperreflexia
Rhythmic movement of trunk and head	Metallic taste
Masklike facies	Urinary incontinence or urgency
Faint, monotonous speech	Lumbosacral pain
Paresthesias	
Sialorrhea	

8-year-old girl with normal mental status but symmetric pallidal lesions and dystonia (Barron et al. 1994). The cause-and-effect relation of increased manganese in the blood with hepatic failure needs further research (Alves et al. 1997; Fell et al. 1996).

PSYCHIATRIC SIGNS AND SYMPTOMS ATTRIBUTED TO MANGANESE POISONING

Manganese damages the globus pallidus, a part of the basal ganglia (Albin 2000). Further injury occurs in the midbrain, substantia nigra, frontal and parietal cortex, cerebellum, and hypothalamus (Goetz 1985; Goyer 1996; Pies 1997). Table 9–3 lists the several resulting psychiatric symptoms. The damage produces extrapyramidal symptoms that may mimic Parkinson's disease, especially because the treatment of psychotic symptoms from manganese poisoning with phenothiazine-derivative drugs can potentiate the parkinsonian symptoms of poisoning (Mehta and Reilly 1990). Phenothiazine intoxication, Parkinson's disease, and manganism equally destroy melanin cells in the substantia nigra (Donaldson and Barbeau 1985).

In serious cases, virtually all the symptoms in Table 9–3 appear, especially uncontrollable laughter or crying, mood disturbances, cognitive and perceptual abnormalities, sleep disturbances, and impulsive or "silly" acts. These symptoms constitute the classic description of "manganese madness." Psychiatric symptoms usually precede neurological symptoms, although neurological symptoms

TABLE 9–3.	Psychiatric signs and symptoms attributed to manganese poisoning
Mood	Irritability, mild euphoria, nervousness or anxiety, depression (rare)
Behavior	Uncontrollable laughing and/or crying, "silliness," social withdrawal, aggression, compulsive running or walking, minor criminal acts, change in personality, hypersexuality (one case)
Cognitive	Poor memory and concentration
Perceptual	Hallucinations, paranoia
Other	Hypersomnia, insomnia, nightmares

can exist without psychiatric disturbance. Symptoms may persist even after normalization of brain imaging studies (Nelson et al. 1993). Milder or subclinical cases may present with only vague sleep or mood complaints.

DIAGNOSIS AND TREATMENT OF MANGANESE POISONING

Parkinsonian symptoms with or without psychiatric symptoms accompanied by elevated blood or urine manganese levels indicate manganese poisoning. Serum manganese levels do not always reflect cerebral levels. Magnetic resonance imaging (MRI) of the brain assists in assessing damage to the basal ganglia (Alves et al. 1997). MRI of the brain often shows bilateral and symmetrical manganese hyperintensities in the globus pallidus in manganese-exposed workers, patients with portal-systemic shunting and liver dysfunction, and patients receiving total parenteral nutrition (Bertinet et al. 2000; Discalzi et al. 2000; Iwase et al. 2000; Lucchini et al. 2000). Expected findings include normal computed tomography scan of the brain and nonspecific electroencephalographic recordings (Barron et al. 1994; Izmerov and Tarasova 1993; Pies 1997; Sjogren et al. 1996). A history of occupational or environmental exposure or parenteral nutrition helps establish the diagnosis. Positron-emission tomography scanning shows a generalized decrease in glucose uptake (Nelson et al. 1993; Wolters et al. 1989).

Preferred treatment involves chelation with edetate calcium disodium followed by treatment with L-dopa (Pies 1997). Symptoms can improve, remain stable, or progress with treatment (Goetz 1985; Huang et al. 1993). MRI of the brain confirms that chelation reverses manganese deposition in the basal ganglia (Discalzi et al. 2000). Symptomatic management of psychotic symptoms with phenothiazine-derivative drugs potentiates the symptoms of manganese poisoning and should be avoided (Donaldson and Barbeau 1985; Mehta and Reilly 1990).

REFERENCES

Albin RL: Basal ganglia neurotoxins. Neurol Clin 18:665–680, 2000

Alves G, Thiebot J, Tracqui A, et al: Neurologic disorders due to brain manganese deposition in a jaundiced patient receiving long-term parenteral nutrition. JPEN J Parenter Enteral Nutr 21:41–45, 1997

Banta RG, Markesbery WR: Elevated manganese levels associated with dementia and extrapyramidal signs. Neurology 27:213–216, 1977

Barron TF, Devenyi AG, Mamourian AC: Symptomatic manganese neurotoxicity in a patient with chronic liver disease: correlation of clinical symptoms with MRI findings. Pediatr Neurol 10:145–148, 1994

Bertinet DB, Tinivella M, Balzola FA, et al: Brain manganese deposition and blood levels in patients undergoing home parenteral nutrition. JPEN J Parenter Enterol Nutr 24:223–227, 2000

Calabrese EJ: Pollutants and High-Risk Groups: The Biological Basis of Increased Human Susceptibility to Environmental and Occupational Pollutants. New York, Wiley-Interscience, 1978

Cawte JE: EMIC accounts of a mystery illness: the Groote Eylandt syndrome. Aust N Z J Psychiatry 18:179–187, 1984

Cawte J: Psychiatric sequelae of manganese exposure in the adult, foetal and neonatal nervous systems. Aust N Z J Psychiatry 19:211–217, 1985

Cawte JE, Florence MT: A manganic milieu in North Australia: ecological manganism: its ecology; diagnosis; individual susceptibility; synergism; therapy; prevention; advice for the community. International Journal of Biosocial and Medical Research 11:43–56, 1989

Discalzi G, Pira E, Hernandez EH, et al: Occupational Mn parkinsonism: magnetic resonance imaging and clinical patterns following CaNa2-EDTA chelation. Neurotoxicology 21:863–866, 2000

Donaldson J: The physiopathologic significance of manganese in brain: its relation to schizophrenia and neurodegenerative disorders. Neurotoxicology 8:451–462, 1987

Donaldson J, Barbeau A: Manganese neurotoxicity: possible clues to the etiology of human brain disorders, in Metal Ions in Neurology and Psychiatry. Edited by Gabay S, Harris J, Ho BT. New York, Alan R Liss, 1985, pp 259–285

Fell JME, Reynolds AP, Meadows N, et al: Manganese toxicity in children receiving long-term parenteral nutrition. Lancet 347:1218–1221, 1996

Ferraz HB, Bertolucci PHF, Pereira JS, et al: Chronic exposure to the fungicide maneb may produce symptoms and signs of CNS manganese intoxication. Neurology 38:550–553, 1988

Frumkin H, Solomon G: Manganese in the U.S. gasoline supply. Am J Ind Med 31:107–115, 1997

Goetz CG: Other metals, in Neurotoxins in Clinical Practice. New York, Medical & Scientific Books, 1985, pp 45–62

Goyer RA: Toxic effects of metals, in Casarett and Doull's Toxicology: The Basic Science of Poisons. Edited by Klaassen CD, Amdur MO. New York, McGraw-Hill, 1996, pp 691–736

Hamilton A, Hardy HL: Manganese, in Industrial Toxicology. Edited by Hamilton A, Hardy HL. Acton, MA, Publishing Sciences Group, 1974, pp 127–130

Huang C-C, Lu C-S, Chu N-S, et al: Progression after chronic manganese exposure. Neurology 43:1479–1483, 1993

Iwase K, Kondoh H, Higaki J, et al: Hyperintense basal ganglia on T1-weighted magnetic resonance images following postoperative parenteral nutrition in a pancreatoduodenectomized patient. Dig Surg 17:190–193, 2000

Izmerov N, Tarasova L: Occupational diseases developed as a result of severely injured nervous system: acute and chronic neurotic effects. Environ Res 62:172–177, 1993

Katz GV: Metals and metalloids other than mercury and lead, in Neurotoxicity of Industrial and Commercial Chemicals, Vol 1. Edited by O'Donoghue JL. Boca Raton, FL, CRC Press, 1985, pp 171–191

Kilburn CJ: Manganese, malformations and motor disorders: findings in a manganese-exposed population. Neurotoxicology 8:421–430, 1987

Kiloh LG, Lethlean AK, Morgan G, et al: An endemic neurological disorder in tribal Australian aborigines. J Neurol Neurosurg Psychiatry 43:661–668, 1980

Lucchini R, Albini E, Placidi D, et al: Brain magnetic resonance imaging and manganese exposure. Neurotoxicology 21:769–775, 2000

Masumoto K, Suita S, Taguchi T, et al: Manganese intoxication during intermittent parenteral nutrition: report of two cases. JPEN J Parenter Enterol Nutr 25:95–99, 2001

Mehta R, Reilly JJ: Manganese levels in a jaundiced long-term total parenteral nutrition patient: potentiation of haloperidol toxicity? Case report and literature review (abstract). JPEN J Parenter Enteral Nutr 14:428–430, 1990

Nelson K, Golnick J, Korn T, et al: Manganese encephalopathy: utility of early magnetic resonance imaging. British Journal of Industrial Medicine 50:510–513, 1993

Pies R: Silly rhymes and stupid crimes. Psychiatric Times 14:10–12, 1997

Sjogren B, Iregren A, Frech W, et al: Effects on the nervous system among welders exposed to aluminium [sic] and manganese. Occup Environ Med 53:32–40, 1996

Wolters EC, Huang C-C, Clark C, et al: Positron emission tomography in manganese intoxication. Ann Neurol 26:647–651, 1989

ADDITIONAL READINGS

Amr M, Allam M, Osmaan AL, et al: Neurobehavioral changes among workers in some chemical industries in Egypt. Environ Res 63:295–300, 1993

Bleich S, Degner D, Sprung R, et al: Chronic manganism: fourteen years of follow-up (letter). J Neuropsychiatry Clin Neurosci 11:117, 1999

Bowler RM, Mergler D, Sassine MP, et al: Neuropsychiatric effects of manganese on mood. Neurotoxicology 20:367–378, 1999

Canavan MM, Cobb S, Drinker CK: Chronic manganese poisoning: report of a case, with autopsy. Archives of Neurology and Psychiatry 32:501–512, 1934

Casamajor L: An unusual form of mineral poisoning affecting the nervous system: manganese? JAMA 60:646–649, 1913

Chandra SV, Seth PK, Mankeshwar JK: Manganese poisoning: clinical and biochemical observations. Environ Res 7:374–380, 1974

Charles JR: Manganese toxaemia; with special reference to the effects of liver feeding. Brain Journal of Neurology 50:30–43, 1927

Chia SE, Foo SC, Gan SL, et al: Neurobehavioral functions among workers exposed to manganese ore. Scand J Work Environ Health 19:264–270, 1993

Cook DG, Fahn S, Brait KA: Chronic manganese intoxication. Arch Neurol 30:59–64, 1974

Crump KS, Rousseau P: Results from eleven years of neurological health surveillance at a manganese oxide and salt producing plant. Neurotoxicology 20:273–286, 1999

Davis GG, Huey WB: Chronic manganese poisoning: two cases. Journal of Industrial Hygiene 3:231–238, 1921

Deschamps FJ, Guillaumot M, Raux S: Neurological effects in workers exposed to manganese. J Occup Environ Med 43:127–132, 2001

Dietz MC, Ihrig A, Wrazidlo W, et al: Results of magnetic resonance imaging in long-term manganese dioxide-exposed workers. Environ Res 85:37–40, 2001

Edsall DL, Wilbur FP, Drinker CK: The occurrence, course and prevention of chronic manganese poisoning. Journal of Industrial Hygiene 1:183–193, 1919

El Naby SA, Hassanein M: Neuropsychiatric manifestations of chronic manganese poisoning. J Neurol Neurosurg Psychiatry 28:282–288, 1965

Emara AM, El-Ghawabi SH, Madkour OI, et al: Chronic manganese poisoning in the dry battery industry. British Journal of Industrial Medicine 28:78–82, 1971

Fitzgerald K, Mikalunas V, Rubin H, et al: Hypermanganesemia in patients receiving total parenteral nutrition. JPEN J Parenter Enterol Nutr 23:333–336, 1999

Gayle RF: Manganese poisoning and its effect on the central nervous system. JAMA 85:2008–2011, 1925

Hua M-S, Huang C-C: Chronic occupational exposure to manganese and neurobehavioral function. J Clin Exp Neuropsychol 13:495–507, 1991

Huang C-C, Chu N-S, Lu C-S, et al: Chronic manganese intoxication. Arch Neurol 46: 1104–1106, 1989

Huang C-C, Chu N-S, Lu C-S, et al: Long-term progression in chronic manganism. Neurology 50:698–700, 1998

Iregren A: Psychological test performance in foundry workers exposed to low levels of manganese. Neurotoxicol Teratol 12:673–675, 1990

Kim Y, Kim KS, Yang JS, et al: Increase in signal intensities on T1-weighted magnetic resonance images in asymptomatic manganese-exposed workers. Neurotoxicology 20:901–907, 1999

Kostadinova GM: Personal characteristics of workers exposed to manganese (abstract), in XX International Congress on Occupational Health, Cairo, Egypt, 1981, p 448

Lucchine R, Apostoli P, Perrone C, et al: Long-term exposure to "low levels" of manganese oxides and neurofunctional changes in ferroalloy workers. Neurotoxicology 20:287–297, 1999

Markesbery WR, Ehmann WD, Hossain TIM, et al: Brain manganese concentrations in human aging and Alzheimer's disease. Neurotoxicology 5:49–58, 1984

McNally WD: Industrial manganese poisoning: with a review of the literature. Industrial Medicine 4:581–599, 1935

Mena I, Marin O, Fuenzalida S, et al: Chronic manganese poisoning: clinical picture and manganese turnover. Neurology 17:128–136, 1967

Mergler D, Huel G, Bowler R, et al: Nervous system dysfunction among workers with long-term exposure to manganese. Environ Res 64:151–180, 1994

Mergler D, Baldwin M, Belanger S, et al: Manganese neurotoxicity, a continuum of dysfunction: results from a community based study. Neurotoxicology 20:327–342, 1999

Naby S, Kayed KS, Aref MA: EEG induced fast activity in chronic manganese poisoning. Acta Neurol Scand 40:259–268, 1964

Penalver R: Manganese poisoning: the 1954 Ramazzini oration. Industrial Medicine and Surgery 24:1–7, 1955

Penalver R: Diagnosis and treatment of manganese intoxication. AMA Archives of Industrial Health 16:64–66, 1957

Racette BA, McGee-Minnich L, Moerlein SM, et al: Welding-related parkinsonism: clinical features, treatment, and pathophysiology. Neurology 56:8–13, 2001

Reimund JM, Dietemann JL, Warter JM, et al: Factors associated to hypermaganesemia patients receiving home parenteral nutrition. Clin Nutr 19:343–348, 2000

Rodier J: Manganese poisoning in Moroccan miners. British Journal of Industrial Medicine 12:21–35, 1955

Roels H, Lauwerys R, Buchet J-P, et al: Epidemiological survey among workers exposed to manganese: effects on lung, central nervous system, and some biological indices. Am J Ind Med 11:307–327, 1987

Roels H, Ghyselen P, Buchet J-P, et al: Assessment of the permissible exposure level to manganese in workers exposed to manganese dioxide dust. British Journal of Industrial Medicine 49:25–34, 1992

Rosenstock HA, Simons DG, Meyer JS: Chronic manganism: neurologic and laboratory studies during treatment with levodopa. JAMA 217:1354–1358, 1971

Sano S, Yamashita N, Kawanishi S, et al: An epidemiological survey and clinical investigations on retired workers from manganese mines and ore grinders in Kyoto prefecture. Japanese Journal of Hygiene 37:566–579, 1982

Santos-Burgoa C, Rios C, Mercado LA, et al: Exposure to manganese: health effects on the general population—a pilot study in central Mexico. Environ Res 85:90–104, 2001

Saric M, Markicevic A, Hrustic O: Occupational exposure to manganese. British Journal of Industrial Medicine 34:114–118, 1977

Schuler P, Oyanguren H, Maturana V, et al: Manganese poisoning: environmental and medical study at a Chilean mine. Industrial Medicine and Surgery 26:167–173, 1957

Sjogren B, Gustavsson P, Hogstedt C: Neuropsychiatric symptoms among welders exposed to neurotoxic metals. British Journal of Industrial Medicine 47:704–707, 1990

Smyth LT, Ruhf RC, Whitman NE, et al: Clinical manganism and exposure to manganese in the production and processing of ferromanganese alloy. J Occup Med 15: 101–109, 1973

Tanaka S, Lieben J: Manganese poisoning and exposure in Pennsylvania. Arch Environ Health 19:674–684, 1969

Wang J-D, Huang C-C, Hwang Y-H, et al: Manganese induced parkinsonism: an outbreak due to an unrepaired ventilation control system in a ferromanganese smelter. British Journal of Industrial Medicine 46:856–859, 1989

Wennberg A, Iregren A, Struwe G, et al: Manganese exposure in steel smelters a health hazard to the nervous system. Scand J Work Environ Health 17:255–262, 1991

Whitlock CM, Amuso SJ, Bittenbender JB: Chronic neurological disease in two manganese steel workers. Am Ind Hyg Assoc J 27:454–459, 1966

Yamada M, Ohno S, Okayasu I, et al: Chronic manganese poisoning: a neuropathological study with determination of manganese distribution in the brain. Acta Neuropathol 70:273–278, 1986

10

Mercury

EPIDEMIOLOGY

Of the heavy metals, mercury has medical, socioeconomic, and environmental importance second only to lead. The most publicized cases of mercury poisoning have occurred in industrial settings. Table 10–1 lists the numerous occupations at risk for mercury exposure. By 1957, 80 industries used mercury for 3,000 purposes (Bidstrup 1964). The expression from Lewis Carroll's *Alice in Wonderland,* "mad as a hatter," likely portrayed erethism, a condition caused by mercury poisoning of European and American hatters who used mercury to pack fur into watertight fabric. Acrodynia was another mercury-associated illness usually diagnosed in children taking mercury-based medications.

The literature describes several mercury poisoning epidemics. Outbreaks occurred in Iraq, Pakistan, and Guatemala from bread made with mercury-contaminated grain. Three separate incidents of mass poisonings occurred in Iraq in 1956, 1960, and 1972 (Bakir et al. 1973). In the 1972 epidemic, 6,530 people were hospitalized, and 450 died (Maghazaji 1974). In 1969, a New Mexico family became ill after they consumed organic mercury-contaminated pork (Roueche 1970).

TABLE 10–1. Past and present occupations at risk for mercury exposure

Adhesive makers/users	Etchers/lithographers/photoengravers	Metallurgists
Amalgam makers/users	Felt hat makers	Mildew proofers of textiles
Artificial flower makers	Fingerprinting equipment users	Milliners
Bacteriostatic agent (glue/pastes) makers	Fire gilding workers (gold/silver platers)	Miners
Barometer makers.users	Fluorescent lamp/bulb makers/users	Neon sign makers
Brewery fermentation equipment makers	Frozen mercury aerospace mold makers	Paper/pulp producers
Bronzers	Fungicide/seed dressing makers/users	Pharmaceutical makers
Carbon brush makers	Gamma globulin preparation makers	Photographic equipment makers
Makers of certain cosmetics: mascaras, wave fixatives, skin lighteners outside the United States	Hazardous waste site workers	Pigment makers
	Herbicide/pesticide makers/users	Plastics workers
	Ink manufacturers	Plumbers
Certain detonator/percussion cap makers	Jewelers	Pottery/chinaware/porcelain makers
Certain dry cell battery makers	Joint compound workers	Repairers of direct current meters
Certain surgical dressing users	Latex paint makers/users	Scientific instrument makers
Chlorine/caustic soda/chlor-alkali workers	Leather tanning good makers	Scientific laboratory workers
Dentists/dental technicians	Marine paint makers/users	Tannery workers
Diaper rinse users	Mercury-cathode cell makers	Tattoo artists and users
Dye makers	Mercury compound makers	Taxidermists
Electrical switch makers	Mercury vapor carbine makers/users	Thermometer manufacturers
Embalmers	Mercury vapor lamp makers/users	Welders
		Wood preservative makers

The most publicized epidemic broke out around Minamata Bay of the Shiranui Sea, an inland sea in Japan. The first cases appeared in 1953 and possibly earlier (Harada 1995). More than 2,200 persons developed what became known as Minamata disease, later attributed to mercury pollution of Minamata Bay by local industry (Harada 1995; Tucker 1972).

Industrial and occupational exposures continue to occur (Bluhm et al. 1992; O'Carroll et al. 1995). The journal *Science* reported the death of a prominent research chemist from mercury poisoning in a laboratory (Holden 1997). Other exposures can result from interior and exterior latex paints, many of which contained mercury-based antibacterials until 1990 and 1991, respectively (Agocs and Clarkson 1995). These paints raise household air mercury concentration 1,000-fold (Agocs and Clarkson 1995). Thermometers still use mercury, and children of thermometer plant workers have mercury levels five times those of other children in the same community (Hudson et al. 1987).

Poisonings of individuals and small groups, some developing psychiatric sequelae, frequently result from unusual sources or irresponsible acts (Lowry et al. 1999). One case of poisoning resulted from a leaking home sphygmomanometer (Rennie et al. 1999). Other recent cases resulted from certain cosmetics (Harada et al. 2001; McRill et al. 2000; Weldon et al. 2000). One case report described the onset of tics as the only symptom of mercury poisoning in a child using an herbal spray for mouth ulcers (Li et al. 2000). In the 1990s, acrodynia, major depression, or psychosis developed in more than one instance of children playing with and spilling jars of elemental mercury (Fagala and Wigg 1992; Yeates and Mortensen 1994). In one case, children contaminated 86 persons, 17 homes, and several classrooms of a local school with five pints of elemental mercury they found in an abandoned van (Malecki and Hopkins 1995). Injury from "swordfights" with tubular fluorescent bulbs also may cause acrodynia (Tunnessen et al. 1987). These bulbs contain mercury that varies with their length.

A 1995 health warning to mental health professionals cautioned that Hispanic spiritualist healers currently sprinkle mercury in homes (Zayas and Ozuah 1996). Some Hispanics practice self-injection of elemental mercury, a practice believed to increase strength (Zillmer et al. 1986). Certain Hindu and Chinese cultures believe in aphrodisiac and immortalizing powers of mercury (Goetz 1985).

A major century-long debate over the safety of mercury dental amalgams seems resolved except for an argument advanced by proponents of "environmental medicine" and multiple chemical sensitivities. They proposed that so-called oral galvanism causes a "smarting," burning, metallic taste associated with headache, eye symptoms, swollen throat, vertigo, and symptoms from the extremities and sinuses (Axell et al. 1983). Debate continues despite consistently negative findings in mercury amalgam studies. Eating tuna causes greater mercury exposure than from amalgam, and amalgam mercury exposes an individual to less than 1% of the daily mercury dose considered occupationally safe (Agocs and Clarkson 1995). Studies performed by the National Bureau of Standards, the Council on Dental Materials and Devices, the Council on Dental Research, and the Public Health Service found no impairment associated with routine use of amalgam (Dodes 1995; Rupp and Paffenbarger 1971). Recent negative studies included "the nun study" of 129 Roman Catholic sisters aged 75–102 years. The surface areas of their existing amalgams had no correlation with eight measures of cognitive performance (Saxe et al. 1995). A study of Swedish twins had the same results (Bjorkman et al. 1996). Undiagnosed periodontal conditions cause most of the symptoms of "oral galvanism" (Johansson et al. 1984). Other studies attribute the symptoms to psychosocial stressors, painful life events, and other psychiatric illnesses (Ekholm et al. 1987; Hammaren and Hugoson 1989; Jontell et al. 1985; Michel et al. 1989; Yontchev et al. 1986).

Emphasis must be placed on the notion of "routine use" of amalgam when discounting its toxic potential. Dentists and their assistants can be poisoned by amalgam, and the resulting psychiatric problems confirm the importance of maintaining proper amalgam handling in dental offices (Cook and Yates 1969; Echeverria et al. 1995; Gonzalez-Ramirez et al. 1995; Hooper 1980; Iyer et al. 1976; Ngim et al. 1992; Pagnotto and Comproni 1976; Smith 1978).

SIGNS AND SYMPTOMS OF MERCURY POISONING

Signs and symptoms of mercury poisoning listed in Table 10–2 appear after inhalation, dermal contact, or ingestion (Agocs and Clarkson 1995). The time of onset varies with the type of exposure and mercury involved. Acute effects appear within hours of inhalation, dermal contact, or ingestion of inorganic mercury (Table 10–2) (Agocs and Clarkson 1995). Chronic inorganic mercury poisoning results from low exposures over time, usually from inhalation or ingestion. Ingestion of elemental mercury from a thermometer has no toxicological importance (Goyer 1996). Inhalation or ingestion of organic mercury produces acute symptoms but primarily causes chronic poisoning. Some authors hypothesize a subpopulation with latent damage from organic mercury who develop chronic, progressive, or delayed symptoms exacerbated by aging (Takeuchi et al. 1979).

Fetuses, infants, and children have increased susceptibility to mercury poisoning. Organic mercury readily crosses the placenta and concentrates in breast milk (Agocs and Clarkson 1995). In Minamata and Iraq, pregnant women did not have symptoms, but their children had severe injury (Winneke 1990). Fetal exposure to organic mercury causes abnormal neuronal migration and disordered layering of neurons in the cortex (Goyer 1996). Neuropathological studies of fatal poisonings show extensive damage to the cerebral cortex with cortical atrophy, neuronal loss, and gliosis (Davis et al. 1994; Takeuchi et al. 1979). The Seychelles Child Development Study examined the effects of maternal consumption of organic mercury on the developmental outcomes of children. At the 9-year point of monitoring, no developmental abnormalities were linked with maternal mercury consumption (Axtell et al. 2000; Davidson et al. 1999, 2000; Myers and Davidson 2000; Myers et al. 2000; Palumbo et al. 2000).

Genetic conditions, including cystinosis, cystinuria, and tyrosinemia, and deficiencies of vitamins C and E or selenium increase the risk for mercury poisoning (Calabrese 1978; Goetz 1985). Vitamin E and selenium reduce the toxic expression but not the accumulation of mercury (Goetz 1985).

PSYCHIATRIC SIGNS AND SYMPTOMS ATTRIBUTED TO MERCURY POISONING

Table 10–3 summarizes the psychiatric signs and symptoms attributed to mercury poisoning. Two syndromes appear frequently in case histories: erethism in adults and acrodynia in children. The psychiatric components of erethism consist of irritability, excitability, timidity and excessive embarrassment, depression, and anxiety. Certain differences between acrodynia and erethism led some investigators to question mercury's role in acrodynia. Acrodynia in infants and children usually lacks the timidity and excessive embarrassment of the adult syndrome. Prominent features of acrodynia include the red, swollen, and cold extremities not usually seen in adult cases. In

TABLE 10–2. Signs and symptoms of mercury poisoning

Inorganic mercury	
Acute	**Chronic**
Pulmonary Cough, dyspnea, chest pain, interstitial pneumonitis, pulmonary edema, necrotizing bronchiolitis	**Neurological** Tremor—fine, rhythmic with coarse jerking movements worsened by voluntary movements (hatter's shakes); distal paresthesias; motor and sensory nerve conduction delay; limb weakness; dyskinesia; convulsions
Gastrointestinal Ashy discoloration of mouth/pharynx, abdominal pain, nausea, vomiting, diarrhea, gastrointestinal bleeding, membranous colitis, hematemesis, intestinal wall necrosis with scarring/fibrosis/stenosis	
Renal Acute nephritis, acute tubular necrosis	**Other** Gingivitis, stomatitis, mercurialentis (haze seen by slit lamp on anterior surface of lens), renal damage, nephrotic syndrome, chronic nephritis, fetid breath, brownish mercurial streak along margin of teeth
Skin Dermatographism, irritation, vesication, corrosion, dermatitis, burning, swelling, erythematous rash	
Other Psychiatric symptoms, tachycardia, hematological changes, enlargement of thyroid, metallic taste, salivation, intense thirst, fetid breath, conjunctivitis, cardiovascular collapse with dehydration, fever, death; acrodynia or pink disease (infants/children): mental disturbances, insomnia, sweating, extremity sensations/pain, peripheral vascular disorders, photophobia, anorexia, weakness, fever, tachycardia, red/swollen/cold/peeling hands and feet, stomatitis, gingivitis, loss of teeth/hair, constipation, tremor, weakness, death	

TABLE 10–2. Signs and symptoms of mercury poisoning *(continued)*

Organic mercury	
Acute	**Chronic**
Skin irritation, mucous membrane irritation, gastrointestinal symptoms, renal damage, nasal septum ulceration/perforation	**Neurological** Generalized ataxia, dysarthria, visual field loss, astereognosis, headache, slight intention tremor, numbness/tingling of lips and fingers, paresthesias, peripheral neuropathy, pain in limbs, hearing/taste/smell disturbance, disturbance of gait, weakness/unsteadiness of legs, falling, exaggerated tendon reflexes, positive Romberg's sign, rigidity, ballismus, chorea, pathological reflexes, athetosis, pyramidal signs, disordered handwriting, contractions, fasciculations, atrophy, coma, death **Other** Mental retardation, cerebral palsy, rashes, hypersalivation, hyperhydrosis, fatigue, metallic taste, gastrointestinal discomfort

TABLE 10–3. Psychiatric signs and symptoms attributed to mercury poisoning

Mood	Irritability, anxiety/nervousness, mood lability, excitability, anhedonia, depression
Behavior	Crying, restlessness, violence, suicidal/homicidal, apathy, timidity, inability to take orders, excessive embarrassment, shyness, social withdrawal
Cognitive	Memory loss, poor concentration
Perceptual	Paranoia, hallucinations
Other	Explosive speech, abusive language, insomnia, nightmares, mental retardation, loss of libido, fatigue, personality change
	Poor attention, academic decline (adolescents)

the past, medications that contained mercury, such as calomel, caused acrodynia in some children but not in others. Although questions remain over why some children appear more vulnerable to acrodynia, current theory attributes it to mercury (Tunnessen et al. 1987).

DIAGNOSIS AND TREATMENT OF MERCURY POISONING

A known history of exposure may not always accompany the presentation. Cases in recent years resulted from unexpected sources. Primary diagnostic tests include urinary and blood mercury levels (Goetz 1985). Whole blood or plasma levels indicate high- or low-dose acute exposures, respectively (Agocs and Clarkson 1995). Urine tests correlate with current exposure to *inorganic* mercury levels but only after reaching steady state. This normally takes 1 year of exposure. Before steady state, urine levels correlate with renal levels (Maroni and Catenacci 1994). The kidneys excrete little *organic* mercury, which forces the use of blood levels for diagnosis (Maroni and Catenacci 1994). Hair concentrations reflect long-term exposure but not dosage (Agocs and Clarkson 1995; Maroni and Catenacci 1994).

Several studies of electroencephalograms in mercury poisoning showed diffuse and background slowing, attenuation, temporal spikes, and sharp waves (Brenner and Snyder 1980; Fagala and Wigg 1992; Piikivi and Tolonen 1989; Vroom and Greer 1972). Magnetic resonance imaging of a case of elemental mercury poisoning showed mild central and cortical atrophy with diffuse and focal white matter disease unlike multiple sclerosis (White et al. 1993). One study that used single photon emission computed tomography (SPECT) detected hypermetabolism of the posterior cingulate (O'Carroll et al. 1995).

DSM-IV-TR (American Psychiatric Association 2000) recognizes three substance-induced disorders associated with mercury poisoning (Table 10–4). The lack of consistency between DSM-IV-TR diagnoses and the medical literature probably reflects developing psychiatric nosology rather than lack of association. The literature supports the addition of mercury-induced psychotic and mood disorders and delirium to DSM-IV-TR.

TABLE 10–4. DSM-IV-TR diagnoses associated with mercury poisoning

Substance-induced anxiety disorder[a]
Substance-induced persisting amnestic disorder
Symptoms of dementia

[a]DSM-IV-TR lists heavy metals as cause.

Treatment of mercury poisoning requires removal from the exposure followed by chelation. New chelation methods that use *N*-acetylpenicillamine, 2,3,-dimercaptopropane-1-sulfonate, or dimercaptosuccinic acid replaced early uses of British Anti-Lewisite and D-penicillamine (Marsh 1985). British Anti-Lewisite (2,3-dimercaptopropanol) increases cerebral organic mercury in some cases (Goetz 1985). Ethylenediaminetetraacetic acid does not displace mercury and worsens the renal toxicity of mercury (Goetz 1985).

REFERENCES

Agocs M, Clarkson T: Mercury toxicity, in Environmental Medicine: Integrating a Missing Element Into Medical Education. Edited by Pope AM, Rall DP. Washington, DC, National Academy Press, 1995, pp 450–472

American Psychiatric Association: Diagnostic and Statistical Manual of Mental Disorders, 4th Edition, Text Revision. Washington, DC, American Psychiatric Association, 2000

Axell T, Nilner K, Nilsson B: Clinical evaluation of patients referred with symptoms related to oral galvanism. Swed Dent J 7:169–178, 1983

Axtell CD, Cox C, Myers GJ, et al: Association between methylmercury exposure from fish consumption and child development at five and a half years of age in the Seychelles Child Development Study: an evaluation of nonlinear relationships. Environ Res 84:71–80, 2000

Bakir F, Damluji SF, Amin-Zaki L, et al: Methylmercury poisoning in Iraq. Science 181:230–241, 1973

Bidstrup PL: Toxicity of Mercury and Its Compounds. Amsterdam, Elsevier, 1964

Bjorkman L, Pedersen NL, Lichtenstein P: Physical and mental health related to dental amalgam fillings in Swedish twins. Community Dent Oral Epidemiol 24:260–267, 1996

Bluhm RE, Bobbitt RG, Welch LW, et al: Elemental mercury vapour toxicity, treatment, and prognosis after acute, intensive exposure in chloralkali plant workers, part 1: history, neuropsychological findings and chelator effects. Hum Exp Toxicol 11:201–210, 1992

Brenner RP, Snyder RD: Late EEG findings and clinical status after organic mercury poisoning. Arch Neurol 37:282–284, 1980

Calabrese EJ: Pollutants and High-Risk Groups: The Biological Basis of Increased Human Susceptibility to Environmental and Occupational Pollutants. New York, Wiley-Interscience, 1978

Cook TA, Yates PO: Fatal mercury intoxication in a dental surgery assistant. Br Dent J 127:553–555, 1969

Davidson PW, Myers GJ, Shamlaye CF, et al: Association between prenatal exposure to methylmercury and developmental outcomes in Seychellois children: effect modification by social and environmental factors. Neurotoxicology 20:833–841, 1999

Davidson PW, Palumbo D, Myers GJ, et al: Neurodevelopmental outcomes of Seychellois children from the pilot cohort at 108 months following prenatal exposure to methylmercury from a maternal fish diet. Environ Res 84:1–11, 2000

Davis LE, Kornfeld M, Mooney HS, et al: Methylmercury poisoning: long-term clinical, radiological, toxicological, and pathological studies of an affected family. Ann Neurol 35:680–688, 1994

Dodes JE: Mercury in dental amalgam. FASEB J 9:1499–1500, 1995

Echeverria D, Heyer NJ, Martin MD, et al: Behavioral effects of low-level exposure to Hg among dentists. Neurotoxicol Teratol 17:161–168, 1995

Ekholm A, Aalberg V, Hampf G: Psychopathology of people seeking treatment for oral galvanism. International Journal of Psychosomatics 34:3–6, 1987

Fagala GE, Wigg CL: Psychiatric manifestations of mercury poisoning. J Am Acad Child Adolesc Psychiatry 31:306–311, 1992

Goetz CG: Mercury, in Neurotoxins in Clinical Practice. New York, Spectrum Publications, 1985, pp 19–35

Gonzalez-Ramirez D, Maiorino RM, Zuniga-Charles M, et al: Sodium 2,3-dimercapto-propane-1-sulfonate challenge test for mercury in humans, II: urinary mercury, porphyrins and neurobehavioral changes of dental workers in Monterrey, Mexico. J Pharmacol Exp Ther 272:264–274, 1995

Goyer RA: Toxic effects of metals, in Casarett and Doull's Toxicology: The Basic Science of Poisons. Edited by Klaassen CD, Amdur MO. New York, McGraw-Hill, 1996, pp 691–736

Hammaren M, Hugoson A: Clinical psychiatric assessment of patients with burning mouth syndrome resisting oral treatment. Swed Dent J 13:77–88, 1989

Harada M: Minamata-disease: methylmercury poisoning in Japan caused by environmental pollution. Crit Rev Toxicol 25:1–24, 1995

Harada M, Nakachi S, Tasaka K, et al: Wide use of skin-lightening soap may cause mercury poisoning in Kenya. Sci Total Environ 269:183–187, 2001

Holden C: Death from lab poisoning (news). Science 276:1797, 1997

Hooper PL: Mercury poisoning in dentistry. Wisconsin Medical Journal 79:35–36, 1980

Hudson PJ, Vogt RL, Brondum J, et al: Elemental mercury exposure among children of thermometer plant workers. Pediatrics 79:935–938, 1987

Iyer K, Goodgold J, Eberstein A, et al: Mercury poisoning in a dentist. Arch Neurol 33:788–790, 1976

Johansson B, Stenman E, Bergman M: Medical study of patients referred for investigation regarding so-called oral galvanism. Scandinavian Journal of Dental Research 92:469–475, 1984

Jontell M, Haraldson T, Persson L-O, et al: An oral and psychosocial examination of patients with presumed oral galvanism. Swed Dent J 9:175–185, 1985

Li AM, Chan MH, Leung TF, et al: Mercury intoxication presenting with tics. Arch Dis Child 83:174–175, 2000

Lowry LK, Rountree PP, Levin JL, et al: The Texarkana mercury incident. Tex Med 95:65–70, 1999

Maghazaji HI: Psychiatric aspects of methylmercury poisoning. J Neurol Neurosurg Psychiatry 37:954–958, 1974

Malecki JM, Hopkins R: Mercury exposure in a residential community—Florida, 1994. MMWR Morb Mortal Wkly Rep 44:436–443, 1995

Maroni M, Catenacci G: Biological monitoring of neurotoxic compounds, in Occupational Neurology and Clinical Neurotoxicology. Edited by Bleecker ML, Hansen JA. Baltimore, MD, Williams & Wilkins, 1994, pp 43–83

Marsh DO: The neurotoxicity of mercury and lead, in Neurotoxicity of Industrial and Commercial Chemicals, Vol 1. Edited by O'Donoghue JL. Boca Raton, FL, CRC Press, 1985, pp 159–169

McRill C, Boyer LV, Flood TJ, et al: Mercury toxicity due to use of a cosmetic cream. J Occup Environ Med 42:4–7, 2000

Michel I, Norback D, Edling C: An epidemiologic study of the relation between symptoms of fatigue, dental amalgam and other factors. Swed Dent J 13:33–38, 1989

Myers GJ, Davidson PW: Does methylmercury have a role in causing developmental disabilities in children? Environ Health Perspect 108 (suppl 3):413–420, 2000

Myers GJ, Davidson PW, Cox C, et al: Twenty-seven years studying the human neurotoxicity of methylmercury exposure. Environ Res 83:275–285, 2000

Ngim CH, Foo SC, Boey KW, et al: Chronic neurobehavioral effects of elemental mercury in dentists. British Journal of Industrial Medicine 49:782–790, 1992

O'Carroll RE, Masterton G, Dougall N, et al: The neuropsychiatric sequelae of mercury poisoning: the Mad Hatter's Disease revisited. Br J Psychiatry 167:95–98, 1995

Pagnotto LD, Comproni EM: The silent hazard: an unusual case of mercury contamination of a dental suite. J Am Dent Assoc 92:1195–1198, 1976

Palumbo DR, Cox C, Davidson PW, et al: Association between prenatal exposure to methylmercury and cognitive functioning in Seychellois children: a reanalysis of the McCarthy Scales of Children's Ability from the main cohort study. Environ Res 84:81–88, 2000

Piikivi L, Tolonen U: EEG findings in chlor-alkali workers subjected to low long term exposure to mercury vapour. British Journal of Industrial Medicine 46:370–375, 1989

Rennie AC, McGregor-Schuerman M, Dale IM, et al: Mercury poisoning after spillage at home from a sphygmomanometer on loan from hospital. BMJ 319:366–367, 1999

Roueche B: Annals of medicine: insufficient evidence. The New Yorker 46:64–79, 1970

Rupp NW, Paffenbarger GC: Significance to health of mercury used in dental practice: a review. J Am Dent Assoc 82:1401–1407, 1971

Saxe SR, Snowdon DA, Wekstein MW, et al: Dental amalgam and cognitive function in older women: findings from the Nun study. J Am Dent Assoc 126:1495–1501, 1995

Smith DL Jr: Mental effects of mercury poisoning. South Med J 71:904–905, 1978

Takeuchi T, Eto N, Eto K: Neuropathology of childhood cases of methylmercury poisoning (Minamata disease) with prolonged symptoms, with particular reference to the decortication syndrome. Neurotoxicology 1:1–20, 1979

Tucker A: Mad cats and dead men at Minamata, in The Toxic Metals. London, Earth Island Limited, 1972, pp 15–45

Tunnessen WW Jr, McMahon KJ, Baser M: Acrodynia: exposure to mercury from fluorescent light bulbs. Pediatrics 79:786–789, 1987

Vroom FQ, Greer M: Mercury vapour intoxication. Brain 95:305–318, 1972

Weldon MM, Smolinski MS, Maroufi A, et al: Mercury poisoning associated with a Mexican beauty cream. West J Med 173:15–18, 2000

White RF, Feldman RG, Moss MB, et al: Magnetic resonance imaging (MRI), neurobehavioral testing, and toxic encephalopathy: two cases. Environ Res 61:117–123, 1993

Winneke G: Neurobehavioral toxicity of selected environmental chemicals: clinical and subclinical aspects, in Behavioral Measures of Neurotoxicity: Report of a Symposium. Edited by Russell RW, Flattau PE, Pope AM. Washington, DC, National Academy Press, 1990, pp 226–242

Yeates KO, Mortensen ME: Acute and chronic neuropsychological consequences of mercury vapor poisoning in two early adolescents. J Clin Exp Neuropsychol 16:209–222, 1994

Yontchev E, Hedegard B, Carlsson GE: Reported symptoms, diseases, and medication of patients with orofacial discomfort complaints. Int J Oral Maxillofac Surg 15: 687–695, 1986

Zayas LH, Ozuah PO: Mercury use in Espiritismo: a survey of botanicas (letter). Am J Public Health 86:111–112, 1996

Zillmer EA, Lucci K-A, Barth JT, et al: Neurobehavioral sequelae of subcutaneous injection with metallic mercury. Clin Toxicol 24:91–110, 1986

ADDITIONAL READINGS

Agate JN, Buckell M: Mercury poisoning from fingerprint photography. Lancet 2:451–454, 1949

Ahlmark A: Poisoning by methyl mercury compounds. British Journal of Industrial Medicine 5:117–119, 1948

Ahlqwist M, Bengtsson C, Lapidus L, et al: A. Serum mercury concentration in relation to survival, symptoms, and diseases: results from the prospective population study of women in Gothenburg, Sweden. Acta Odontol Scand 57:168–174, 1999

Aks SE, Erichson T, Branches FJP, et al: Fractional mercury levels in Brazilian gold refiners and miners. Clin Toxicol 33:1–10, 1995

Amr M, Allam M, Osmaan AL, et al: Neurobehavioral changes among workers in some chemical industries in Egypt. Environ Res 63:295–300, 1993

Angotzi G, Camerino D, Carboncini F, et al: Neurobehavioral follow-up study of mercury exposure, in Neurobehavioral Methods in Occupational Health. Edited by Gilioli R, Cassitto MG, Foa V. Oxford, UK, Pergamon, 1983, pp 247–253

Bailer J, Rist F, Rudolf A, et al: Adverse health effects related to mercury exposure from dental amalgam fillings: toxicological or psychological causes? Psychol Med 31:255–263, 2001

Benning D: Outbreak of mercury poisoning in Ohio. Industrial Medicine and Surgery 27:354–363, 1958

Bidstrup PL, Bonnell JA, Harvey DG, et al: Chronic mercury poisoning in men repairing direct-current meters. Lancet 2:856–861, 1951

Branches FJP, Erickson TB, Aks SE, et al: The price of gold: mercury exposure in the Amazonian rain forest. Clin Toxicol 31:295–306, 1993

Buckell M, Hunter D, Milton R, et al: Chronic mercury poisoning. British Journal of Industrial Medicine 3:55–63, 1946

Camerino D, Cassitto MG, Desideri E, et al: Behavior of some psychological parameters in a population of a Hg extraction plant. Clin Toxicol 18:1299–1309, 1981

Cassitto MG, Foa V: Assessment of behavioral toxicity in occupational health, in Application of Behavioral Pharmacology in Toxicology. Edited by Zbinden G, Cuomo V, Racagni G, et al. New York, Raven, 1983, pp 319–344

Cernichiari E, Toribara TY, Liang L, et al: The biological monitoring of mercury in the Seychelles study. Neurotoxicology 16:613–628, 1995

Davidson PW, Myers GJ, Cox C, et al: Longitudinal neurodevelopmental study of Seychellois children following in utero exposure to methylmercury from maternal fish ingestion: outcomes at 19 and 29 months. Neurotoxicology 16:677–688, 1995a

Davidson PW, Myers GJ, Cox C, et al: Neurodevelopmental test selection, administration, and performance in the main Seychelles child development study. Neurotoxicology 16:665–676, 1995b

Davis LE, Wands JR, Weiss SA, et al: Central nervous system intoxication from mercurous chloride laxatives. Arch Neurol 30:428–431, 1974

Dembert ML: Occupational chemical exposures and psychiatric disorders. Jefferson Journal of Psychiatry 9:57–69, 1991

Dinman BD, Chaffin DB: Surface electromyography in chronic inorganic mercury intoxication, in Adverse Effects of Environmental Chemicals and Psychotropic Drugs: Quantitative Interpretation of Functional Tests, Vol 1. Edited by Horvath M. Amsterdam, Elsevier, 1973, pp 155–169

Dodes JE: The amalgam controversy: an evidence-based analysis J Am Dent Assoc 132:348–356, 2001

Dyall-Smith DJ, Scurry JP: Mercury pigmentation and high mercury levels from the use of a cosmetic cream. Med J Aust 153:409–415, 1990

Ehmann WD, Markesbery WR, Alauddin M, et al: Brain trace elements in Alzheimer's disease. Neurotoxicology 7:197–206, 1986

Ehrenberg RL, Vogt RL, Smith AB, et al: Effects of elemental mercury exposure at a thermometer plant. Am J Ind Med 19:495–507, 1991

Ellingsen DG, Bast-Pettersen R, Efskind J, et al: Neuropsychological effects of low mercury vapor exposure in chloralkali workers. Neurotoxicology 22:249–258, 2001

El-Sadik YM, El-Dakhakhny A-A: Effects of exposure of workers to mercury at a sodium hydroxide producing plant. Am Ind Hyg Assoc J 31:705–710, 1970

Engleson G, Herner T: Alkyl mercury poisoning. Acta Paediatr 41:289–294, 1952

Fieldler N, Udasin I, Gochfeld M, et al: Neuropsychological and stress evaluation of a residential mercury exposure. Environ Health Perspect 107:343–347, 1999

Frumkin H, Letz R, Williams PL, et al: Health effects of long-term mercury exposure among chloralkali plant workers. Am J Ind Med 39:1–18, 2001

Fung YK, Meade AG, Rack EP, et al: Determination of blood mercury concentrations in Alzheimer's patients. Clin Toxicol 33:243–247, 1995

Gilewski MJ: Probable behavioral side effects of a mercury preparation. Clin Gerontol 3:69–70, 1984

Goldwater LJ, Kleinfeld M, Berger AR: Mercury exposure in a university laboratory. AMA Archives of Industrial Health 13:245–249, 1956

Gowdy JM, Demers FX: Whole blood mercury levels in mental hospital patients. Am J Psychiatry 135:115–117, 1978

Grandjean P, Weihe P, White RF: Milestone development in infants exposed to methylmercury from human milk. Neurotoxicology 16:27–34, 1995

Grandjean P, Weihe P, White RF, et al: Cognitive deficit in 7-year-old children with prenatal exposure to methylmercury. Neurotoxicol Teratol 19:417–428, 1997

Grandjean P, Budtz-Jorgensen E, White RF, et al: Methylmercury exposure biomarkers as indicators of neurotoxicity in children aged 7 years. Am J Epidemiol 150:301–305, 1999

Grandjean P, White RF, Nielsen A, et al: Methylmercury neurotoxicity in Amazonian children downstream from gold mining. Environ Health Perspect 107:587–591, 1999

Haq IU: Agrosan poisoning in man. BMJ 1:1579–1582, 1963

Hassan A, Velasquez E, Belmar R, et al: Mercury poisoning in Nicaragua: a case study of the export of environmental and occupational health hazards by a multinational corporation. International Journal of Health Service 11:221–226, 1981

Haut MW, Morrow LA, Pool D, et al: Neurobehavioral effects of acute exposure to inorganic mercury vapor. Applied Neuropsychology 6:193–200, 1999

Hay WJ, Rickards AG, McMenemey WH, et al: Organic mercurial encephalopathy. J Neurol Neurosurg Psychiatry 26:199–202, 1963

Hill WH: A report on two deaths from exposure to the fumes of a di-ethyl mercury. Can J Public Health 34:158–160, 1943

Hook O, Lundgren K-D, Swensson A: On alkyl mercury poisoning: with a description of two cases. Acta Medica Scandinavica 150:131–137, 1954

Hua M-S, Huang C-C, Yang Y-Y: Chronic elemental mercury intoxication: neuropsychological follow-up case study. Brain Inj 10:377–384, 1995

Hunter D, Bomford RR, Russell DS: Poisoning by methyl mercury compounds. Quarterly Journal of Medicine 33:193–213, 1940

Kark RAP, Poskanzer DC, Bullock JD, et al: Mercury poisoning and its treatment with n-acetyl-d,l-penicillamine. N Engl J Med 285:10–16, 1971

Kishi R, Doi R, Fukuchi Y, et al: Subjective symptoms and neurobehavioral performances of ex-mercury miners at an average of 18 years after the cessation of chronic exposure to mercury vapor. Environ Res 62:289–302, 1993

Kishi R, Doi R, Fukuchi Y, et al: Residual neurobehavioural effects associated with chronic exposure to mercury vapour. Occup Environ Med 51:35–41, 1994

Koos BJ, Longo LD: Mercury toxicity in the pregnant woman, fetus, and newborn infant: a review. Am J Obstet Gynecol 126:390–409, 1976

Korten AE, Jorm AF, Henderson AS, et al: Control-informant agreement on exposure history in case-control studies of Alzheimer's disease. Int J Epidemiol 21:1121–1131, 1992

Langolf GD, Smith PJ, Henderson R, et al: Measurements of neurological functions in the evaluation of exposure to neurotoxic agents. Ann Occup Hyg 24:293–296, 1981

Lebel J, Mergler D, Branches F, et al: Neurotoxic effects of low-level methylmercury contamination in the Amazonian Basin. Environ Res 79:20–32, 1998

Letz R, Gerr F, Cragle D, et al: Residual neurologic deficits 30 years after occupational exposure to elemental mercury. Neurotoxicology 21:459–474, 2000

Lewis M, Worobey J, Ramsay DS, et al: Prenatal exposure to heavy metals: effect on childhood cognitive skills and health status. Pediatrics 89:1010–1015, 1992

Liang Y-X, Sun R-K, Sun Y, et al: Psychological effects of low exposure to mercury vapor: application of a computer-administered neurobehavioral evaluation system. Environ Res 60:320–327, 1993

Marsh DO, Clarkson TW, Myers GJ, et al: The Seychelles study of fetal methylmercury exposure and child development: introduction. Neurotoxicology 16:583–596, 1995a

Marsh DO, Turner MD, Smith JC, et al: Fetal methylmercury study in a Peruvian fish-eating population. Neurotoxicology 16:717–726, 1995b

Mastromatteo E: Recent occupational health experiences in Ontario. J Occup Med 7: 502–511, 1965

Mathiesen T, Ellingsen DG, Kjuus H: Neuropsychological effects associated with exposure to mercury vapor among former chloralkali workers. Scand J Work Environ Health 25:342–350, 1999

McFarland RB, Reigel H: Chronic mercury poisoning from a single brief exposure. J Occup Med 20:532–534, 1978

McKeown-Eyssen GE, Ruedy J: Methyl mercury exposure in northern Quebec, I: neurologic findings in adults. Am J Epidemiol 118:461–469, 1983

McKeown-Eyssen GE, Ruedy J, Neims A: Methyl mercury exposure in northern Quebec, II: neurologic findings in children. Am J Epidemiol 118:470–479, 1983

Miller G, Chamlin R, McCormack WM: An outbreak of neuromyasthenia in a Kentucky factory—the possible role of a brief exposure to organic mercury. Am J Epidemiol 86:756–764, 1967

Myers GJ, Davidson PW, Cox C, et al: Neurodevelopmental outcomes of Seychellois children sixty-six months after in utero exposure to methylmercury from a maternal fish diet: pilot study. Neurotoxicology 16:639–652, 1995a

Myers GJ, Davidson PW, Cox C, et al: Summary of the Seychelles child development study on the relationship of fetal methylmercury exposure to neurodevelopment. Neurotoxicology 16:711–716, 1995b

Myers GJ, Marsh DO, Cox C, et al: A pilot neurodevelopmental study of Seychellois children following in utero exposure to methylmercury from a maternal fish diet. Neurotoxicology 16:629–638, 1995c

Myers GJ, Marsh DO, Davidson PW, et al: Main neurodevelopmental study of Seychellois children following in utero exposure to methylmercury from a maternal fish diet: outcome at six months. Neurotoxicology 16:653–664, 1995d

Neal PA, Jones RR: Chronic mercurialism in the hatters' fur-cutting industry. JAMA 110:337–343, 1938

Neal PA, Flinn RH, Edwards TI, et al: Mercurialism and Its Control in the Felt-Hat Industry. Washington, DC, U.S. Government Printing Office, 1941

Nitschke I, Muller F, Smith J, et al: Amalgam fillings and cognitive abilities in a representative sample of the elderly population. Gerodontology 17:39–44, 2000

Peled N, Richter E, Luria M, et al: Mercury exposures and effects in a thermometer factory (abstract), in XX International Congress on Occupational Health, September 25–October 1, 1981, Cairo, Egypt. 1981, p 131

Piikivi L, Hanninen H, Martelin T, et al: Psychological performances and long-term exposure to mercury vapors. Scand J Work Environ Health 10 35–41, 1984

Powell TJ: Chronic neurobehavioural effects of mercury poisoning on a group of Zulu chemical workers. Brain Inj 14:797–814, 2000

Rice DC: Identification of functional domains affected by developmental exposure to methylmercury: Faroe Islands and related studies. Neurotoxicology 21:1039–1044, 2000

Richter ED: Mercury exposure and effects at a thermometer factory. Scand J Work Environ Health 8 (suppl 1):161–166, 1982

Rosenman KD, Valciukas JA, Glickman L, et al: Sensitive indicators of inorganic mercury toxicity. Arch Environ Health 41:208–215, 1986

Ross WD, Kehoe RA: Industrial intoxications, in Practical Psychiatry for Industrial Physicians. Springfield, IL, Charles C Thomas, 1956, pp 239–254

Ross WD, Sholiton MC: Specificity of psychiatric manifestations in relation to neurotoxic chemicals. Acta Psychiatr Scand Suppl 303:100–104, 1983

Ross WD, Gechman AS, Sholiton MC, et al: Need for alertness to neuropsychiatric manifestations of inorganic mercury poisoning. Compr Psychiatry 18:595–598, 1977

Rossini SR, Reimao R, Lefevre BH, et al: Chronic insomnia in workers poisoned by inorganic mercury: psychological and adaptive aspects. Arq Neuropsiquiatr 58:32–38, 2000

Sexton DJ, Powell KE, Liddle J, et al: A nonoccupational outbreak of inorganic mercury vapor poisoning. Arch Environ Health 33:186–191, 1978

Sherman JD: Case reports based on the review-of-systems approach, in Chemical Exposure and Disease. Edited by Sherman JD. New York, Van Nostrand Reinhold, 1988, pp 97–137

Smith PJ, Langolf GD, Goldberg J: Effects of occupational exposure to elemental mercury on short term memory. British Journal of Industrial Medicine 40:413–419, 1983

Smith RG, Vorwald AJ, Patil LS, et al: Effects of exposure to mercury in the manufacture of chlorine. Am Ind Hyg Assoc J 31:687–700, 1970

Soleo L, Urbano ML, Petrera V, et al: Effects of low exposure to inorganic mercury on psychological performance. British Journal of Industrial Medicine 47:105–109, 1990

Steuerwald U, Weihe P, Jorgensen PJ, et al: Maternal seafood diet, methylmercury exposure, and neonatal neurologic function. J Pediatr 136:599–605, 2000

Stewart P, Reihman J, Lonky E, et al: Prenatal PCB exposure and Neonatal Behavioral Assessment Scale (NBAS) performance. Neurotoxicol Teratol 22:21–29, 2000

Stromberg R, Langworth S, Soderman E: Mercury inductions in persons with subjective symptoms alleged to dental amalgam fillings. Eur J Oral Sci 107:208–214, 1999

Thompson CM, Markesbery WR, Ehmann WD, et al: Regional brain trace-element studies in Alzheimer's disease. Neurotoxicology 9:1–7, 1988

Triebig G, Schaller K-H: Neurotoxic effects in mercury-exposed workers. Neurobehavioral Toxicology and Teratology 4:717–720, 1982

Turner MD, Marsh DO, Smith JC, et al: Methylmercury in populations eating large quantities of marine fish. Arch Environ Health 35:367–378, 1980

Urban P, Lukas E, Benicky L, et al: Neurological and electrophysiological examination on workers exposed to mercury vapors. Neurotoxicology 17:191–196, 1996

Urban P, Lukas E, Nerudova J, et al: Neurological and electrophysiological examinations on three groups of workers with different levels of exposure to mercury vapors. Eur J Neurol 6:571–577, 1999

Uzzell BP, Oler J: Chronic low-level mercury exposure and neuropsychological functioning. J Clin Exp Neuropsychol 8:581–593, 1986

Valciukas JA, Levin SM, Nicholson WJ, et al: Neurobehavioral assessment of Mohawk Indians for subclinical indications of methyl mercury neurotoxicity. Arch Environ Health 41:269–272, 1986

Weihe P, Grandjean P, Debes F, et al: Health implications for Faroe Islanders of heavy metals and PCBs from pilot whales. Sci Total Environ 186:141–148, 1996

West I, Lim J: Mercury poisoning among workers in California's mercury mills: a preliminary report. J Occup Med 10:697–701, 1968

White RF, Feldman RG, Travers PH: Neurobehavioral effects of toxicity due to metals, solvents and insecticides. Clin Neuropharmacol 13:392–412, 1990

Williamson AM, Teo RKC, Sanderson J: Occupational mercury exposure and its consequences for behavior. Int Arch Occup Environ Health 50:273–286, 1982

Yang Y-J, Huang C-C, Shih T-S, et al: Chronic elemental mercury intoxication: clinical and field studies in lampsocket manufacturers. Occup Environ Med 51:267–270, 1994

Zillmer EA, Lucci K-A, Barth JT, et al: Neurobehavioral sequelae of subcutaneous injection with metallic mercury. Clin Toxicol 24:91–110, 1986

Epidemic Mercury Poisoning in Iraq

Al-Damluji SF, The Clinical Committee on Mercury Poisoning: Intoxication due to alkylmercury-treated seed—1971–72 outbreak in Iraq: clinical aspects. Bull World Health Organ 53:65–81, 1976

Amin-Zaki L, Elhassani S, Majeed MA, et al: Intra-uterine methylmercury poisoning in Iraq. Pediatrics 54:587–595, 1974

Amin-Zaki L, Majeed MA, Clarkson TW, et al: Methylmercury poisoning in Iraqi children: clinical observations over two years. BMJ 1:613–616, 1978

Amin-Zaki L, Majeed MA, Elhassani S, et al: Prenatal methylmercury poisoning: clinical observations over five years. American Journal of Diseases of Children 133: 172–177, 1979
Jalili MA, Abbasi AH: Poisoning by ethyl mercury toluene sulphonanilide. British Journal of Industrial Medicine 18:303–308, 1961
Kantarjian AD: A syndrome clinically resembling amyotrophic lateral sclerosis following chronic mercurialism. Neurology 11:639–644, 1961
Marsh DO, Myers GJ, Clarkson TW, et al: Fetal methylmercury poisoning: clinical and toxicological data on 29 cases. Ann Neurol 7:348–353, 1980
Rustam H, Hamdi T: Methyl mercury poisoning in Iraq. Brain 97:499–510, 1974

Mercury Poisoning in New Mexico

Brenner RP, Snyder RD: Late EEG findings and clinical status after organic mercury poisoning. Arch Neurol 37:282–284, 1980
Davis LE, Kornfeld M, Mooney HS, et al: Methylmercury poisoning: long-term clinical, radiological, toxicological, and pathological studies of an affected family. Ann Neurol 35:680–688, 1994
Pierce PE, Thompson JF, Likosky WH, et al: Alkyl mercury poisoning in humans: report of an outbreak. JAMA 220:1439–1442, 1972
Snyder RD: Congenital mercury poisoning. N Engl J Med 284:1014–1016, 1971

Minamata Disease

Eto K: Minamata disease. Neuropathology 20(suppl):S14–S19, 2000
Kinjo Y, Higashi H, Nakano A, et al: Profile of subjective complaints and activities of daily living among current patients with Minamata disease after 3 decades. Environ Res 63:241–251, 1993
Kondo K: Congenital Minamata disease: warnings from Japan's experience. J Child Neurol 15:458–464, 2000
Kurland LT, Faro SN, Siedler H: Minamata disease: the outbreak of a neurologic disorder in Minamata, Japan, and its relationship to the ingestion of seafood contaminated by mercuric compounds. World Neurology 1:370–391, 1960
McAlpine D, Araki S: Minamata disease. AMA Archives of Neurology 1:522–530, 1959
Tamashiro H, Arakaki M, Futatsuka M, et al: Methylmercury exposure and mortality in southern Japan: a close look at causes of death. J Epidemiol Community Health 40:181–185, 1986
Tsubaki T, Irukayama K: Minamata Disease: Methylmercury Poisoning in Minamata and Niigata, Japan. Amsterdam, Elsevier Scientific, 1977

11

Thallium

EPIDEMIOLOGY

Soon after its discovery in 1861, thallium, like arsenic, assumed the conflicted role of both a medicine and a tool for murder and suicide. In recent years, political assassins in certain countries used thallium (Goetz 1985).

In the 1920s and 1930s, pediatricians prescribed thallium acetate for its depilatory action to treat ringworm of the scalp, especially in children (Prick et al. 1955). Thallium-based pesticides included a paste or pellet called Zelio (or Celio in some references) and thalgrain (Chamberlain et al. 1958; Mutch et al. 1992).

Even during the height of thallium product use, no formal studies investigated the epidemiology of thallium poisonings. Many reports made general statements such as "cases in the hundreds" or "scores of cases with many deaths" when describing clinical experiences. By the 1930s, more than 400 cases of thallium poisoning resulted in the United States from depilatory uses alone (Munch 1934). European literature during the same time reflected a similar, if not greater, morbidity (Prick et al. 1955). In the 1950s, thallium poisoning from pesticides in children became a serious problem, especially in southern states (Reed et al. 1963). Consumers often placed thallium insecticide "doughnuts" or "cookies" in their houses, offering irresistible temptation to young children (Reed et al. 1963). A mass poisoning in California resulted after victims ate thalgrain unknowingly used to make flour (Chamberlain et al. 1958; Reed et al. 1963; Smith and Doherty 1964).

During the 1970s, medical guidelines recommended thallium testing for any cases of unexplained neurological symptoms and peripheral joint pains ("Toxicity of Thallium" 1972). In recent years, implanted surgical thallium wires and Chinese herbal preparations caused unexpected poisonings (Marrubini et al. 1987; Schaumburg and Berger 1992). One report described three thallium poisonings from adulteration of illicit cocaine (Insley et al. 1986). In some cases, the source remains unknown (McMillan et al. 1997). Table 11–1 lists the occupations with the highest risk for thallium exposure.

TABLE 11–1. Occupational settings at risk for thallium exposure
Alloys (mercury and silver)
Fireworks
Fungicides
Highly refractive index glass
Infrared optical instruments
Insecticides
Jewelry
Photoelectric cells
Separation of industrial diamonds from other minerals
Tungsten filaments
Waste products from production of sulfuric acid
Waste products of lead/zinc plants

SIGNS AND SYMPTOMS OF THALLIUM POISONING

Symptoms result from inhalation, ingestion, or skin absorption (Bank 1980). The numerous possible symptoms include a classical presentation consisting of gastrointestinal distress followed by sensory changes in the distal limbs and dramatic scalp hair loss (Schaumburg and Berger 1992). The hair loss does not always occur but can involve the eyebrows, lashes, beard, axillae, trunk, and extremities (Prick et al. 1955). Poisoning presents with acute symptoms followed by death in 1–2 days or can be subacute or chronic with residual symptoms (Goetz 1985). Thallium causes prominent psychiatric symptoms in subacute and chronic poisonings. Table 11–2 lists the physical signs and symptoms reported from thallium poisoning. Table 11–3 lists the reported psychiatric complaints.

TABLE 11–2. Signs and symptoms of thallium poisoning

Acute	Hemorrhagic gastroenteritis, pain, rhinorrhea/conjunctivitis, fever, nausea, vomiting, diarrhea, delirium, convulsions, death
Subacute or chronic	
Neurological	Polyneuritis, tremors, paresthesias of hands and feet, retrobulbar neuritis, painful extremities, cranial nerve palsies, optic neuropathy, flaccid paralysis, choreiform movements, myoclonic movements of head and extremities, sensory neuropathy, ascending weakness, optic neuritis and blindness, abnormal reflexes, Babinski's reflex, residual weakness, visual problems
Other	Skin eruptions, hepatorenal injury, bone marrow depression, alopecia, hypertension, achlorhydria, stomatitis, excessive salivation, gingival discoloration, tachycardia, arrhythmias, weakness

TABLE 11–3. Psychiatric signs and symptoms attributed to thallium poisoning

Mood	Depression, anxiety, irritability, nervousness
Behavior	Restlessness, crying spells, personality changes, rage, hysteria
Cognitive	Delirium, dementia, confusion, Korsakoff's syndrome, poor memory
Perceptual	Psychosis, paranoia
Other	Insomnia, sleep-wake reversal, diffuse electroencephalogram abnormalities, mental retardation

PSYCHIATRIC SIGNS AND SYMPTOMS ATTRIBUTED TO THALLIUM POISONING

As in all cases of suicide by poisoning, separation of the toxic effects of the poison from the underlying mental condition leading to the suicide presents a challenge. Table 11–3 excludes, when known, psychiatric symptoms reported after suicidal uses of thallium or withdrawal from alcohol intoxication. The remaining signs and symptoms occurred in homicidal, accidental, and industrial poisonings. Irritability, rage, and sleep-wake reversals appear most frequently. The onset of delirium in many poisonings may account for confusion, restlessness, and nervousness. Several reports consistently found prolonged or permanent psychosis, dementia, or mental retardation following thallium poisoning (Bedville and Spragg 1956; Gefel et al. 1970; Moeschlin 1980; Munch et al. 1933; Reed et al. 1963). The association of any signs and symptoms in Table 11–3 with hair loss should raise suspicions of thallium poisoning, even in the twenty-first century.

DIAGNOSIS AND TREATMENT OF THALLIUM POISONING

Finding thallium in the blood and/or urine with expected symptoms establishes the diagnosis of thallium poisoning (McMillan et al. 1997). Past treatments consisted of chelation with British Anti-Lewisite (2,3-dimercaptopropanol). Medical management of a recent poisoning in China through telemedicine and Internet e-mail led to an international consensus that the preferred treatment uses Prussian blue (potassium ferric hexacyanoferrate) and hemodialysis (Noyes 1996). The only study that recommends specific psychiatric treatment of thallium poisoning suggests fluoxetine for irritability or rage (McMillan et al. 1997). Investigation of any case of thallium poisoning should include an assessment to rule out suicidal or homicidal intent, even in industrial settings.

REFERENCES

Bank WJ: Thallium, in Experimental and Clinical Neurotoxicology. Edited by Spencer PS, Schaumburg HH. Baltimore, MD, Williams & Wilkins, 1980, pp 570–577

Bedville BL, Spragg GS: Report of a case of thallium poisoning treated with thiouracil. Med J Aust 2:222–223, 1956

Chamberlain PH, Stavinoha WB, Davis H, et al: Thallium poisoning. Pediatrics 22: 1170–1182, 1958

Gefel A, Liron M, Hirsch W: Chronic thallium poisoning. Isr J Med Sci 6:380–382, 1970

Goetz CG: Other metals, in Neurotoxins in Clinical Practice. New York, Medical & Scientific Books, 1985, pp 45–62

Insley BM, Grufferman S, Ayliffe HE: Thallium poisoning in cocaine abusers. Am J Emerg Med 4:545–548, 1986

Marrubini MLB, Manzo L, Montagna M, et al: Iatrogenic thallium poisoning: report of two cases, in Heavy Metals and the Environment, Vol 2: New Orleans—September 1987. Edited by Lindberg SE, Hutchinson TC. Edinburgh, CEP Consultants, 1987, pp 115–117

McMillan TM, Jacobson RR, Gross M: Neuropsychology of thallium poisoning. J Neurol Neurosurg Psychiatry 63:247–250, 1997

Moeschlin S: Thallium poisoning. Clin Toxicol 17:133–146, 1980

Munch JC: Human thallotoxicosis. JAMA 102:1929–1934, 1934

Munch JC, Ginsburg HM, Nixon CE: The 1932 thallotoxicosis outbreak in California. JAMA 100:1315–1319, 1933

Mutch E, Blain PG, Williams FM: Interindividual variations in enzymes controlling organophosphate toxicity in man. Hum Exp Toxicol 11:109–116, 1992

Noyes H: Internet telemedicine saves woman's life (news). The Mercury (U.S. Army Medical Department, Houston, TX) 24:6, 1996

Prick JJG, Smitt WGS, Muller L: Thallium Poisoning. Amsterdam, Elsevier, 1955

Reed D, Crawley J, Faro SN, et al: Thallotoxicosis: acute manifestations and sequelae. JAMA 183:516–522, 1963

Schaumburg HH, Berger A: Alopecia and sensory polyneuropathy from thallium in a Chinese herbal medication (letter). JAMA 268:3430–3431, 1992

Smith DH, Doherty RA: Thallitoxicosis: report of three cases in Massachusetts. Pediatrics 34:480–490, 1964

Toxicity of thallium (editorial). BMJ 3:717–717, 1972

ADDITIONAL READINGS

Duncan WS, Crosby EH: A case of thallium poisoning following the prolonged use of a depilatory cream. JAMA 96:1866–1868, 1931

Fairweather MJ, Stovall V, Santiago P, et al: Thallium poisoning of children in Texas: report of 3 cases. Texas State Journal of Medicine 51:466–468, 1955

Grunfeld O, Hinostroza G: Thallium poisoning. Arch Intern Med 114:132–138, 1964

Hubler WR: Hair loss as a symptom of chronic thallotoxicosis. South Med J 59:436–442, 1966

Lehman J, Gaffney L: Thallium poisoning: a report of three cases. Ann Intern Med 6:60–64, 1933

Richeson EM: Industrial thallium intoxication. Industrial Medicine and Surgery 27:607–619, 1958

Schamberg JF: Reports of thallium acetate poisoning following the use of Koremlu (letter). JAMA 96:1868, 1931

Schenk VWD, Stolk PJ: Psychosis following arsenic (possibly thallium) poisoning. Psychiatria, Neurologia, Neurochirurgia 70:31–37, 1967

Steinberg HJ: Accidental thallium poisoning in adults. South Med J 54:6–9, 1961

Thompson C, Dent J, Saxby P: Effects of thallium poisoning on intellectual function. Br J Psychiatry 153:396–399, 1988

12

Tin

EPIDEMIOLOGY

The first reports of inorganic tin toxicity appeared in the early nineteenth century (Kimbrough 1976). Only after the disastrous medicinal use of Stalinon, a medication consisting of triethyltin and trimethyltin, in France in 1954 did the toxic properties of organotins become known. Stalinon, allegedly a cure for various infections, poisoned 217 individuals. One hundred of the victims died (Barnes and Stoner 1959; Piver 1973). Most of the deaths resulted from cerebral edema, a finding consistent with animal studies (Duncan 1985; Hartman 1988). The belief that Stalinon would cure infectious diseases resulted from two errors. First, a nineteenth-century idea existed that tin miners developed immunity to boils. Second, some clinicians overinterpreted the mildly positive results of an early twentieth-century animal study that successfully treated bacterial infections with tin (Barnes and Stoner 1959).

Poisoning by neurotoxic organotins now occurs rarely in industrial or laboratory settings. Occupations with the highest risk for neurotoxic organotin poisoning include chemists, chemical workers, and chemical engineers.

SIGNS AND SYMPTOMS OF TIN POISONING

Delayed symptoms frequently develop 1–3 days after exposure, especially a nearly universal headache or other severe pain complaint. Severity correlates with urinary organotin output (Besser et al. 1987). Severe exposures have poor long-term prognosis, often with permanent residual symptoms. Clusters of symptoms frequently mimic Klüver-Bucy syndrome or temporal lobe dysfunction with seizures or electroencephalogram abnormalities. Table 12–1 lists the physical signs and symptoms reported from organotin poisoning.

TABLE 12–1. Signs and symptoms of organotin poisoning

Gastrointestinal	Nausea, vomiting, abdominal pain
Neurological	Headache, pain—generalized and dental, visual disturbance, vertigo or syncope, tinnitus, deafness, cerebellar signs, ataxia, gaze-evoked nystagmus, paresthesias, electroencephalogram abnomalities—diffuse and focused, seizures, paralysis, papilledema, death
Other	Weight loss or gain, chemical skin burns, neurogenic bladder dysfunction

PSYCHIATRIC SIGNS AND SYMPTOMS ATTRIBUTED TO ORGANOTIN POISONING

The few dramatic incidents of organotin poisoning show consistent psychiatric findings in most victims. Table 12–2 lists the reported psychiatric complaints. Typical symptoms of mood lability, rage, and sexual and physical aggression with hyperphagia indicate temporal lobe or limbic system injury. Neuropathological and electroencephalogram studies support a physiological basis of psychiatric sequelae. Victims of Stalinon poisoning experienced persistent neurological and psychiatric symptoms for years after exposure (Kimbrough 1976). This conforms to case studies in the 1990s (Barnes and Stoner 1959; Feldman et al. 1993).

DIAGNOSIS AND TREATMENT OF ORGANOTIN POISONING

A toxic level of urinary organotin accompanied by expected symptoms indicates organotin poisoning. In fatal cases, cerebral edema

TABLE 12–2. Psychiatric signs and symptoms attributed to organotin poisoning

Mood and affect	Depression, irritability, inappropriate affect, rapid cycles (hours) of depression and rage
Behavior	Aggression (physical and sexual) and rage, hyperphagia or anorexia, amotivation, indifference, hyperactivity
Cognitive	Memory loss, loss of vigilance, disorientation, cognitive dysfunction
Perceptual	Psychotic behavior
Other	Insomnia and other sleep disturbances, loss of libido, fatigue/weakness

causes irreversible neuronal damage (Besser et al. 1987; Rey et al. 1984; Watanabe 1980). Electron microscopy shows cytoplasmic lamellated inclusions or "zebra bodies" (Besser et al. 1987). Magnetic resonance imaging findings were normal in one case study (Feldman et al. 1993).

Standard treatment consists of British Anti-Lewisite (2,3-dimercaptopropanol) (Boyer 1989), although D-penicillamine also may be used (Rey et al. 1984). The residual impairments observed in many victims result from the ineffectiveness of many chelating agents in these intoxications. No specific psychiatric treatments are used for the sequelae.

REFERENCES

Barnes JM, Stoner HB: The toxicology of tin compounds. Pharmacol Rev 11:211–231, 1959

Besser R, Kramer G, Thumler R, et al: Acute trimethyltin limbic-cerebellar syndrome. Neurology 37:945–950, 1987

Boyer IJ: Toxicity of dibutyltin, tributyltin and other organotin compounds to humans and to experimental animals. Toxicology 55:253–298, 1989

Duncan ID: Toxic myelinopathies, in Neurotoxicity of Industrial and Commercial Chemicals, Vol 1. Edited by O'Donoghue JL. Boca Raton, FL CRC Press, 1985, pp 15–50

Feldman RG, White RF, Eriator II: Trimethyltin encephalopathy. Arch Neurol 50: 1320–1324, 1993

Hartman DE: Neuropsychological toxicology of metals, in Neuropsychological Toxicology: Identification and Assessment of Human Neurotoxic Syndromes. New York, Pergamon, 1988, pp 55–107

Kimbrough RD: Toxicity and health effects of selected organotin compounds: a review. Environ Health Perspect 14:51–56, 1976

Piver WT: Organotin compounds: industrial applications and biological investigation. Environ Health Perspect 4:61–79, 1973

Rey C, Reinecke HJ, Besser R: Methyltin intoxication in six men: toxicologic and clinical aspects. Vet Hum Toxicol 26:121–122, 1984

Watanabe I: Organotins (triethyltin), in Experimental and Clinical Neurotoxicology. Edited by Spencer PS, Schaumburg HH. Baltimore, MD, Williams & Wilkins, 1980, pp 545–556

ADDITIONAL READINGS

Brown AW, Aldridge WN, Street BW, et al: The behavioral and neuropathologic sequelae of intoxication by trimethyltin compounds in the rat. Am J Pathol 97:59–76, 1979

Fortemps E, Amand G, Bomboir A, et al: Trimethyltin poisoning: report of two cases. Int Arch Occup Environ Health 41:1–6, 1978

Ross WD, Sholiton MC: Specificity of psychiatric manifestations in relation to neurotoxic chemicals. Acta Psychiatr Scand Suppl 303:100–104, 1983

Ross WD, Emmett EA, Steiner J, et al: Neurotoxic effects of occupational exposure to organotins. Am J Psychiatry 138:1092–1095, 1981

IV

Solvents

13

Solvents

EPIDEMIOLOGY

Solvents include numerous chemical classes: alcohols, ketones, ethers, esters, glycols, aldehydes, saturated and unsaturated aliphatic and aromatic hydrocarbons, halogenated hydrocarbons, carbon disulfide, and mixtures (Lilis 1992). These chemicals extract, dissolve, or suspend insoluble materials such as fats and polymers (Joint WHO/Nordic Council of Ministers Working Group 1985). Solvents most associated with psychiatric illness are carbon disulfide, halogenated hydrocarbons, aromatic hydrocarbons, and mixtures.

Solvent manufacturing is an important part of the economy. Annual productions of carbon disulfide and xylene range in the millions of tons (Arlien-Soborg 1992; Snyder and Andrews 1996). The annual production of 1,1,1-trichloroethane, found in 250 household chemicals, exceeds 700 million tons (Kurt and Buffler 1995). With this level of production, a significant number of workers are at risk for exposure. More than 450,000 workers have exposure risks to perchloroethylene or tetrachloroethylene in the dry cleaning industry (White et al. 1990). Various sources indicate possible exposures of 3.5 million workers to trichloroethylene and 140,000 potentially exposed to xylene (Lilis 1992). Table 13–1 lists the higher-risk industrial, environmental, and household settings for exposure.

Solvent exposures also can occur in environmental settings. Major oil spills can induce symptoms from both stress and solvent exposure (Lyons et al. 1999). The novel and movie *A Civil Action* (Harr 1995) portrays the effect of a trichloroethylene contamination on the community of Woburn, Massachusetts. Hundreds of such hazardous waste sites on the Environmental Protection Agency's National Priorities List contain solvents. Solvents constitute 6 of the 10 most common substances at these sites (Committee on Environmental Epidemiology 1991).

Carbon Disulfide

Beginning in the 1850s, the French used carbon disulfide in "cold" vulcanizaton of rubber, during which rubber was softened and spread thin for making balloons and condoms (Davidson and Feinleib 1972). The appearance of large numbers of psychiatric illnesses among rubber workers prompted Auguste-Louis Delpech to study the outbreak. Carbon disulfide induced mania and psychosis in workers who subsequently jumped from heights to kill themselves in the factories (Hartman 1988). Delpech later authored the first report of the psychiatric symptoms of carbon disulfide poisoning. In recent times, industrial exposures to carbon disulfide are possible in several settings but especially in rayon manufacturing.

Halogenated Hydrocarbons

Several neurotoxic solvents are halogenated hydrocarbons. Methyl bromide is discussed separately as a fumigant in Chapter 5. Methyl chloride initially was used as an anesthetic, but the practice ended after its toxicity became apparent (Repko and Lasley 1979). In the 1920s, refrigerators used methyl chloride for the cooling process. Before long, leaking refrigerators caused numerous poisonings of refrigerator repairpersons and consumers. Government restrictions banned methyl chloride in refrigerators by the 1940s and 1950s (Arlien-Soborg 1992).

Early uses of trichloroethylene included degreasing, and by 1940, a formulation of trichloroethylene named Trilene had widespread use as an anesthetic. Toxicity soon became apparent, especially after cranial nerve injuries and activated latent herpes infections resulted from anesthesia (Defalque 1961; Humphrey and McClelland 1944). Other important halogenated hydrocarbons include methylene chlo-

TABLE 13–1. Occupational and environmental sources of solvent exposure

AROMATIC HYDROCARBONS			
Benzene (including nitrobenzene, dinitrobenzene, hydroxybenzene, and aminobenzene derivatives)			
Adhesives	Engravers	Insecticides	Rotogravures
Aniline dyes	Explosives	Lacquers	Rubber
Art supplies	Floor polishes	Landfills	Shoe dyes
Bronzers	Food containers	Leather (artificial)	Soaps
Celluloid	Food preservatives	Leather dressings	Solvents
Chemical industry	Fungistats	Linoleum	Stains
Degreasing	Gasoline	Lithography	Underground gasoline tanks
Deodorizers	Glues	Lubricating oils	Varnishes
Dry batteries	Heat transfer fluid	Paint	Vehicle exhaust
Drying/packing	Herbicides	Paint strippers	Waxes
Dyes	Household cleaners	Plastics	Wood preservatives
Enamelers	Inks	Resins	
Styrene			
Acrylonitrile-butradiene-styrene (ABS)	Electrical devices	Polymers and copolymers	Shower stalls
	Foam	Polystyrene	Swimming pools
Bathtubs	Food packaging	Reinforced plastic boats	Thermal insulation
Carton coatings	Motor vehicles	Rosins	Toys
Containers	Paper coatings	Rubber	

TABLE 13–1. Occupational and environmental sources of solvent exposure *(continued)*

Toluene			
Chemical manufacturing	Fuels	Lumber	Rubber
Cigarette smoke	Gasoline	Paint	Service station attendants
Coke ovens	Glues	Paint thinners	Solvents
Color printing	Hazardous waste sites	Photogravure	Spray paints
Dyes	Lacquers	Pigments	Tank truck drivers
Explosives	Linoleum	Refinery workers	Underground gasoline tanks
Xylene			
Adhesives	Lacquers	Photogravure	Spray paints
Color printing	Leather (artificial)	Rubber	Thinners
Degreasing	Paint	Silk manufacturing	Varnishes
Histology laboratories			
HALOGENATED HYDROCARBONS			
Methyl chloride			
Chemical manufacturing	Methyl silicone polymers	Polystyrene	Rubber
Dewaxing	Oils	Polyurethane	Tetramethyl lead
Insecticides			
Methylene chloride			
Adhesives	Fire extinguishers	Pharmaceuticals	Printed circuit boards
Aerosols	Inks	Photo film	Thinners
Fibers	Paint	Plastics	Varnish
Methylchloroform			
Computer chip manufacturing	Typewriter correction fluid		

TABLE 13–1. Occupational and environmental sources of solvent exposure *(continued)*

Perchloroethylene (tetrachloroethylene)			
Brake cleaners	Lubricants	Pharmaceuticals	Textiles
Degreasing	Metal cleaners	Spot removers	Water repellents
Dry cleaning	Paint removers	Suede protectors	Wood cleaners
1,1,1-Trichloroethane			
Adhesives	Degreasing	Inks	Videocassette recorder cleaners
Automobile door lock lubricant	Household products	Spot removers	
Trichloroethylene			
Adhesives	Dyes	Metal fabricating	Printing
Anesthesia (old)	Flame retardants	Paint	Resins
Caffeine extraction	Fluorocarbon production	Paint removers	Rubber
Cleaners	Fumigants	Perfumes	Shoemaking
Degreasing	Lacquers	Pet foods	Soaps
Disinfectants	Landfills	Pharmaceuticals	Tobacco denicotinizing
Dry cleaning	Mechanics		
ORGANIC SULFUR-CONTAINING COMPOUNDS			
Carbon disulfide			
Adhesives	Flotation devices	Pesticides	Solvents for sulfur, iodine, bromine, phosphorus, and selenium
Artificial silk	Fumigation	Pharmaceuticals	
Chemical manufacturing	Neoprene cement	Rayon	
Corrosion inhibitors	Paint	Resins	Tires
Electroplating	Paint removers	Rubber	

TABLE 13–1. Occupational and environmental sources of solvent exposure *(continued)*

MIXTURES (GASOLINE, WHITE SPIRITS, AND COMBINATIONS OF SOLVENTS)			
Adhesives	Electron microscopy	Metal polishers	Printing ink
Anodizers	Electronics	Metal workers	Refineries
Artists	Engravers	Office workers	Roofers
Automobile body workers	Fuels	Optical technicians	Semiconductors
Automobile mechanics	Glaziers	Paint	Service stations
Cabinetmakers	Foundry workers	Painters	Shoe repair
Candle makers	Fur processing	Paperhangers	Silk screening
Carpenters	Lacquers	Papermaking	Tattoo artists
Caulkers	Locksmiths	Pest control workers	Underground gasoline tanks
Dental laboratories	Machinists		
ETHYLENE OXIDE			
Chemical industry	Hospital sterilant	Lubricants	
Fur fumigants	Industrial sterilant		

ride, tetrachloroethylene, methylchloroform or 1,1,1-trichloroethane, vinyl chloride, and trichloroethylene (Lilis 1992).

Aromatic Hydrocarbons

The most important neurotoxic aromatic hydrocarbons are benzene and its derivatives. The numerous derivatives of benzene include nitrobenzenes, toluene, xylene, aniline, creosote, phenols, salicylates, tannic acid, sulfa drugs, dinitrobenzenes, diphenyl, formaldehyde, and tetryl, a booster for high explosives (A.B. Baker and Tichy 1953). Yearly production of benzene in 1976 amounted to 11 billion pounds, and 2 million workers held occupations with potential benzene exposure (Lilis 1992).

Until modern techniques allowed better purification, toluene and xylene contained significant amounts of benzene. Gasoline still contains significant quantities of benzene (Gosselin et al. 1984). Little commercial interest existed for styrene until World War II, when the development of synthetic rubber required styrene in the production process (Miller et al. 1994). Outside of applications in the plastics and rubber industries, few other uses of styrene exist.

Mixtures

Mixtures constitute a category of solvents produced by distillation and cracking of petroleum. The group includes gasoline, petroleum ether, rubber solvent, petroleum naphtha, mineral spirits, white spirits, Stoddard solvent, kerosene, and jet fuels (Lilis 1992). Gasolines are mixtures of alkanes, cycloalkanes, alkenes, aromatic hydrocarbons, and antiknock additives.

SYMPTOMS OF SOLVENT POISONING

Table 13–2 lists the physical signs and symptoms attributed to various solvents. Some of the physical symptoms attributed to toluene or other benzene derivatives could result from residual benzene. Several genetic and medical conditions increase the susceptibility to solvent poisoning. These include glucose-6-phosphate dehydrogenase (G6PD) deficiency, sickle cell trait, thalassemias, NADH (the reduced form of nicotinamide-adenine dinucleotide) dehydrogenase deficiency, inadequate carbon disulfide metabolism, hyperlipidemia, homocystinuria, high aryl hydrocarbon hydroxylase inducibility, alcohol use, and renal disease (Calabrese 1991).

TABLE 13–2. Signs and symptoms of solvent poisoning

Carbon disulfide	
Gastrointestinal	Epigastric pain, nausea, anorexia, liver necrosis
Cardiovascular	Coronary artery disease, hypertension, hypercholesterolemia
Vascular	Vascular changes, cerebrovascular disease, retinal microaneurysms
Renal	Nephrosclerosis, renal disease
Neurological	Weakness, paresthesias, peripheral neuritis, cranial nerve injury, pain, footdrop, abnormal gait, tremor, choreiform movements, optic neuritis, polyneuropathy, parkinsonism, headache, electroencephalogram changes, retrobulbar neuritis
Special senses	Blindness, hearing loss, corneal sensitivity, visual disturbances
Other	Oily skin, skin and mucous membrane irritation, chronic cough
Trichloroethylene	
Gastrointestinal	Nausea, vomiting, liver necrosis
Renal	Acute renal failure, kidney necrosis
Cardiovascular	Blood pressure changes, arrhythmias, sudden death
Pulmonary	Tachypnea, pulmonary edema, dyspnea
Skin	Skin and mucous membrane irritation, activation of herpes simplex, contact dermatitis, "degreaser's flush" when consuming alcohol, burns, conjunctivitis, dermatographism, rash
Neurological	Anesthesia, analgesia, seizures, headache, trigeminal neuropathy, weakness, hemiparesis, cranial nerve damage, neuritis, paralysis, tremor, ataxia, vertigo
Other	Hot flashes, perspiration, increased blood lipids, mild anemia
Methyl chloride	
Gastrointestinal	Jaundice, nausea, anorexia, vomiting, weight loss, dysphagia, hiccups, abdominal pain
Neurological	Tremor, headache, delirium, amblyopia, vertigo, footdrop, weakness, incoordination, staggering, ataxia, death
Other	Excessive perspiration

TABLE 13–2. Signs and symptoms of solvent poisoning *(continued)*

Benzene (including nitrobenzenes and dinitrobenzenes)	
Gastrointestinal	Nausea, vomiting, hepatic dysfunction
Neurological	Headache, ataxia, fasciculations, seizures, tremor, coma, weakness, electroencephalogram abnormalities, peripheral neuropathy, tinnitus, vertigo, polyneuritis, retrobulbar neuritis, spinal cord involvement, death
Hematological	Erythropenia, leukopenia, anemia, thrombocytopenia, purpura, aplastic anemia, leukemia
Special senses	Hearing loss, visual field contraction, decreased visual acuity, cataracts
Skin	Mucous membrane irritation, yellow staining, profuse perspiration, icterus
Styrene	
Gastrointestinal	Nausea
Neurological	Light-headedness, dizziness, drunkenness, incoordination
Skin	Mucous membrane irritation, contact dermatitis
Toluene	
Gastrointestinal	Hepatic dysfunction, nausea
Cardiovascular	Dysrhythmias
Pulmonary	Respiratory tract irritation
Neurological	Headache, dizziness, ataxia, tremor, drunkenness, encephalopathy, coma, death
Special senses	Metallic taste, scotomata
Skin	Corneal burns, mucous membrane irritation
Other	Metabolic acidosis, electrolyte imbalances
Xylene	
Gastrointestinal	Nausea, vomiting, hepatic dysfunction
Cardiovascular	Sudden death, dysrhythmias
Pulmonary	Chemical pneumonitis, pulmonary edema
Neurological	Weakness, fatigue, dizziness, paresthesias, tremor, polyneuropathy, headache, disturbed vision, confusion, coma
Skin	Keratitis, dermatitis, mucous membrane irritation, flushing, erythema, blistering

TABLE 13–2. Signs and symptoms of solvent poisoning *(continued)*

Mixtures	
Gastrointestinal	Nausea, vomiting, diarrhea
Cardiovascular	Sudden death
Pulmonary	Chemical pneumonitis, pulmonary edema, hemorrhage, necrosis
Neurological	Incoordination, restlessness, ataxia, delirium, headache, vertigo, headache, blurred vision, slurred speech, dysphagia, peripheral neuropathy, coma
Skin	Chronic dermatitis, mucous membrane irritation, flushing
Hematological	Bone marrow depression, erythropenia, leukopenia, thrombocytopenia
Other	Anemia, salivation, hypokalemia
Perchloroethylene or tetrachloroethylene	
Gastrointestinal	Nausea, hepatic dysfunction
Renal	Renal dysfunction
Neurological	Dizziness, incoordination
Skin	Mucous membrane and skin irritation
Ethylene oxide	
Gastrointestinal	Nausea, vomiting, flu symptoms
Pulmonary	Pulmonary edema, dyspnea
Neurological	Headache, drowsiness, aphonia, seizures, sensory problems, abnormal gait, death
Skin	Burns, mucous membrane irritation, frostbite (liquid)
1,1,1-Trichloroethane	
Gastrointestinal	Hepatic dysfunction
Renal	Renal dysfunction
Cardiovascular	Sudden death, dysrhythmias
Pulmonary	Respiratory depression
Neurological	Anesthetic effects, peripheral sensory neuropathy
Methylene chloride	
Metabolized to carbon monoxide: see Chapter 14 for symptoms	
Additional symptoms	
Gastrointestinal	Hepatic dysfunction
Skin	Mucous membrane irritation, corneal burns, dermatitis

SUMMARY OF PSYCHIATRIC SYMPTOMS OF SOLVENT POISONING

Table 13–3 lists the psychiatric signs and symptoms attributed to accidental or occupational exposure to various solvents. No doubt exists over the neurotoxicity of carbon disulfide, even at low doses, or of many other solvents at high doses. Significant controversy surrounds the neurotoxicity of low levels of occupational exposure.

In the 1960s, Swedish and Finnish researchers performed the earliest epidemiological studies on occupational disabilities from solvents (Iregren 1996). The Danish government awarded the first solvent disability pension in 1976 (Cohr 1983). The proposed solvent-induced syndrome had several names, including psycho-organic syndrome, neurasthenic syndrome, painter's syndrome, Scandinavian solvent syndrome, and chronic toxic encephalopathy (Rosenberg 1995). Patients with these syndromes allegedly had personality, mood, and cognitive changes and various somatic complaints. The proposed disorders gained recognition from the World Health Organization in 1985.

The Scandinavian and later American medical literature contained serious faults in methodology. The greatest problem arose from not controlling for workers' compensation. Some workers selected for testing received total disability as a result of the tests. Conclusions drawn from certain case reports also showed "litigation effect" (Bowler et al. 1991; Dretchen et al. 1992). Other errors included poor control for the following: dose, duration of exposure, consistent use of tests, nutrition, other diseases, psychiatric disorders, solvent type, alcohol use, litigation, misinterpretation of data, variable diagnostic labels, comparison bias, and other confounders (Harrington 1987; Rebert and Hall 1994; Rosenberg 1995). Well-controlled studies of exposures to solvents other than carbon disulfide found fewer neuropsychiatric impairments than did the Scandinavian studies (Hooisma et al. 1993; Maizlish et al. 1985).

While the psychiatric effects of high-dose exposure to solvents remain unquestioned, the most recent reviews of the effects of low-level, chronic exposures to solvents reflect an ongoing debate (Filley and Kleinschmidt-Demasters 2001; Gamble 2000; Ritchie et al. 2001). The majority of recently performed controlled studies support a deleterious effect of low-level exposures (Condray et al. 2000; LoSasso et al. 2001; Morrow et al. 2001; Nasterlack et al. 1999). Other studies attribute subjective complaints in workers exposed to low-

TABLE 13–3. Psychiatric signs and symptoms attributed to accidental solvent poisoning

Carbon disulfide	
Mood	Depression, irritability, anxiety
Behavior	Mania, suicidal, homicidal, bizarre/odd, hilarity/weeping, violence
Cognitive	Memory loss, poor concentration
Perceptual	Hallucinations, delusions
Other	Insomnia, loss of libido, somnolence, sleep apnea
Trichloroethylene	
Mood	Mood changes, anxiety, irritability
Behavior	Agitation, mania, restlessness, suicidal, homicidal, aggression, behavior problems (children)
Cognitive	Poor concentration, cognitive impairment, memory loss, confusion, Pick's disease (one case report), learning problems (children)
Perceptual	Psychosis, delusions, hallucinations
Other	Sleep disturbance, catalepsy, lethargy, sleep apnea
Methyl chloride	
Mood	Nervousness, emotional lability, depression, irritability, euphoria
Behavior	Violence, personality changes
Cognitive	Memory loss, delirium, loss of concentration, confusion
Other	Insomnia, somnolence, nightmares, impotence
Benzene	
Mood	Nervousness
Other	Somnolence, insomnia
Styrene	
Mood	Irritability, depression
Cognitive	Memory loss, poor concentration
Other	Somnolence, sleep problems, insomnia, fatigue
Toluene	
Mood	Irritability, depression, mood lability
Behavior	Personality change
Cognitive	Poor memory, poor concentration
Other	Sleep problems, sexual problems, fatigue
Xylene	
Mood	Mood problems
Cognitive	Memory problems
Other	Sleep problems

TABLE 13–3. Psychiatric signs and symptoms attributed to accidental solvent poisoning *(continued)*

Mixtures	
Mood	Anxiety, irritability, depression, mood lability
Behavior	Lack of initiative
Cognitive	Memory loss, confusion
Other	Insomnia, somnolence, fatigue, other sleep disturbances
Perchloroethylene or tetrachloroethylene	
Mood	Irritability
Cognitive	Poor memory, poor concentration
Other	Fatigue
Ethylene oxide	
Mood	Irritability, depression, anxiety
Behavior	Agitation
Cognitive	Poor concentration, poor memory
Perceptual	Hallucinations
Other	Fatigue
1,1,1-Trichloroethane	
Mood	Anxiety, irritability, depression
Cognitive	Poor memory, poor concentration
Other	Insomnia

levels of solvents to personality characteristics or other conditions unrelated to solvent exposure (Albers et al. 2000; Seeber et al. 2000). Imaging studies of exposed workers have also failed to reach a consensus opinion (Aaserud et al. 2000; Haut et al. 2000; Varelas et al. 1999).

SOLVENT ABUSE

Epidemiology

Ancient Greeks allegedly inhaled carbon dioxide for "trance-inducing" effects (Hartman 1988; King 1983). Columbus observed inhalation of mind-altering snuffs by West Indian tribes. The inhalation of gases became a widespread American practice in the late eighteenth century after the discoveries of nitrous oxide, chloroform, and ether (Hartman 1988). Following the development of gasolines and aerosols in the twentieth century, inhalant abuse rapidly grew and reached medical awareness in 1951 when Clinger and Johnson (1951) described the first psychiatric cases. Early in the "epidemic" of twentieth-century solvent abuse, referrals to the New York City Bureau of Child Guidance discovered solvent abuse in 14 of 30 children with neurosis, behavior disorder, conduct disorder, or mental retardation (Telisman et al. 1983). In recent years, individuals desiring "orgasm extension" abused preparations of isobutyl nitrate, isobutyl alcohol, and isopentyl nitrite (Cohen 1977).

Table 13–4 lists important commercial solvents of abuse. Methylchloroform, the solvent in typewriter correction fluid, caused 30 deaths by 1988 (Lilis 1992). Ethyl chloride more recently became an inhalant of abuse (Hersh 1991). Chlorofluorocarbons, used as refrigerants and in the past as insecticide propellants and in deodorants, breath fresheners, hair spray, and other personal care products, caused hundreds of deaths after intentional inhalation (Maximilian et al. 1982).

TABLE 13–4. Commercial solvents of abuse

Aerosols	Marking pencils
Antifreeze	Nonstick frying pan aerosols
Cleaning fluid	Paints and removers
Computer cleaners	Personal hygiene products
Deodorants	Refrigerants
Disinfectants	Room deodorizers
Fingernail polish	Shoe polishes
Gasoline	Spot removers
Glues	Transmission fluid
Lighter fluid	Typewriter correction fluid

1,4-Butanediol, an industrial solvent, is metabolized to γ-hydroxybutyrate, a drug of abuse. One report described the potential mortality and psychiatric morbidity from the intentional ingestion of 1,4-butanediol for bodybuilding or self-treatment of depression or insomnia (Zvosec et al. 2001).

The paucity of literature on solvent abuse compared with other drug abuse contrasts with its prevalence and medical importance. In New York State, adolescent solvent abuse approximated that of lysergic acid diethylamide (LSD) (Stephens et al. 1978). Solvent abuse parallels marijuana use until the eighth grade, when solvent use declines and marijuana use increases (Beauvais 1992). Solvent use appears on the rise, reflected by a 1991 study that found greater use of solvents than cocaine by adolescents (Beauvais 1992). One study in the United States found that 11.2% of high school students tried solvents, and 4.3% had tried them within the past year (Beauvais 1992). The 1988 National High School Senior Survey found lifetime rates of 19.5% and 14.0% for males and females, respectively (Beauvais 1992). Hispanic Americans and African Americans had lower rates than did Anglo-Americans. American Indians had lifetime prevalence rates exceeding 30% for both sexes. Solvent abuse tends to occur most frequently in the user's home, although use can also take place on the street, at parties, or in school (McGarvey et al. 1999). The importance of these findings increases with the recognition that adult polysubstance use frequently develops from adolescent solvent abuse. Many adults choose solvents and alcohol (also a solvent) as their preferred substances (Beauvais 1992; Stephens et al. 1978).

Prevalence of adolescent experimentation with solvents in the United Kingdom averages 3.5%–10%, with approximately 100 deaths per year from solvent intoxication (Ramsey et al. 1989). Despite the lower Hispanic American rate in the United States, solvent abuse remains the most common adolescent addiction in Mexico City, Mexico. Mexican public psychiatric hospitals report frequent cases of inhalant-induced psychotic disorder (Doon 1990; Hernandez-Avila et al. 1998).

Case reports of solvent abuse present a wide array of unusual or unexpected circumstances. Patients on psychiatric wards may inhale aerosol deodorants (Reid and Turner 1994). Sniffing of cleaning liquids containing methanol results in complications from methanol poisoning (McCormick et al. 1990). Inhalation of metallic spray paints causes depositions of copper and zinc particles in the lungs (Wilde 1975). Abusers of *n*-hexane or methyl *N*-butyl ketone glues can develop peripheral neuropathy without psychiatric manifestations (O'Donoghue 1985). Some poisonings present with atypical symptoms mimicking parkinsonism or causing stroke from vascular spasm (Parker et al. 1984; Uitti et al. 1994). One case report described an adolescent who moved to a tent in his backyard to continuously inhale gasoline through a self-constructed device (Brown 1968). Members of an isolated Canadian Indian community developed widespread gasoline addiction. Families passed gasoline at dinner tables for drinking; some injected it; parents gave it as a reward; and others prostituted for it or died from gasoline burning or drowning (Boeckx and Cooding 1978).

Poor methodology restricts the use of most epidemiological studies of solvent abuse. Several major issues remain unresolved, especially whether solvent abuse causes or results from the psychiatric dysfunctions observed in solvent abusers, their families, and their communities. Table 13–5 lists family and community characteristics often associated with solvent abuse. Most reviews agree that the psychosocial findings in Table 13–5 predate the use of solvents.

TABLE 13–5. Individual, family, and community characteristics associated with solvent abuse

Alcohol misuse
Antisocial behavior; more deviant than other drug users
Family dysfunction
Limited recreation
Mental retardation
Neuropsychiatric impairment
Other drug involvement; specific associations unclear
Poor academic performance
Poor supervision of children
Poverty, but any socioeconomic background possible
Transitional states in ethnic communities (American Indians)
Unemployment

Source. Edeh 1989; Goldstein 1978; Oetting and Webb 1992; Westermeyer 1987.

Psychiatric Signs and Symptoms of Solvent Abuse

Table 13–6 lists the psychiatric signs and symptoms attributed to intentional inhalation of solvents. One important review concluded that permanent brain damage with psychiatric manifestations does not result from solvent abuse (Ron 1986). In support of this opinion, individuals without neurological signs may have other conditions, including substance abuse or psychiatric illness, that cause their dysfunction (Chadwick and Anderson 1989). Contrary to that opinion, nearly 20 computed tomography, magnetic resonance imaging, positron emission tomography, and single photon emission computed tomography studies of solvent users and others with occupational or hobby exposures found brain abnormalities from solvent abuse, especially in individuals with neuropsychological test abnormalities or neurological signs (Chadwick and Anderson 1989) (Table 13–7). Other findings in solvent abusers include abnormal brain stem auditory evoked potentials and neuropathological studies (Kornfeld et al. 1994; Metrick and Brenner 1982). Electroencephalograms may show episodic slowing or spikes (Brozovsky and Winkler 1965; Satran and Dodson 1963)

TABLE 13–6. Psychiatric signs and symptoms attributed to intentional solvent inhalation

Mood	Depression, anxiety, irritability, mood swings
Behavior	Laughter, suicidality, violence, behavior problems, personality changes
Cognitive	Encephalopathy
Perceptual	Hallucinations, delusions
Other	Academic problems

ANESTHETICS

Many of the industrial solvents were originally used as anesthetics. Anesthetic exposure occurs through both occupational and intentional use. Abused anesthetics include ether, nitrous oxide, chloroform, and halothane (Chenoweth 1977). Ketamine abusers represent a growing population presenting to emergency rooms with hallucinations and agitation (Weiner et al. 2000). One case report of an anesthesiologist who was addicted to Pentrane described him as a gasoline sniffer as a child who developed anxiety, decreased libido, and insomnia from his Pentrane dependence (de Francisco 1971). Although perhaps not related to anesthetic exposure, anesthesiologists have twice the death rate from suicide than do a comparable socioeconomic group (Bruce et al. 1968). One concerned observer reported unpublished evidence of decreased psychological performance of anesthesiology residents from the start of residency to the end of 1 year (Chang and Katz 1976). Recent surveys of mortality risks of anesthesiologists have substantiated the increased risk of suicide for this profession (Alexander et al. 2000).

Other psychiatric studies of anesthetic use evaluated psychiatric symptoms in outpatient or volunteer exposures. Experimental exposure to halothane or isoflurane resulted in significant dysphoria and intellectual dysfunction lasting at least 4 days but resolving by 30 days (Davison et al. 1975). Voluntary cyclopropane exposure resulted in 24-hour symptoms of decreased concentration, fatigue, depression, abnormal thoughts, nervousness, and sleep disturbance (James 1969). Subjective complaints and decreased intellectual function measured by objective testing persisted for 1–6 days. A study of 408 outpatients receiving anesthetics found that 45% developed symptoms including drowsiness and headache within 24 hours (Fahy and Marshall 1969). Postanesthetic morbidity was correlated with female sex and higher neuroticism scores on psychological testing.

TABLE 13–7. Brain imaging findings in solvent abusers or nonintentional exposures

Finding	Study
Computed tomography	
Widening of cortical/cerebellar sulci	Boor and Hurtig 1977
Pontomedullary atrophy	Metrick and Brenner 1982
Diffuse cerebral/cerebellar atrophy	Escobar and Aruffo 1980
	Huang et al. 1996
Temporal lobe demyelination	Gatley et al. 1991
Magnetic resonance imaging	
Cerebral, cerebellar, brain stem white matter abnormalities	Caldemeyer et al. 1993
	Filley et al. 1990
	Kojima et al. 1993
	Sodeyama et al. 1993
	Suzuki et al. 1992
	Xiong et al. 1993
	Yamanouchi et al. 1995
Brain atrophy	Hirai and Ikeuchi 1993
	Ikeda and Tsukagoshi 1990
	Ohnuma et al. 1995
	Sodeyama et al. 1993
	Xiong et al. 1993
	Yamanouchi et al. 1995
Basal ganglia abnormalities	Unger et al. 1994
Positron emission tomography	
Striatal dopaminergic dysfunction	Uitti et al. 1994
Single photon emission computed tomography	
Hypoperfusion in dorsal frontal/parietal lobes	Heuser et al. 1993; Kucuk et al. 2000; Okada et al. 1999

DIAGNOSIS AND TREATMENT OF ACCIDENTAL AND INTENTIONAL SOLVENT EXPOSURE

DSM-IV-TR (American Psychiatric Association 2000) recognizes inhalant-, anesthetic-, and solvent-related disorders (Table 13–8). Anesthetics are associated with substance-induced anxiety disorder. Inhalant-related disorders include intoxication, delirium, persisting dementia, psychotic disorders with delusions or hallucinations, mood or anxiety disorders, and disorders not otherwise specified. Diagnosis depends on history or laboratory studies described earlier in this chapter. Physical signs such as deposits from inhalants around the mouth or nose or on hands and clothing may indicate recent use (Westermeyer 1987). Nasal membranes may be inflamed (Westermeyer 1987).

TABLE 13–8. DSM-IV-TR inhalant-induced disorders

Inhalant intoxication
Inhalant intoxication delirium[a]
Inhalant-induced persisting dementia[a]
Inhalant-induced psychotic disorder,[a] with delusions
Inhalant-induced psychotic disorder, with hallucinations
Inhalant-induced mood disorder
Inhalant-induced anxiety disorder[b]
Inhalant-related disorder not otherwise specified

[a]DSM-IV-TR attributes an equivalent substance-induced disorder to "solvent" exposure.
[b]DSM-IV-TR attributes an equivalent substance-induced disorder to "solvent" and anesthetic exposure.

Most inhalants or volatile substances are solvents, but the DSM-IV-TR text attributes only five of the eight disorders associated with inhalants to solvents: substance-induced psychotic disorder, anxiety disorder, delirium, persisting amnestic disorder, and symptoms of dementia. The association of solvents with dementia is more controversial than their association with mood disorders, but DSM-IV-TR does not recognize mood disorder resulting from solvent exposure. These inconsistencies probably reflect incomplete fidelity between the literature and the psychiatric nosology rather than current opinion.

The nosology of solvent poisoning proposed by a 1987 international consensus meeting (Table 13–9) on the occupational effects of solvent exposures complicates the application of DSM-IV-TR to med-

TABLE 13–9. Proposed classification of occupational solvent poisoning

Type 1	Symptoms only with objective findings=neurasthenic syndrome
Type 2A	Sustained personality or mood changes; not reversible
Type 3A	Impairment of intellectual functions=mild dementia=psycho-organic syndrome Minor neurological signs Usually from solvent abuse, a one-time high Exposure or long-term, chronic exposure
Type 4	Dementia, neurological signs

ical literature (E. L. Baker and Seppalainen 1987; Morrow et al. 1994; Rosenberg 1995). DSM-IV-TR–based diagnoses should replace the World Health Organization diagnostic categories to facilitate standardized research.

Solvent abuse and occupational exposures result in numerous physical problems that need assessment with a complete physical examination, including chest X ray, electrocardiogram, electroencephalogram, complete blood count, urinalysis, chemistry, and liver function tests (Comstock and Comstock 1977; Jumper-Thurman and Beauvais 1992). Significant overlap exists between solvent-induced symptoms and malingering, somatoform, factitious, and other psychiatric disorders. Certain cases need evaluation with neuropsychological testing, electromyography, nerve conduction velocity, computed tomography, or magnetic resonance imaging (Rosenberg 1995; Snyder and Andrews 1996). Specific laboratory tests exist for most of the major solvents (Table 13–10) (Maroni and Catenacci 1994). Methyl chloride and gasoline have no specific laboratory tests.

TABLE 13–10. Specific laboratory tests for certain solvents

Solvent	Test
Carbon disulfide	Iodine-azide test: the speed of reduction of iodine by sodium azide is accelerated
Trichloroethylene	Urinary excretion of trichloroacetic acid and trichloroethanol
Styrene	Urinary mandelic acid and phenylglyoxylic acid
Toluene	Urinary hippuric acid and *o*-cresol; blood toluene can result from certain food additives
Xylene	Urinary ortho-, meta-, and para-methyl hippuric acid
Perchloroethylene	Urinary trichloroacetic acid and blood perchloroethylene
1,1,1-Trichloroethane	Blood or breath levels
Methylene chloride	Carboxyhemoglobin level; levels of methylene chloride in blood or breath

Treatment consists primarily of abstinence and symptomatic management of withdrawal or related disorders. Carbamazepine and haloperidol have equal efficacy for treating inhalant-induced psychotic disorder (Hernandez-Avila et al. 1998). Risperidone may effectively treat the psychotic symptoms and craving for inhalants (Misra et al. 1999).

REFERENCES

Aaserud O, Nakstad PH, Bakke SJ, et al: Failure to confirm neurotoxic impairment using cerebral magnetic resonance imaging on solvent-exposed workers. Scand J Work Environ Health 26:346–352, 2000

Albers JW, Wald JJ, Garabrant DH, et al: Neurologic evaluation of workers previously diagnosed with solvent-induced toxic encephalopathy. J Occup Environ Med 42:410–423, 2000

Alexander BH, Checkoway H, Nagahama SI, et al: Cause-specific mortality risks of anesthesiologists. Anesthesiology 93:922–930, 2000

American Psychiatric Association: Diagnostic and Statistical Manual of Mental Disorders, 4th Edition, Text Revision. Washington, DC, American Psychiatric Association, 2000

Arlien-Soborg P: Solvent Neurotoxicity. Boca Raton, FL, CRC Press, 1992

Baker AB, Tichy FY: The effects of the organic solvents and industrial poisonings on the central nervous system. Research Publication of the Association for Research of Nervous and Mental Diseases 32:475–505, 1953

Baker EL, Seppalainen AM: Human aspects of solvent neurobehavioral effects. Neurotoxicology 7:43–56, 1987

Beauvais F: Volatile solvent abuse: trends and patterns, in Inhalant Abuse: A Volatile Research Agenda. Edited by Sharp CW, Beauvais F, Spence R. Washington, DC, U.S. Government Printing Office, 1992, pp 13–42

Boeckx RL, Cooding FJ: An epidemic of gasoline sniffing, in Voluntary Inhalation of Industrial Solvents. Edited by Sharp CW, Carroll LT. Rockville, MD, U.S. Government Printing Office, 1978, pp 179–186

Boor JW, Hurtig HI: Persistent cerebellar ataxia after exposure to toluene. Ann Neurol 2:440–442, 1977

Bowler RM, Mergler D, Harrison R, et al: Affective and personality disturbances among female former microelectronics workers. J Clin Psychol 47:41–52, 1991

Brown NW: Gasoline inhalation. J Med Assoc Ga 57:217–221, 1968

Brozovsky M, Winkler EG: Glue sniffing in children and adolescents. New York State Journal of Medicine 85 (part 2):1984–1989, 1965

Bruce DL, Eide KA, Linde HW, et al: Causes of death among anesthesiologists: a 20-year survey. Anesthesiology 29:565–569, 1968

Calabrese EJ: Genetic predisposition to occupationally related diseases: current status and future directions, in Ecogenetics: Genetic Predisposition to the Toxic Effects of Chemicals. Edited by Grandjean P. London, Chapman & Hall, 1991, pp 21–55

Caldemeyer KS, Pascuzzi RM, Moran CC, et al: Toluene abuse causing reduced MR signal intensity in the brain. American Journal of Radiology 161:1259–1261, 1993

Chadwick OFD, Anderson HR: Neuropsychological consequences of volatile substance abuse: a review. Hum Toxicol 8:307–312, 1989

Chang LW, Katz J: Pathologic effects of chronic halothane inhalation: an overview. Anesthesiology 45:640–653, 1976

Chenoweth MB: Abuse of inhalation anesthetic drugs, in Review of Inhalants: Euphoria to Dysfunction. Edited by Sharp CW, Brehm ML. Washington, DC, U.S. Government Printing Office, 1977, pp 102–111

Clinger OW, Johnson NA: Purposeful inhalation of gasoline vapors. Psychiatr Q 25: 557–567, 1951

Cohen S: Inhalant abuse: an overview of the problem, in Review of Inhalants: Euphoria to Dysfunction. Edited by Sharp CW, Brehm ML. Washington, DC, U.S. Government Printing Office, 1977, pp 2–11

Cohr K-H: Danish experience with white spirit, in The Neuropsychological Effects of Solvent Exposures. Edited by Cherry N, Waldron HA. Havant, Hampshire, Colt Foundation, 1983, pp 51–62

Committee on Environmental Epidemiology: Dimensions of the problem: exposure assessment, in Environmental Epidemiology, Vol 1: Public Health and Hazardous Wastes. Washington, DC, National Academy Press, 1991, pp 101–153

Comstock EG, Comstock BS: Medical evaluation of inhalant abusers, in Review of Inhalants: Euphoria to Dysfunction. Edited by Sharp CW, Brehm ML. Washington, DC, U.S. Government Printing Office, 1977, pp 54–80

Condray R, Morrow LA, Steinhauer SR, et al: Mood and behavioral symptoms in individuals with chronic solvent exposure. Psychiatry Res 97:191–206, 2000

Davidson M, Feinleib M: Carbon disulfide poisoning: a review. Am Heart J 83:100–114, 1972

Davison LA, Steinhelber JC, Eger EI, et al: Psychological effects of halothane and isoflurane anesthesia. Anesthesiology 43:313–324, 1975

de Francisco CP: Pentrane dependence: a case report. Br J Psychiatry 119:609–610, 1971

Doon R: Caribbean industry with potential impact on human health, in Advances in Neurobehavioral Toxicology: Applications in Environmental and Occupational Health. Edited by Johnson BL. Chelsea, MI, Lewis Publishers, 1990, pp 29–34

Defalque RJ: Pharmacology and toxicology of trichloroethylene: a critical review of the world literature. Clin Pharmacol Ther 2:665–688, 1961

Dretchen KL, Balter NJ, Schwartz SL, et al: Cognitive dysfunction in a patient with long-term occupational exposure to ethylene oxide. J Occup Med 34:1106–1113, 1992

Edeh J: Volatile substance abuse in relation to alcohol and illicit drugs: psychosocial perspectives. Hum Toxicol 8:313–317, 1989

Escobar A, Aruffo C: Chronic thinner intoxication: clinico-pathologic report of a human case. J Neurol Neurosurg Psychiatry 43:986–994, 1980

Fahy A, Marshall M: Postanaesthetic morbidity in out-patients. Br J Anaesth 41:433–438, 1969

Filley CM, Kleinschmidt-Demasters BK: Toxic leukoencephalopathy. N Engl J Med 344:425–432, 2001

Filley CM, Heaton RK, Rosenberg NL: White matter dementia in chronic toluene abuse. Neurology 40:532–534, 1990

Gamble JG: Low-level hydrocarbon solvent exposure and neurobehavioural effects. Occup Med (Lond) 50:81–102, 2000

Gatley MS, Kelly GA, Turnbull IW: A case of organic solvent exposure and temporal lobe demyelination. Journal of Social and Occupational Medicine 41:83–85, 1991

Goldstein GS: Inhalant abuse among the Pueblo tribes of New Mexico, in Voluntary Inhalation of Industrial Solvents. Edited by Sharp CW, Carroll LT. Rockville, MD, U.S. Government Printing Office, 1978, pp 90–94

Gosselin RE, Smith RP, Hodge HC, et al: Clinical Toxicology of Commercial Products. Baltimore, MD, Williams & Wilkins, 1984

Harr J: A Civil Action. New York, Vintage, 1995

Harrington JM: Health experience of workers in the petroleum manufacturing and distribution industry: a review of the literature. Am J Ind Med 12:475–497, 1987

Hartman DE: Neuropsychological toxicology of solvents, in Neuropsychological Toxicology: Identification and Assessment of Human Neurotoxic Syndromes. New York, Pergamon, 1988, pp 108–159

Haut MW, Leach S, Kuwabara H, et al: Verbal working memory and solvent exposure: a positron emission tomography study. Neuropsychology 14:551–558, 2000

Hernandez-Avila CA, Ortega-Soto HA, Jasso A, et al: Treatment of inhalant-induced psychotic disorder with carbamazepine versus haloperidol. Psychiatr Serv 49: 812–815, 1998

Hersh R: Abuse of ethyl chloride. Am J Psychiatry 148:270–271, 1991

Heuser G, Mena I, Goldstein J, et al: Neurospect findings in patients (PTS) exposed to neurotoxic chemicals (abstract). Clin Nucl Med 18:923, 1993

Hirai H, Ikeuchi Y: [MRI of chronic toluene intoxication] (English abstract). Rinsho Shinkeigaku 33:552–555, 1993

Hooisma J, Hanninen H, Emmen HH, et al: Behavioral effects of exposure to organic solvents in Dutch painters. Neurotoxicol Teratol 15:397–406, 1993

Huang CC, Chu CC, Chen RS, et al: Chronic carbon disulfide encephalopathy. Eur Neurol 36:364–368, 1996

Humphrey JH, McClelland M: Cranial-nerve palsies with herpes following general anaesthesia: a report from the central Middlesex County Hospital. BMJ 1:315–318, 1944

Ikeda M, Tsukagoshi H: Encephalopathy due to toluene sniffing. Eur Neurol 30:347–349, 1990

Iregren A: Behavioral methods and organic solvents: questions and consequences. Environ Health Perspect 104 (suppl 2):361–366, 1996

James FM: The effects of cyclopropane anesthesia without surgical operation on mental functions of normal man. Anesthesiology 30:264–272, 1969

Joint WHO/Nordic Council of Ministers Working Group: Chronic effects of organic solvents on the central nervous system and diagnostic criteria, in Organic Solvents and the Central Nervous System, Copenhagen, World Health Organization, 1985

Jumper-Thurman P, Beauvais F: Treatment of volatile solvent abusers, in Inhalant Abuse: A Volatile Research Agenda. Edited by Sharp CW, Beauvais F, Spence R. Washington, DC, U.S. Government Printing Office, 1992, pp 203–213

King M: Long term neuropsychological effects of solvent abuse, in The Neuropsychological Effects of Solvent Exposure. Edited by Cherry N, Waldron HA. Havant, Hampshire, Colt Foundation, 1983, pp 75–84

Kojima S, Hirayama K, Furumoto H, et al: [Magnetic resonance imaging in chronic toluene abuse, and volitional hyperkinesia] (English abstract). Rinsho Shinkeigaku 33:477–482, 1993

Kornfeld M, Moser AB, Moser HW, et al: Solvent vapor abuse leukoencephalopathy: comparison to adrenoleukodystrophy. J Neuropathol Exp Neurol 53:389–398, 1994

Kucuk NO, Kilic EO, Ibis E, et al: Brain SPECT findings in long-term inhalant abuse. Nucl Med Commun 21:769–773, 2000

Kurt TL, Buffler P: 1,1,1-Trichloroethane, in Environmental Medicine: Integrating a Missing Element Into Medical Education. Edited by Pope AM, Rall DP. Washington, DC, National Academy Press, 1995, pp 750–766

Lilis R: Diseases associated with exposure to chemical substances: organic compounds, in Public Health and Preventive Medicine. Edited by Last JM, Wallace RB. Norwalk, CT, Appleton & Lange, 1992, pp 403–454

LoSasso GL, Rapport LJ, Axelrod BN: Neuropsychological symptoms associated with low-level exposure to solvents and (meth)acrylates among nail technicians. Neuropsychiatry Neuropsychol Behav Neurol 14:183–189, 2001

Lyons RA, Temple JM, Evans D, et al: Acute health effects of the Sea Empress oil spill. J Epidemiol Community Health 53:306–310, 1999

Maizlish NA, Langolf GD, Whitehead LW, et al: Behavioural evaluation of workers exposed to mixtures of organic solvents. British Journal of Industrial Medicine 42:579–590, 1985

Maroni M, Catenacci G: Biological monitoring of neurotoxic compounds, in Occupational Neurology and Clinical Neurotoxicology. Edited by Bleecker ML, Hansen JA. Baltimore, MD, Williams & Wilkins, 1994, pp 43–83

Maximilian VA, Risberg J, Prohovnik I, et al: Regional cerebral blood flow and verbal memory after chronic exposure to organic solvents. Brain Cogn 1:196–205, 1982

McCormick MJ, Mogabgab E, Adams SL: Methanol poisoning as a result of inhalational solvent abuse. Ann Emerg Med 19:639–642, 1990

McGarvey EL, Clavet GJ, Mason W, et al: Adolescent inhalant abuse: environments of use. Am J Drug Alcohol Abuse 25:731–741, 1999

Metrick SA, Brenner RP: Abnormal brainstem auditory evoked potentials in chronic paint sniffers. Ann Neurol 12:553–556, 1982

Miller RR, Newhook R, Poole A: Styrene production, use, and human exposure. Crit Rev Toxicol 24(S1):S1–S10, 1994

Misra LK, Kofoed L, Fuller W: Treatment of inhalant abuse with risperidone (letter). J Clin Psychiatry 60:620, 1999

Morrow LA, Steinhauer SR, Ryan CM: The utility of psychophysiological measures in assessing the correlates and consequences of organic solvent exposure. Toxicol Ind Health 10:537–544, 1994

Morrow LA, Stein L, Bagovich GR, et al: Neuropsychological assessment, depression, and past exposure to organic solvents. Appl Neuropsychol 8:65–73, 2001

Nasterlack M, Dietz MC, Frank KH, et al: A multidisciplinary cross-sectional study on solvent-related health effects in painters compared with construction workers. Int Arch Occup Environ Health 72:205–214, 1999

O'Donoghue JL: Alkanes, alcohols, ketones, and ethylene oxide, in Neurotoxicity of Industrial and Commercial Chemicals, Vol II. Edited by O'Donoghue JL. Boca Raton, FL, CRC Press, 1985, pp 61–97

Oetting ER, Webb J: Psychosocial characteristics and their links with inhalants: a research agenda, in Inhalant Abuse: A Volatile Research Agenda. Edited by Sharp CW, Beauvais F, Spence R. Washington, DC, U.S. Government Printing Office, 1992, pp 59–97

Ohnuma A, Kimura I, Saso S: MRI in chronic paint-thinner intoxication. Neuroradiology 37:445–446, 1995

Okada S, Yamanouchi N, Kodama K, et al: Regional cerebral blood flow abnormalities in chronic solvent abusers. Psychiatry Clin Neurosci 53:351–356, 1999

Parker MJ, Tarlow MJ, Anderson JM: Glue sniffing and cerebral infarction. Arch Dis Child 59:675–677, 1984

Ramsey J, Anderson HR, Bloor K, et al: An introduction to the practice, prevalence and chemical toxicology of volatile substances abuse. Hum Toxicol 8:261–269, 1989

Rebert CS, Hall TA: The neuroepidemiology of styrene: a critical review of representative literature. Crit Rev Toxicol 24(S1):S57–S106, 1994

Reid S, Turner J: Solvent abuse in psychiatric settings. Br J Psychiatry 165:414–415, 1994

Repko JD, Lasley SM: Behavioral, neurological, and toxic effects of methyl chloride: a review of the literature. CRC Critical Reviews in Toxicology 6:283–302, 1979

Ritchie GD, Still KR, Alexander WK, et al: A review of the neurotoxicity risk of selected hydrocarbon fuels. J Toxicol Environ Health B Crit Rev 4:223–312, 2001

Ron MA: Volatile substance abuse: a review of possible long-term neurological, intellectual and psychiatric sequelae. Br J Psychiatry 148:235–246, 1986

Rosenberg NL: Occupational and Environmental Neurology. Boston, MA, Butterworth-Heinemann, 1995

Satran R, Dodson VN: Toluene habituation: report of a case. N Engl J Med 268:719–721, 1963

Seeber A, Demes P, Golka K, et al: Subjective symptoms due to solvent mixtures, dioxin, and toluene: impact of exposure versus personality factors. Neurotoxicology 21:677–684, 2000

Snyder R, Andrews LS: Toxic effects of solvents and vapors, in Casarett and Doull's Toxicology: The Basic Science of Poison. Edited by Klassen CD, Amdur MO, Doull J. New York, McGraw-Hill, 1996, pp 737–771

Sodeyama N, Orimo S, Okiyama R, et al: [A case of chronic thinner intoxication developing hyperkinesie volitionnelle three years after stopping thinner abuse] (English abstract). Rinsho Shinkeigaku 33:213–215, 1993

Stephens RC, Diamond SC, Spielman CR, et al: Sniffing from Suffolk to Syracuse: a report of youthful solvent use in New York State, in Voluntary Inhalation of Industrial Solvents. Edited by Sharp CW, Carroll LT. Rockville, MD, U.S. Department of Health, Education, and Welfare, 1978, pp 23–40

Suzuki K, Wakayama Y, Takada H, et al: [A case of chronic toluene intoxication with abnormal MRI findings: abnormal intensity areas in cerebral white matter, basal ganglia, internal capsule, brain stem and middle cerebellar peduncle] (English abstract). Rinsho Shinkeigaku 32:84–87, 1992

Telisman S, Prpic-Majic D, Beritic T: PbB and ALAD in mentally retarded and normal children. Int Arch Occup Environ Health 52:361–369, 1983

Uitti RJ, Snow BJ, Shinotoh H, et al: Parkinsonism induced by solvent abuse. Ann Neurol 35:616–619, 1994

Unger E, Alexander A, Fritz T, et al: Toluene abuse: physical basis for hypointensity of the basal ganglia on T2-weighted MR images. Radiology 193:473–476, 1994

Varelas PN, Syrigou AI, Kotoulas G, et al: Cortical atrophy detected by computed tomography in gasoline station attendants. Sci Total Environ 239:143–149, 1999

Weiner AL, Vieira L, McKay CA, et al: Ketamine abusers presenting to the emergency department: a case series. J Emerg Med 18:447–451, 2000

Westermeyer J: The psychiatrist and solvent-inhalant abuse: recognition, assessment, and treatment. Am J Psychiatry 144:903–907, 1987

White RF, Feldman RG, Travers PH: Neurobehavioral effects of toxicity due to metals, solvents and insecticides. Clin Neuropharmacol 13:392–412, 1990

Wilde C: Aerosol metallic paints: deliberate inhalation: a study of inhalation and/or ingestion of copper and zinc particles. International Journal of the Addictions 10:127–134, 1975

World Health Organization: Organic Solvents and the Central Nervous System. Copenhagen, World Health Organization, 1985

Xiong L, Matthes JD, Li J, et al: MR imaging of "spray heads": toluene abuse via aerosol paint inhalation. AJNR Am J Neuroradiol 14:1195–1199, 1993

Yamanouchi N, Okada S, Kodama K, et al: White matter changes caused by chronic solvent abuse. AJNR Am J Neuroradiol 16:1643–1649, 1995

Zvosec DL, Smith SW, McCutcheon JR, et al: Adverse events, including death, associated with the use of 1,4-butanediol. New Engl J Med 344:87–94, 2001

ADDITIONAL READINGS

Carbon Disulfide

Aaserud O, Gjerstad L, Nakstad P, et al: Neurological examination, computerized tomography, cerebral blood flow and neuropsychological examination in workers with long-term exposure to carbon disulfide. Toxicology 49:277–282, 1988

Aaserud O, Hommeren OJ, Tvedt B, et al: Carbon disulfide exposure and neurotoxic sequelae among viscose rayon workers. Am J Ind Med 18:25–37, 1990

Bard CL: Cases in practice: malignant pustule: and insanity due to bisulphide of carbon. Southern California Practitioner 7:476–485, 1892

Braceland FJ: Mental symptoms following carbon disulphide absorption and intoxication. Ann Intern Med 16:246–261, 1942

Cassitto MG, Bertazzi PA, Camerino D, et al: Subjective and objective behavioural alterations in carbon disulphide workers. Med Lav 69:144–150, 1978

Cassitto MG, Camerino D, Imbriani M, et al: Carbon disulfide and the central nervous system: a 15-year neurobehavioral surveillance of an exposed population. Environ Res 63:252–263, 1993

Feldman RG, Ricks NL, Baker EL: Neuropsychological effects of industrial toxins: a review. Am J Ind Med 1:211–227, 1980

Francine AP: Acute carbon bisulfide poisoning (letter). American Medicine 9:871, 1905

Gilioli R, Bulgheroni C, Bertazzi PA, et al: Study of neurological and neurophysiological impairment in carbon disulphide workers. Med Lav 69:130–143, 1978

Gordy ST, Trumper M: Carbon disulfide poisoning: with a report of six cases. JAMA 110:1543–1549, 1938

Gordy ST, Trumper M: Carbon disulfide poisoning: report of 21 cases. Industrial Medicine 9:231–234, 1940

Hakky U: Five-year follow-up of psychological manifestations after exposure to carbon disulphide (abstract). XX International Congress on Occupational Health, September 25–October 1, 1982. Cairo, Egypt, p 589

Hanninen H: Psychological picture of manifest and latent carbon disulphide poisoning. British Journal of Industrial Medicine 28:374–381, 1971

Hanninen H, Nurminen M, Tolonen M, et al: Psychological tests as indicators of excessive exposure to carbon disulfide. Scand J Psychol 19:163–174, 1978

Huang CC, Chu CC, Chen RS, et al: Chronic carbon disulfide encephalopathy. Eur Neurol 36:364–368, 1996

Johnson BL, Putz-Anderson VR, Boyd JA, et al: A neurobehavioral examination of workers occupationally exposed to low levels of carbon disulfide (abstract). XX International Congress on Occupational Health, September 25–October 1, 1982. Cairo, Egypt, p 579

Kane FJ: Carbon disulfide intoxication from overdosage of disulfiram. Am J Psychiatry 127:690–694, 1970

Kruse A, Borch-Johnsen K, Pedersen LM: Cerebral damage following a single high exposure to carbon disulphide. Journal of Social and Occupational Medicine 32: 44–45, 1982

Lewey FH: Neurological, medical and biochemical signs and symptoms indicating chronic industrial carbon disulphide absorption. Ann Intern Med 15:869–883, 1941

Lilis R: Behavioral effects of occupational carbon disulfide exposure, in Behavioral Toxicology: Early Detection of Occupational Hazards. Edited by Xintaras C, Johnson BL, de Groot I. Washington, DC, U.S. Government Printing Office, 1974, pp 51–59

Liss GM, Finkelstein MM: Mortality among workers exposed to carbon disulfide. Arch Environ Health 51:193–200, 1996

Mancuso TF, Locke BZ: Carbon disulphide as a cause of suicide: epidemiological study of viscose rayon workers. J Occup Med 14:595–606, 1972

Niculcea-Gherase C: Psychological changes in workers exposed to atmospheres containing carbon disulphide (abstract). XX International Congress on Occupational Health, September 25–October 1, 1982. Cairo, Egypt, p 456

Paluch EA: Two outbreaks of carbon disulfide poisoning in rayon staple fiber plants in Poland. Journal of Industrial Hygiene and Toxicology 30:37–42, 1948

Peters HA, Levine RL, Matthews CG, et al: Carbon disulfide-induced neuropsychiatric changes in grain storage workers. Am J Ind Med 3:373–391, 1982

Peters HA, Levine RL, Matthews CG, et al: Synergistic neurotoxicity of carbon tetrachloride/carbon disulfide (80/20 fumigants) and other pesticides in grain storage workers. Acta Pharmacologica et Toxicologica (Copenhagen) 59 (suppl 6–7):535–546, 1986

Peters HA, Levine RL, Matthews CG, et al: Extrapyramidal and other neurologic manifestations associated with carbon disulfide fumigant exposure. Arch Neurol 45: 537–540, 1988

Peterson F: Three cases of acute mania from inhaling carbon bisulphide. Boston Medical and Surgical Journal 127:325–326, 1892

Putz-Anderson V, Albright BE, Lee ST, et al: A behavioral examination of workers exposed to carbon disulfide. Neurotoxicology 4:67–78, 1983

Rubin HH, Arieff AJ: Carbon disulfide and hydrogen sulfide clinical study of chronic low-grade exposures. Journal of Industrial Hygiene and Toxicology 27:123–129, 1945

Rubin HH, Arieff AJ, Tauber FW: Carbon disulfide and hydrogen sulfide, II: a follow-up clinical study of low grade exposures. AMA Archives of Industrial Hygiene and Occupational Medicine 2:529–533, 1950

Sugimura K, Kabashima K, Tatetsu S, et al: [Computerized tomography in chronic carbon disulfide poisoning] (English abstract). No To Shinkei [Brain and Nerve] 31:1245–1253, 1979

Triebig G, Lehrl S, Weltle D, et al: Clinical and neurobehavioural study of the acute and chronic neurotoxicity of styrene. British Journal of Industrial Medicine 46:799–804, 1989

Tuttle TC, Wood GD, Grether CB: Behavioral and Neurological Evaluation of Workers Exposed to Carbon Disulfide (CS2) (Contract No HSM 99-73-35). Washington, DC, U.S. Government Printing Office, 1976

Vanhoorne M: Study on toxicity of carbon disulphide and hydrogen disulphide in the Belgian viscose industry (abstract), in XX International Congress on Occupational Health, September 25–October 1, 1982. Cairo, Egypt, p 579

Vigliani EC: Clinical observations on carbon disulfide intoxication in Italy. Industrial Medicine and Surgery 19:240–242, 1950

Vigliani EC: Carbon disulphide poisoning in viscose rayon factories. British Journal of Industrial Medicine 11:235–244, 1954

Methyl Chloride

Baker HM: Intoxication with commercial methyl chloride. JAMA 88:1137–1138, 1927

Gudmundsson G: Methyl chloride poisoning 13 years later (letter). Arch Environ Health 32:236–237, 1977

Hansen H, Weaver NK, Venable FS: Methyl chloride intoxication: report of fifteen cases. AMA Archives of Industrial Hygiene and Occupational Medicine 8:328–334, 1953

Jones AM: Methyl chloride poisoning. Q J Med 35:29–43, 1942

Kegel AH, McNally WD, Pope AS: Methyl chloride poisoning from domestic refrigerators. JAMA 93:353–358, 1929

Macdonald JDC: Methyl chloride intoxication: report of 8 cases. J Occup Med 6:81–84, 1964

Mackie IJ: Methyl chloride intoxication. Med J Aust 1:203–205, 1961

McNally WD: Eight cases of methyl chloride poisoning with three deaths. Journal of Industrial Hygiene and Toxicology 28:94–97, 1946

Scharnweber HC, Spears GN, Cowles SR: Chronic methyl chloride intoxication in six industrial workers. J Occup Med 16:112–113, 1974

Thordarson O, Gudmundsson G, Bjarnason O, et al: [Methyl-chloride poisoning] (English abstract). Norkisk Medicin 18:150–154, 1965

Van der Kloot A: Methyl chloride poisoning. IMJ Illinois Medical Journal 65:508–509, 1934

Trichloroethylene

Bardodej Z, Vyskocil J: The problem of trichloroethylene in occupational medicine. AMA Archives of Industrial Hygiene and Occupational Medicine 13:581–592, 1956

Bernad PG, Spyker NS: Neurotoxicity and behavior abnormalities in a cohort chronically exposed to trichloroethylene (abstract). Vet Hum Toxicol 29:475, 1987

Eichert H: Trichloroethylene intoxication. JAMA 106:1652–1654, 1936

Feldman RG, Mayer RM, Taub A: Evidence for peripheral neurotoxic effect of trichloroethylene. Neurology 20:599–606, 1970

Feldman RG, White RF, Currie JN, et al: Long-term follow-up after single toxic exposure to trichloroethylene. Am J Ind Med 8:119–126, 1985

Grandjean E, Munchinger R, Turrian V, et al: Investigations into the effects of exposure to trichloroethylene in mechanical engineering. British Journal of Industrial Medicine 12:131–142, 1955

Harenko A: Two peculiar instances of psychotic disturbance in trichloroethylene poisoning. Acta Neurol Scand Suppl 31:139–140, 1967

Landrigan PJ, Stein GF, Kominsky JR, et al: Common-source community and industrial exposure to trichloroethylene. Arch Environ Health 42:327–332, 1987

Lilis R, Stanescu D, Muica N, et al: Chronic effects of trichloroethylene exposure. Med Lav 60:595–601, 1969

McCunney RJ: Diverse manifestations of trichloroethylene. British Journal of Industrial Medicine 45:122–126, 1988

Mitchell ABS, Parsons-Smith BG: Trichloroethylene neuropathy. BMJ 1:422–423, 1969

Monstad P, Nissen T, Sulg IA, et al: Sleep apnoea and organic solvent exposure. J Neurol 234:152–154, 1987

Rasmussen K, Jeppesen HJ, Sabroe S: Solvent-induced chronic toxic encephalopathy. Am J Ind Med 23:779–792, 1993

Rickles NK: Cerebral intoxication the result of trichloroethylene. Northwest Medicine 44:286–287, 1945

Salvini M, Binaschi S, Riva M: Evaluation of the psychophysiological functions in humans exposed to trichloroethylene. British Journal of Industrial Medicine 28: 293–295, 1971

Seppalainen AM: Neuropsychological indices in carbon disulfide exposure, in Behavioral Toxicology: Early Detection of Occupational Hazards. Edited by Xintaras C, Johnson BL, de Groot I. Washington, DC, U.S. Government Printing Office, 1974, pp 64–72

Shibayama H, Kitoh J, Marui Y, et al: An unusual case of Pick's disease. Acta Neuropathol (Berl) 59:79–87, 1983

Singer R: Neurotoxicity Guidebook. New York, Van Nostrand Reinhold, 1990

Smith GF: The investigation of the mental effects of trichloroethylene. Ergonomics 13:580–586, 1970

Steinberg W: Residual neuropsychological effects following exposure to trichloroethylene (TCE): a case study. Clin Neuropsychol 2:1–4, 1981

Stracciari A, Gallassi R, Ciardulli C, et al: Neuropsychological and EEG evaluation in exposure to trichloroethylene. J Neurol 232:120–122, 1985

Todd J: Trichloroethylene poisoning with paranoid psychosis and Lilliputian hallucination. BMJ 7:439–440, 1954

Triebig G, Schaller KH, Erzigkeit H, et al: [Biochemical investigations and psychological studies of persons chronically exposed to trichloroethylene with regard to non-exposure intervals]. Int Arch Occup Environ Health 38:149–162, 1977

Wise MG, Fisher JG, de la Pena AM: Trichloroethane (TCE) and central sleep apnea: a case study. J Toxicol Environ Health 11:101–104, 1983

Benzene

Bond BB, McLaren EA, Baldwin CL, et al: An update of mortality among chemical workers exposed to benzene. British Journal of Industrial Medicine 43:685–691, 1986

Helmer KJ: Accumulated cases of chronic benzene poisoning in the rubber industry. Acta Medica Scandinavica 118:354–375, 1944

Styrene

Baker EL, White RF, Murawski BJ: Clinical evaluation of neurobehavioral effects of occupational exposure to organic solvents and lead. International Journal of Mental Health 14:135–158, 1985

Bergamaschi E, Smargiassi A, Mutti A, et al: Peripheral markers of catecholaminergic dysfunction and symptoms of neurotoxicity among styrene-exposed workers. Int Arch Occup Environ Health 69:209–214, 1997

Challenor J, Wright D: Aggression in boat builders: a search for altered mood states in boat builders exposed to styrene. Occup Med (Lond) 50:185–192, 2000

Cherry N, Rodgers B, Venables H, et al: Acute behavioural effects of styrene exposure: a further analysis. British Journal of Industrial Medicine 38:346–350, 1981

Cherry N, Hutchins H, Pace T, et al: Neurobehavioural effects of repeated occupational exposure to toluene and paint solvents. British Journal of Industrial Medicine 42: 291–300, 1985

Edling C, Ekberg K: No acute behavioural effects of exposure to styrene: a safe level of exposure? British Journal of Industrial Medicine 42:301–304, 1985

Edling C, Anundi H, Johanson G, et al: Increase in neuropsychiatric symptoms after occupational exposure to low levels of styrene. British Journal of Industrial Medicine 50:843–850, 1993

Flodin U, Ekberg K, Andersson L: Neuropsychiatric effects of low exposure to styrene. British Journal of Industrial Medicine 46:805–808, 1989

Harkonen H: Relationship of symptoms to occupational styrene exposure and to the findings of electroencephalographic and psychological examinations. Int Arch Occup Environ Health 40:231–239, 1977

Harkonen H, Lindstrom K, Seppalainen AM, et al: Exposure-response relationship between styrene exposure and central nervous functions. Scand J Work Environ Health 4:53–59, 1978

Jegaden D, Amann D, Simon JF, et al: Study of the neurobehavioural toxicity of styrene at low levels of exposure. Int Arch Occup Environ Health 64:527–531, 1993

Lindelof B, Almkvist O, Gothe C-J: Sleep disturbances and exposure to organic solvents. Arch Environ Health 47:104–106, 1992

Lindstrom K, Harkonen H, Hernberg S: Disturbances in psychological functions of workers occupationally exposed to styrene. Scand J Work Environ Health 3:129–139, 1976

Lundberg I, Gustavsson A, Hogberg M, et al: Diagnoses of alcohol abuse and other neuropsychiatric disorders among house painters compared with house carpenters. British Journal of Industrial Medicine 49:409–415, 1992

Matikainen E, Forsman-Gronholm F, Pfaffli P, et al: Nervous system effects of occupational exposure to styrene: a clinical and neuropsychological study. Environ Res 61:84–92, 1993

Morrow LA, Robin N, Hodgson MJ, et al: Assessment of attention and memory efficiency in persons with solvent neurotoxicity. Neuropsychology 30:911–922, 1992a

Morrow LA, Steinhauer SR, Hodgson MJ: Delay in P300 latency in patients with organic solvent exposure. Arch Neurol 49:315–320, 1992b

Mutti A, Mazzucchi A, Frigeri G, et al: Neuropsychological investigation on styrene exposed workers, in Neurobehavioral Methods in Occupational Health. Edited by Gilioli R, Cassitto MG, Foa V. Oxford, UK, Pergamon, 1983, pp 271–281

Mutti A, Mazzucchi A, Rustichelli P, et al: Exposure-effect and exposure-response relationships between occupational exposure to styrene and neuropsychological functions. Am J Ind Med 5:275–286, 1984

Ng TP, Ong G, Lam WK, et al: Neurobehavioral effects of industrial mixed solvent exposure in Chinese printing and paint workers. Neurotoxicol Teratol 12:661–664, 1990

Rabovsky J, Fowles J, Hill MD, et al: A health risk benchmark for the neurologic effects of styrene: comparison with NAEL/LOAEL approach. Risk Anal 21:117–126, 2001

Schoenhuber R, Gentilini M: Influence of occupational styrene exposure on memory and attention. Neurotoxicol Teratol 11:585–586, 1989

Seppalainen AM, Harkonen H: Neurophysiological findings among workers occupationally exposed to styrene. Scand J Work Environ Health 3:140–146, 1976

Spurgeon A, Gray CN, Sims J, et al: Neurobehavioral effects of long-term occupational exposures to organic solvents: two comparable studies. Am J Ind Med 22:325–335, 1992

Triebig G, Lehrl S, Weltle D, et al: Clinical and neurobehavioural study of the acute and chronic neurotoxicity of styrene. British Journal of Industrial Medicine 46: 799–804, 1989

Viaene MK, Pauwels W, Veulemans H, et al: Neurobehavioural changes and persistence of complaints in workers exposed to styrene in a polyester boat building plant: influence of exposure characteristics and microsomal epoxide hydrolase phenotype. Occup Environ Med 58:103–112, 2001

Welp E, Kogevinas M, Andersen A, et al: Exposure to styrene and mortality from nervous system diseases and mental disorders. Am J Epidemiol 144:623–633, 1996

White DM, Daniell WE, Maxwell JK, et al: Psychosis following styrene exposure: a case report of neuropsychological sequelae. J Clin Exp Neuropsychol 12:798–806, 1990

Yokoyama K, Araki S, Murata K: Effects of low level styrene exposure on psychological performance in FRP boat laminating workers. Neurotoxicology 13:551–556, 1992

Toluene

Antti-Poika M, Juntunen J, Matikainen E, et al: Occupational exposure to toluene: neurotoxic effects with special emphasis on drinking habits. Int Arch Occup Environ Health 56:31–40, 1985

Boor JW, Hurtig HI: Persistent cerebellar ataxia after exposure to toluene. Ann Neurol 2:440–442, 1977

Cherry N, Venables H, Waldron HA: British studies on the neuropsychological effects of solvent exposure. Scand J Work Environ Health 10 (suppl 1):10–12, 1984

Cherry N, Hutchins H, Pace T, et al: Neurobehavioural effects of repeated occupational exposure to toluene and paint solvents. British Journal of Industrial Medicine 42:291–300, 1985

Eller N, Netterstrom B, Laursen P: Risk of chronic effects on the central nervous system at low toluene exposure. Occup Med 49:389–395, 1999

Foo SC, Jeyaratnam J, Koh D: Chronic neurobehavioral effects of toluene. British Journal of Industrial Medicine 47:480–484, 1990

Foo SC, Ngim CH, Salleh I, et al: Neurobehavioral effects in occupational chemical exposure. Environ Res 60:267–273, 1993

Foo SC, Phoon WO, Lee J: Neurobehavioral symptoms among workers occupationally exposed to toluene. Asia Pac J Public Health 2:192–197, 1988

Goldbloom D, Chouinard G: Schizophreniform psychosis associated with chronic industrial toluene exposure: case report. J Clin Psychiatry 46:350–351, 1985

Iregren A: Effects on psychological test performance of workers exposed to a single solvent (toluene)—a comparison with effects of exposure to a mixture of organic solvents. Neurobehavioral Toxicology and Teratology 4:695–701, 1982

Jeyaratnam J, Foo SC, Boey KW, et al: Neurophysiological and neurobehavioral studies on workers exposed to toluene, in Progress in Occupational Epidemiology: Proceedings of the Sixth International Symposium on Epidemiology in Occupational Health. Edited by Hogstedt C, Reuterwall C. Amsterdam, Excerpta Medica, 1988, pp 263–267

Juntunen J, Matikainen E, Antti-Poika M, et al: Nervous system effects of long-term occupational exposure to toluene. Acta Neurol Scand 72:512–517, 1985

Larsen F, Leira HL: Organic brain syndrome and long-term exposure to toluene: a clinical, psychiatric study of vocationally active printing workers. J Occup Med 30: 875–878, 1988

Le Quesne PM, Axford AT, McKerrow CB, et al: Neurological complications after a single severe exposure to toluene di-isocyanate. British Journal of Industrial Medicine 33:72–78, 1976

Mastromatteo E: Recent occupational health experiences in Ontario. J Occup Med 7: 502–511, 1965

Orbaek P, Lindgren M: Prospective clinical and psychometric investigation of patients with chronic toxic encephalopathy induced by solvents. Scand J Work Environ Health 14:37–44, 1988

Orbaek P, Nise G: Neurasthenic complaints and psychometric function of toluene-exposed rotogravure printers. Am J Ind Med 16:67–77, 1989

Singer R, Scott NE: Progression of neuropsychological deficits following toluene di-isocyanate exposure. Archives of Clinical Neuropsychology 2 135–144, 1987

Triebig G, Claus D, Csuzda I, et al: Cross-sectional epidemiological study on neurotoxicity of solvents in paints and lacquers. Int Arch Occup Environ Health 60:233–241, 1988

Ukai H, Watanabe T, Nakatsuka H, et al: Dose-dependent increase in subjective symptoms among toluene-exposed workers. Environ Res 60:274–289, 1993

Xylene

Hipolito R: Xylene poisoning in laboratory workers: case reports and discussion. Laboratory Medicine 11:593–595, 1980

Kilburn KH, Seidman BC, Warshaw R: Neurobehavioral and respiratory symptoms of formaldehyde and xylene exposure in histology technicians. Arch Environ Health 40:229–233, 1985

Ruijten MWMM, Hooisma J, Brons JT, et al: Neurobehavioral effects of long-term exposure to xylene and mixed organic solvents in shipyard spray painters. Neurotoxicology 15:613–620, 1994

Mixtures

Ahmed FE: Toxicology and human health effects following exposure to oxygenated or reformulated gasoline. Toxicol Lett 123:89–113, 2001

Baker EL, Feldman RG: Paraoccupational exposure to mixed solvents. J Toxicol Clin Toxicol 19:27–34, 1982

Cherry N, Venables H, Waldron HA: British studies on the neuropsychological effects of solvent exposure. Scand J Work Environ Health 10 (suppl 1):10–12, 1984

Hayhurst ER: Poisoning by petroleum distillates. Industrial Medicine 5:53–63, 1936

Kilburn KH: Neurobehavioral and respiratory findings in jet engine repair workers: a comparison of exposed and unexposed volunteers. Environ Res 80:244–252, 1999

Knave B, Persson HE, Goldberg JM, et al: Long-term exposure to jet fuel: an investigation on occupationally exposed workers with special reference to the nervous system. Scand J Work Environ Health 3:152–164, 1976

Knave B, Olson BA, Elofsson S, et al: Long-term exposure to jet fuel, II: a cross-sectional epidemiologic investigation on occupationally exposed industrial workers with special reference to the nervous system. Scand J Work Environ Health 4:19–45, 1978

Knave B, Mindus P, Struwe G: Neurasthenic symptoms in workers occupationally exposed to jet fuel. Acta Psychiatr Scand 60:39–49, 1979

Kumar P, Gupta BN, Pandya KP, et al: Behavioral studies in petrol pump workers. Int Arch Occup Environ Health 61:35–38, 1988

Lindstrom K, Wickstrom G: Psychological function changes among maintenance house painters exposed to low levels of organic solvent mixtures. Acta Psychiatr Scand Suppl 303:81–91, 1983

Porter HO: Aviators intoxicated by inhalation of JP-5 fuel vapors. Aviat Space Environ Med 61:654–656, 1990

Spencer OM: The effect of gasoline fumes on dispensary attendance and output in a group of workers. Public Health Rep 37:2305–2307, 1922

Sterner JH: Study of hazards in spray painting with gasoline as a diluent. Journal of Industrial Hygiene and Toxicology 23:437–448, 1941

Struwe G, Knave B, Mindus P: Neuropsychiatric symptoms in workers occupationally exposed to jet fuel—a combined epidemiological and casuistic study. Acta Psychiatr Scand Suppl 303:55–67, 1983

White RF, Robins TG, Proctor S, et al: Neuropsychological effects of exposure to naphtha among automotive workers. Occup Environ Med 51:102–112, 1994

General

Albers JW, Wald JJ, Werner RA, et al: Absence of polyneuropathy among workers previously diagnosed with solvent-induced toxic encephalopathy. J Occup Environ Med 41:500–509, 1999

Antti-Poika M: Overall prognosis of patients with diagnosed chronic organic solvent intoxication. Int Arch Occup Environ Health 51:127–138, 1982a

Antti-Poika M: Prognosis of symptoms in patients with diagnosed chronic organic solvent intoxication. Int Arch Occup Environ Health 51:81–89, 1982b

Arlien-Soborg P: Chronic toxic encephalopathy in house painters. Acta Neurol Scand Suppl 99:105–113, 1984

Arlien-Soborg P, Bruhn P, Gyldensted C, et al: Chronic painters' syndrome: chronic toxic encephalopathy in house painters. Acta Neurol Scand 60:149–156, 1979

Arlien-Soborg P, Henriksen L, Gade A, et al: Cerebral blood flow in chronic toxic encephalopathy in house painters exposed to organic solvents. Acta Neurol Scand 66:34–41, 1982

Axelson O, Hane M, Hogstedt C: A case-referent study on neuropsychiatric disorders among workers exposed to solvents. Scand J Work Environ Health 2:14–20, 1976

Baelum J, Andersen I, Molhave L: Acute and subacute symptoms among workers in the printing industry. British Journal of Industrial Medicine 39:70–75, 1982

Baker EL, White RF, Murawski BJ: Clinical evaluation of neurobehavioral effects of occupational exposure to organic solvents and lead. International Journal of Mental Health 14:135–158, 1985

Baker EL, Letz RE, Eisen EA, et al: Neurobehavioral effects of solvents in construction painters. J Occup Med 30:116–123, 1988

Bleecker ML, Bolla KI, Agnew J, et al: Dose-related subclinical neurobehavioral effects of chronic exposure to low levels of organic solvents. Am J Ind Med 19:715–728, 1991

Bolla KI, Schwartz BS, Agnew J, et al: Subclinical neuropsychiatric effects of chronic low-level solvent exposure in US paint manufacturers. J Occup Med 32:671–677, 1990

Bolla KI, Schwartz BS, Stewart W, et al: Comparison of neurobehavioral function in workers exposed to a mixture of organic and inorganic lead and in workers exposed to solvents. Am J Ind Med 27:231–246, 1995

Bowler RM, Mergler D, Harrison R, et al: Affective and personality disturbances among female former microelectronics workers. J Clin Psychol 47:41–52, 1991a

Bowler RM, Mergler D, Heul G, et al: Neuropsychological impairment among former microelectronics workers. Neurotoxicology 12:87–104, 1991b

Bowler RM, Mergler D, Rauch SS, et al: Stability of psychological impairment: two year follow-up of former microelectronics workers' affective and personality disturbance. Women Health 18:27–48, 1992a

Bowler RM, Mergler D, Schwarzer R, et al: Analysis of MMPI-2 and POMS in solvent-exposed and referents (abstract). Clinical Neuropsychologist 6:347, 1992b

Brackbill RM, Maizlish NA, Fischbach T: Risk of neuropsychiatric disability among painters in the United States. Scand J Work Environ Health 16:182–188, 1990

Broadwell DK, Darcey DJ, Hudnell HK, et al: Work-site clinical and neurobehavioral assessment of solvent-exposed microelectronics workers. Am J Ind Med 27:677–698, 1995

Bruhn P, Arlien-Soborg C, Gyldensted C, et al: Prognosis in chronic toxic encephalopathy: a two-year follow-up study in 26 house painters with occupational encephalopathy. Acta Neurol Scand 64:259–272, 1981

Callender T, Morrow LA, Subramanian K, et al: Three-dimensional brain metabolic imaging in patients with toxic encephalopathy. Environ Res 60:295–319, 1993

Chen R, Dick F, Seaton A: Health effects of solvent exposure among dockyard painters: mortality and neuropsychological symptoms. Occup Environ Med 56:383–387, 1999a

Chen R, Wei L, Seaton A: Neuropsychological symptoms in Chinese male and female painters: an epidemiological study in dockyard workers. Occup Environ Med 56: 388–390, 1999b

Chen R, Dick F, Semple S, et al: Exposure to organic solvents and personality. Occup Environ Med 58:14–18, 2001

Cherry N, Waldron HA: The prevalence of psychiatric morbidity in solvent workers in Britain. Int J Epidemiol 13:197–200, 1984

Cherry N, Waldron HA, Wells GG, et al: An investigation of the acute behavioral effects of styrene on factory workers. British Journal of Industrial Medicine 37:234–240, 1980

Cherry N, Venables H, Waldron HA: The acute behavioural effects of solvent exposure. Journal of Social and Occupational Medicine 33:13–18, 1983

Cherry N, Hutchins H, Pace T, et al: Neurobehavioural effects of repeated occupational exposure to toluene and paint solvents. British Journal of Industrial Medicine 42:291–300, 1985

Cherry N, Labreche F, McDonald C: Dementia and solvent exposure at work, in Progress in Occupational Epidemiology: Proceedings of the Sixth International Symposium on Epidemiology in Occupational Health. Edited by Hogstedt C, Reuterwall C. Amsterdam, Excerpta Medica, 1988, pp 247–248

Cherry NM, Labreche FP, McDonald JC: Organic brain damage and occupational solvent exposure. British Journal of Industrial Medicine 49:776–781, 1992

Colvin M, Myers J, Nell V, et al: A cross-sectional survey of neurobehavioral effects of chronic solvent exposure on workers in a paint manufacturing plant. Environ Res 63:122–132, 1993

Dager SR, Holland JP, Cowley DS, et al: Panic disorder precipitated by exposure to organic solvents in the work place. Am J Psychiatry 144:1056–1058, 1987

Daniell W, Stebbins A, O'Donnell J, et al: Neuropsychological performance and solvent exposure among car body repair shop workers. British Journal of Industrial Medicine 50:368–377, 1993

Daniell WE, Claypoole KH, Checkoway H, et al: Neuropsychological function in retired workers with previous long-term occupational exposure to solvents. Occup Environ Med 56:93–105, 1999

Dick F, Semple S, Chen R, et al: Neurological deficits in solvent-exposed painters: a syndrome including impaired colour vision, cognitive defects, tremor and loss of vibration sensation. QJM 93:655–661, 2000

Donoghue AM, Dryson EW, Wynn-Williams G: Contrast sensitivity in organic-solvent-induced chronic toxic encephalopathy. J Occup Environ Med 37:1357–1363, 1995

Dryson EW, Ogden JA: Organic solvent induced chronic toxic encephalopathy: extent of recovery, and associated factors, following cessation of exposure. Neurotoxicology 21:659–665, 2000

Edling C, Ekberg K, Ahlborg G, et al: Long term follow up of workers exposed to solvents. British Journal of Industrial Medicine 47:75–82, 1990

Ekberg K, Barregard L, Hagberg S, et al: Chronic and acute effects of solvents on central nervous system functions in floorlayers. British Journal of Industrial Medicine 43:101–106, 1986

El Massioui F, Leserve N, Fournier L: An event-related potential assessment of attention impairment after occupational exposure to organic solvents, in Evoked Potentials III: The Third International Evoked Potentials Symposium. Edited by Barber C, Blum T. Boston, MA, Butterworths, 1987, pp 346–350

Elofsson S-A, Gamberale F, Hindmarsh T, et al: Exposure to organic solvents: a cross-sectional epidemiologic investigation on occupationally exposed car and industrial spray painters with special reference to the nervous system. Scand J Work Environ Health 6:239–273, 1980

Escalona E, Yanes L, Feo O, et al: Neurobehavioral evaluation of Venezuelan workers exposed to organic solvent mixtures. Am J Ind Med 27:15–27, 1995

Eskenazi B, Gaylord L, Bracken MB, et al: In utero exposure to organic solvents and human neurodevelopment. Dev Med Child Neurol 30:492–501, 1988

Feldman RG, Ratner MH, Ptak T: Chronic toxic encephalopathy in a painter exposed to mixed solvents. Environ Health Perspect 107:417–422, 1999

Fidler AT, Baker EL, Letz RE: Neurobehavioural effects of occupational exposure to organic solvents among construction painters. British Journal of Industrial Medicine 44:292–308, 1987

Flodin U, Edling C, Axelson O: Clinical studies of psychoorganic syndromes among workers with exposure to solvents. Am J Ind Med 5:287–295, 1984

Foo SC, Ngim CH, Salleh I, et al: Neurobehavioral effects in occupational chemical exposure. Environ Res 60:267–273, 1993

French LR, Schuman LM, Mortimer JA, et al: A case-control study of dementia of the Alzheimer type. Am J Epidemiol 121:414–421, 1985

Gade A, Mortensen EL, Bruhn P: "Chronic painters syndrome": a reanalysis of psychological test data in a group of diagnosed cases, based on comparisons with matched controls. Acta Neurol Scand 77:293–306, 1988

Gatley MS, Kelly GA, Turnbull IW: A case of organic solvent exposure and temporal lobe demyelination. Journal of Social and Occupational Medicine 41:83–85, 1991

Graves AB, Van Duijn CM, Chandra V, et al: Occupational exposures to solvents and lead as risk factors for Alzheimer's disease: a collaborative re-analysis of case-control studies. Int J Epidemiol 20 (suppl):S58–S61, 1991

Gregersen P: Neurotoxic effects of organic solvents in exposed workers: two controlled follow-up studies after 5.5 and 10.6 years. Am J Ind Med 14:681–701, 1988

Gregersen P, Angelso B, Nielsen TE, et al: Neurotoxic effects of organic solvents in exposed workers: an occupational, neuropsychological, and neurological investigation. Am J Ind Med 5:201–225, 1984

Gregersen P, Klausen H, Elsnab CU: Chronic toxic encephalopathy in solvent-exposed painters in Denmark 1976–1980: clinical cases and social consequences after a 5-year follow-up. Am J Ind Med 11:399–417, 1987

Greve E: Computerized tomography findings among workers with chronic intoxication of the brain. Scand J Soc Med 17:147–159, 1989

Gun RT, Korten AE, Jorm AF, et al: Occupational risk factors for Alzheimer disease: a case-control study. Alzheimer Dis Assoc Disord 11:21–27, 1997

Hageman G, van der Hoeck J, van Hout M, et al: Parkinsonism, pyramidal signs, polyneuropathy, and cognitive decline after long-term occupational solvent exposure. J Neurol 246:198–206, 1999

Hagstadius S, Risberg J: Regional cerebral blood flow in subjects occupationally exposed to organic solvents, in Neurobehavioral Methods in Occupational Health. Edited by Gilioli R, Cassitto MG, Foa V. Oxford, UK, Pergamon, 1983, pp 211–217

Hagstadius S, Orbaek P, Risberg J, et al: Regional cerebral blood flow at the time of diagnosis of chronic toxic encephalopathy induced by organic-solvent exposure and after the cessation of exposure. Scand J Work Environ Health 15:130–135, 1989

Hakkola M: Neuropsychological symptoms among tanker drivers with exposure to solvents. Occup Med 44:243–246, 1994

Hane M, Axelson O, Blume J, et al: Psychological function changes among house painters. Scand J Work Environ Health 3:91–99, 1977

Hanninen H, Eskelinen L, Husman K, et al: Behavioral effects of long-term exposure to a mixture of organic solvents. Scand J Work Environ Health 4:240–255, 1976

Hanninen H, Antti-Poika M, Savolainen P: Psychological performance, toluene exposure and alcohol consumption in rotogravure printers. Int Arch Occup Environ Health 59:475–483, 1987

Hanninen H, Antti-Poika M, Juntunen J, et al: Exposure to organic solvents and neuropsychological dysfunction: a study on monozygotic twins. British Journal of Industrial Medicine 48:18–25, 1991

Hein HO, Suadicani P, Gyntelberg F: Mixed solvent exposure and cerebral symptoms among active and retired workers: an epidemiological investigation of 3387 men aged 53–75 years. Acta Neurol Scand 81:97–102, 1990

Heuser G, Mena I, Goldstein J, et al: Neurospect findings in patients (PTS) exposed to neurotoxic chemicals (abstract). Clin Nucl Med 18:923, 1993

Hodgson MJ, Furman J, Ryan C, et al: Encephalopathy and vestibulopathy following short-term hydrocarbon exposure. J Occup Med 31:51–54, 1989

Hotz P, Tschopp A, Soderstrom D, et al: Smell or taste disturbances, neurological symptoms, and hydrocarbon exposure. Int Arch Occup Environ Health 63:525–530, 1992

Husman K: Symptoms of car painters with long-term exposure to a mixture of organic solvents. Scand J Work Environ Health 6:19–32, 1980

Husman K, Karli P: Clinical neurological findings among car painters exposed to a mixture of organic solvents. Scand J Work Environ Health 6:33–39, 1980

Iregren A: Subjective and objective signs of organic solvent toxicity among occupationally exposed workers. Scand J Work Environ Health 12:469–475, 1986

Juntunen J, Hernberg S, Eistola P, et al: Exposure to industrial solvents and brain atrophy: a retrospective study of pneumoencephalographic findings among 37 patients with exposure to industrial solvents. Eur Neurol 19:366–375, 1980a

Juntunen J, Hupli V, Hernberg S, et al: Neurological picture of organic solvents poisoning in industry: a retrospective clinical study of 37 patients. Int Arch Occup Environ Health 46:219–231, 1980b

Juntunen J, Antti-Poika M, Tola S, et al: Clinical prognosis of patients with diagnosed chronic solvent intoxication. Acta Neurol Scand 65:488–503, 1982

Kandel E, Freed D: Long term exposure to industrial solvents (letter). British Journal of Industrial Medicine 46:750, 1989

Karlson B, Seger L, Osterberg K, et al: Stress management in men with solvent-induced chronic toxic encephalopathy. J Occup Environ Med 42:670–675, 2000

Kiesswetter E, Sietmann B, Zupanic M, et al: Neurobehavioral study on the interactive effects of age and solvent exposure. Neurotoxicology 21:685–695, 2000

Kilburn KH, Warshaw RH: Neurobehavioral effects of formaldehyde and solvents on histology technicians: repeated testing across time. Environ Res 58:134–146, 1992

Kilburn KH, Warshaw RH: Neurotoxic effects from residential exposure to chemicals from an oil reprocessing facility and superfund site. Neurotoxicol Teratol 17:89–102, 1995

Kishi R, Harabuchi I, Katakura Y, et al: Neurobehavioral effects of chronic occupational exposure to organic solvents among Japanese industrial painters. Environ Res 62:303–313, 1993

Kishi R, Tozaki S, Gong YY: Impairment of neurobehavioral function and color vision loss among workers exposed to low concentration of styrene—a review of literature. Industrial Health 38:120–126, 2000

Klinken L, Arlien-Soborg P: Brain autopsy in organic solvent syndrome. Acta Neurol Scand 87:371–375, 1993

Kraut A, Lilis R, Marcus M, et al: Neurotoxic effects of solvent exposure on sewage treatment workers. Arch Environ Health 43:263–268, 1988

Kukull WA, Larson EB, Bowen JD, et al: Solvent exposure as a risk factor for Alzheimer's disease: a case-control study. Am J Epidemiol 141:1059–1071, 1995

Labreche FP, Cherry NM, McDonald JC: Psychiatric disorders and occupational exposure to solvents. British Journal of Industrial Medicine 49:820–825, 1992

Lagakos SW, Wessen BJ, Zelen M: An analysis of contaminated well water and health effects in Woburn, Massachusetts. Journal of the American Statistical Association 81:583–596, 1986

Lang CJ: The use of neuroimaging techniques for clinical detection of neurotoxicty: a review. Neurotoxicology 21:847–855, 2000

Lee S-H, Lee SH: A study on the neurobehavioral effects of occupational exposure to organic solvents in Korean workers. Environ Res 60:227–232, 1993

Lidberg L, Tael T, Wiklund N: Violent crime and occupational exposure to organic solvents (letter). Lancet 2:1080, 1987

Lindberg N, Basch-Kahre E, Lindberg E: Psychotherapeutic examination of patients with suspected chronic solvent intoxication. Psychother Psychosom 37:36–63, 1982

Lindstrom K: Changes in psychological performances of solvent-poisoned and solvent-exposed workers. Am J Ind Med 1:69–84, 1980

Lindstrom K, Martelin T: Personality and long term exposure to organic solvents. Neurobehavioral Toxicology and Teratology 2:89–100, 1980

Lindstrom K, Antti-Poika M, Tola S, et al: Psychological prognosis of diagnosed chronic organic solvent intoxication. Neurobehavioral Toxicology and Teratology 4:581–588, 1982

Lindstrom K, Riihimaki H, Hanninen K: Occupational solvent exposure and neuropsychiatric disorders. Scand J Work Environ Health 10:321–323, 1984

Linz DH, de Garmo PL, Morton WE, et al: Organic solvent-induced encephalopathy in industrial painters. J Occup Med 28:119–125, 1986

Lundberg I, Michelsen H, Nise G, et al: Neuropsychiatric function of housepainters with previous long-term heavy exposure to organic solvents. Scand J Work Environ Health 21 (suppl 1):1–44, 1995

Maximilian VA, Risberg J, Prohovnik I, et al: Regional cerebral blood flow and verbal memory after chronic exposure to organic solvents. Brain Cogn 1:196–205, 1982

McCrank E, Rabheru K: Four cases of progressive supranuclear palsy in patients exposed to organic solvents. Can J Psychiatry 34:934–935, 1989

Mikkelsen S: A cohort study of disability pension and death among painters with special regard to disabling presenile dementia as an occupational disease. Scand J Soc Med Suppl 16:34–43, 1980

Mikkelsen S, Jorgensen M, Browne E, et al: Mixed solvent exposure and organic brain damage: a study of painters. Acta Neurol Scand Suppl 118:1–143, 1988

Milanovic L, Spilich G, Vucinic G, et al: Effects of occupational exposure to organic solvents upon cognitive performance. Neurotoxicol Teratol 12:657–660, 1990

Moen BE, Riise T, Todnem K, et al: Seamen exposed to organic solvents: a cross-sectional study with special reference to the nervous system. Acta Neurol Scand 78:123–135, 1988

Moen BE, Riise T, Haga EM, et al: Reduced performance in tests of memory and visual abstraction in seamen exposed to industrial solvents. Acta Psychiatr Scand 81: 114–119, 1990

Monstad P, Nissen T, Sulg IA, et al: Sleep apnoea and organic solvent exposure. J Neurol 234:152–154, 1987

Monstad P, Mellgren SI, Sulg IA: The clinical significance of sleep apnoea in workers exposed to organic solvents: implications for the diagnosis of organic solvent encephalopathy (abstract). J Neurol 239:195–198, 1992

Morrow LA, Ryan CM, Godstein G, et al: A distinct pattern of personality disturbance following exposure to mixtures of organic solvents. J Occup Med 31:743–746, 1989

Morrow LA, Ryan CM, Hodgson M, et al: Alterations in cognitive and psychological functioning after organic solvent exposure. J Occup Med 32:444–450, 1990

Morrow LA, Ryan CM, Hodgson MJ, et al: Risk factors associated with persistence of neuropsychological deficits in persons with organic solvent exposure. J Nerv Ment Dis 179:540–545, 1991

Morrow LA, Kamis H, Hodgson M: Psychiatric symptomatology in persons with organic solvent exposure. J Consult Clin Psychol 61:171–174, 1993

Morrow LA, Condray R, Steinhauer SR: Neuropsychiatric sequelae following chemical exposure. Arch Environ Health 50:390–391, 1995

Morrow LA, Steinhauer SR, Condray R, et al: Neuropsychological performance of journeymen painters under acute solvent exposure and exposure-free conditions. J Int Neuropsychol Soc 3:269–275, 1997

Morrow LA, Gibson C, Bagovich GR, et al: Increased incidence of anxiety and depressive disorders in persons with organic solvent exposure. Psychosom Med 62: 746–750, 2000

Myers JE, Nell V, Colvin M, et al: Neuropsychological function in solvent-exposed South African paint makers. J Occup Environ Med 41:1011–1018, 1999

Nelson NA, Robins TG, White RF, et al: A case-control study of chronic neuropsychiatric disease and organic solvent exposure in automobile assembly plant workers. Occup Environ Med 51:302–307, 1994

Nijem J, Kristensen P, Al-Khatib A, et al: Prevalence of neuropsychiatric and mucous membrane irritation complaints among Palestinian shoe factory workers exposed to organic solvents and plastic compounds. Am J Ind Med 40:192–198, 2001

Nijem K, Kristensen P, Al-Khatib A, et al: Prevalence of self-reported health complaints among shoe workers of small workshop exposed to organic solvents in Hebron City, West Bank: a cross-sectional survey. Med Lav 91:206–216, 2000

Noraberg J, Arlien-Soborg P: Neurotoxic interactions of industrially used ketones. Neurotoxicology 21:409–418, 2000

O'Flynn RR, Monkman SM, Waldron HA: Organic solvents and presenile dementia: a case referent study using death certificates. British Journal of Industrial Medicine 44:259–262, 1987

Olsen J, Sabroe S: A case-reference study of neuropsychiatric disorders among workers exposed to solvents in the Danish wood and furniture industry. Scand J Soc Med Suppl 16:44–49, 1980

Olson BA: Effects of organic solvents on behavioral performance of workers in the paint industry. Neurobehavioral Toxicology and Teratology 4:703–708, 1982

Orbaek P, Risberg J, Rosen I, et al: Effects of long-term exposure to solvents in the paint industry. Scand J Work Environ Health 11 (suppl 2):1–28, 1985

Orbaek P, Lindgren M, Olivechrona H, et al: Computed tomography and psychometric test performances in patients with solvent induced chronic toxic encephalopathy and healthy controls. British Journal of Industrial Medicine 44:175–179, 1987

Orbaek P, Rosen I, Svensson K: Power spectrum analysis of EEG at diagnosis and follow up of patients with solvent induced chronic toxic encephalopathy. British Journal of Industrial Medicine 45:476–482, 1988

Osterberg K, Orbaek P, Karlson B, et al: Psychological test performance during experimental challenge toluene and n-butyl acetate in cases of solvent-induced toxic encephalopathy. Scand J Work Environ Health 26:219–226, 2000

Parkinson DK, Bromet EJ, Cohen S, et al: Health effects of long-term solvent exposure among women in blue-collar occupations. Am J Ind Med 17:661–675, 1990

Prockop LD: Nervous system damage secondary to inhalation of industrial solvents, in Voluntary Inhalation of Industrial Solvents. Edited by Sharp CW, Carroll LT. Rockville, MD, U.S. Government Printing Office, 1978, pp 198–209

Rasmussen K, Sabroe S: Neuropsychological symptoms among metal workers exposed to halogenated hydrocarbons. Scand J Soc Med 14:161–168, 1986

Rasmussen H, Olsen J, Lauritsen J: Risk of encephalopathia among retired solvent-exposed workers. J Occup Med 27:561–566, 1985

Reinvang I, Borchgrevink HM, Aaserud O, et al: Neuropsychological findings in a non-clinical sample of workers exposed to solvents. J Neurol Neurosurg Psychiatry 57:614–616, 1994

Riise T, Moen BE: A case-control study of disability pension among seamen, with special reference to neuropsychiatric disorders and solvent exposure (abstract). Acta Neurol Scand Suppl Suppl 116:104, 1988

Riise T, Moen BE: A nested case-control study of disability pension among seamen, with special reference to neuropsychiatric disorders and exposure to solvents. Neuroepidemiology 9:88–94, 1990

Riise T, Kyvik KR, Moen B: A cohort study of disability pensioning among Norwegian painters, construction workers, and workers in food processing. Epidemiology 6:132–136, 1995

Risberg J, Hagstadius S: Effects on the regional cerebral blood flow of long-term exposure to organic solvents. Acta Psychiatr Scand Suppl 303:92–99, 1983

Rodezno RA, Lundberg I, Escalona E: Development of a questionnaire in Spanish on neurotoxic symptoms. Am J Ind Med 28:505–520, 1995

Ryan CM, Morrow LA, Hodgson M: Casosmia and neurobehavioral dysfunction associated with occupational exposure to mixtures of organic solvents. Am J Psychiatry 145:1442–1445, 1988

Schwartz BS, Ford DP, Bolla KI, et al: Solvent-associated olfactory dysfunction: not a predictor of deficits in learning and memory. Am J Psychiatry 148:751–756, 1991

Seppalainen AM, Antti-Poika M: Time course of electrophysiological findings for patients with solvent poisoning. Scand J Work Environ Health 9:15–24, 1983

Seppalainen AM, Lindstrom K, Martelin T: Neurophysiological and psychological picture of solvent poisoning. Am J Ind Med 1:31–42, 1980

Serra C, Rossi A, Mozzillo A, et al: Quantitative EMG and EEG findings in patients exposed to chronic intoxication from industrial adhesives. Acta Neurologica 2:276–284, 1980

Shalat SL, Seltzer B, Baker EL Jr: Occupational risk factors and Alzheimer's disease: a case-control study. J Occup Med 30:934–936, 1988

Sherman JE: Inherently dangerous industry approach, in Chemical Exposure and Disease: Diagnostic and Investigative Techniques. Edited by Sherman JD. New York, Van Nostrand Reinhold, 1988, pp 72–96

Silverman JS: Hyperosmia and depression following exposure to toxic vapors (letter). JAMA 264:2803, 1990

Simon TR, Hickey DC, Rea WJ, et al: Breast implants and organic solvent exposure can be associated with abnormal cerebral SPECT studies in clinically impaired patients (abstract). Radiology 185:234, 1992

Skjodt T, Torfing KF, Teisen H: Computed tomography in patients with dementia probably due to toxic encephalopathy. Acta Radiol 29:495–496, 1988

Spurgeon A, Glass DC, Calvert IA, et al: Investigation of dose related neurobehavioural effects in paintmakers exposed to low levels of solvents. Occup Environ Med 51:626–630, 1994

Steinhauer SR, Morrow LA, Condray R, et al: Respiratory sinus arrhythmia in persons with organic solvent exposure: comparisons with anxiety patients and controls. Arch Environ Health 56:175–180, 2001

Stollery BT, Flindt LH: Memory sequelae of solvent intoxication. Scand J Work Environ Health 14:45–48, 1988

Struwe G, Wennberg A: Psychiatric and neurological symptoms in workers occupationally exposed to organic solvents, in Biological Psychiatry 1981: Proceedings of the IIIrd World Congress of Biological Psychiatry. Edited by Perris C, Struwe G, Jansson B. Amsterdam, Elsevier, 1981, pp 126–133

Struwe G, Wennberg A: Psychiatric and neurological symptoms in workers occupationally exposed to organic solvents—results of a differential study. Acta Psychiatr Scand Suppl 303:68–80, 1983

Struwe G, Mindus P, Jonsson B: Psychiatric ratings in occupational health research: a study of mental symptoms in lacquerers. Am J Ind Med 1:23–30, 1980

Till C, Koren G, Rovet JF: Prenatal exposure to organic solvents and child neurobehavioral performance. Neurotoxicol Teratol 23:235–245, 2001

Triebig G, Hallermann J: Survey of solvent related chronic encephalopathy as an occupational disease in European countries. Occup Environ Med 58:575–581, 2001

Triebig G, Lang C: Brain imaging techniques applied to chronically solvent-exposed workers: current results and clinical evaluation. Environ Res 61:239–250, 1993

Triebig G, Barocka A, Erbguth F, et al: Neurotoxicity of solvent mixtures in spray painters 2: neurologic, psychiatric, psychological, and neuroradiologic findings. Int Arch Occup Environ Health 64:361–372, 1992

Triebig G, Nasterlack M, Hacke W, et al: Neuropsychiatric symptoms in active construction painters with chronic solvent exposure. Neurotoxicology 21:791–794, 2000

Valciukas JA, Lilis R, Singer RM, et al: Neurobehavioral changes among shipyard painters exposed to solvents. Arch Environ Health 40:47–52, 1985

van der Hoek JA, Verberk MM, Hageman G: Criteria for solvent-induced chronic toxic encephalopathy: a systematic review. Int Arch Occup Environ Health 73:362–368, 2000

van der Hoek JA, Verberk MM, van der Laan G, et al: Routine diagnostic procedures for chronic encephalopathy induced by solvents: survey of experts. Occup Environ Med 58:382–385, 2001

van Vliet C, Swaen GMH, Slangen JJM, et al: The organic solvent syndrome: a comparison of cases with neuropsychiatric disorders among painters and construction workers. Int Arch Occup Environ Health 59:493–501, 1987

van Vliet C, Swaen GMH, Meijers JMM, et al: Prenarcotic and neuraesthenic symptoms among Dutch workers exposed to organic solvents. British Journal of Industrial Medicine 46:586–590, 1989a

van Vliet C, Swaen GMH, Volovics A, et al: Exposure-outcome relationships between organic solvent exposure and neuropsychiatric disorders: results from a Dutch case-control study. Am J Ind Med 16:707–718, 1989b

van Vliet C, Swaen GMH, Volovics A, et al: Neuropsychiatric disorders among solvent-exposed workers: first results from a Dutch case-control study. Int Arch Occup Environ Health 62:127–132, 1990

Wang J-D, Chen J-D: Acute and chronic neurological symptoms among paint workers exposed to mixtures of organic solvents. Environ Res 61:107–116, 1993

White RF: Differential diagnosis of Alzheimer's disease and solvent encephalopathy in older workers, in Advances in Neurobehavioral Toxicology: Applications in Environmental and Occupational Health. Edited by Anger WK, Durao A, Xintaras C. Chelsea, MI, Lewis Publishers, 1998, pp 183–188

White RF, Proctor SP, Echeverria D, et al: Neurobehavioral effects of acute and chronic mixed-solvent exposure in the screen printing industry. Am J Ind Med 28:221–231, 1995

Williamson AM, Winder C: A prospective cohort study of the chronic effects of solvent exposure. Environ Res 62:256–271, 1993

Winchester RV, Madjar VM: Solvent effects on workers in the paint, adhesive and printing industries. Ann Occup Hyg 30:307–317, 1986

Miscellaneous

Baader EW, Bauer HJ: Industrial intoxication due to pentachlorophenol. Industrial Medicine and Surgery 20:286–290, 1951

Baker EL, White RF, Murawski BJ: Clinical evaluation of neurobehavioral effects of occupational exposure to organic solvents and lead. International Journal of Mental Health 14:135–158, 1985

Barrowcliff DF, Knell AJ: Cerebral damage due to endogenous chronic carbon monoxide poisoning caused by exposure to methylene chloride. Journal of Social and Occupational Medicine 29:12–14, 1979

Chalupa B, Synkova J, Sevcik M: The assessment of electroencephalographic changes and memory disturbances in acute intoxications with industrial poisons. British Journal of Industrial Medicine 17:238–241, 1960

Cherry N, Venables H, Waldron HA, et al: Some observations on workers exposed to methylene chloride. British Journal of Industrial Medicine 38:351–355, 1981

Crystal HA, Schaumburg HH, Grober E, et al: Cognitive impairment and sensory loss associated with chronic low-level ethylene oxide exposure. Neurology 38:567–569, 1988

Donley DE: Toxic encephalopathy and volatile solvents in industry: report of a case. Journal of Industrial Hygiene and Toxicology 18:571–577, 1936

Echeverria D, White RF, Sampaio C: A behavioral evaluation of PCE exposure in patients and dry cleaners: a possible relationship between clinical and preclinical effects. Occup Environ Med 37:667–680, 1995

Endo M, Sata T, Umaki I, et al: Ethylene oxide withdrawal delirium. Biol Psychiatry 19:1731–1734, 1984

Estrin WJ, Cavalieri SA, Wald P, et al: Evidence of neurologic dysfunction related to long-term ethylene oxide exposure. Arch Neurol 44:1283–1286, 1987

Estrin WJ, Bowler RM, Lash A, et al: Neurotoxicological evaluation of hospital sterilizer workers exposed to ethylene oxide. Clin Toxicol 28:1–20, 1990

Fukushima T, Abe K, Nakagawa A, et al: Chronic ethylene oxide poisoning in a factory manufacturing medical appliances. Journal of Social and Occupational Medicine 36:118–123, 1986

Garland A, Camps FE: Methyl iodide poisoning. British Journal of Industrial Medicine 2:209–211, 1945

Gold JH: Chronic perchloroethylene poisoning. Canadian Psychiatric Association Journal 14:627–630, 1969

Grant AP: Acute ethylene glycol poisoning treated with calcium salts. Lancet 2:1252–1253, 1952

Greenburg L, Mayers MR, Goldwater LJ, et al: Health hazards in the manufacture of "fused collars," I: exposure to ethylene glycol monomethyl ether. Journal of Industrial Hygiene and Toxicology 20:134–147, 1938

Gross JA, Haas ML, Swift TR: Ethylene oxide neurotoxicity: report of four cases and review of the literature. Neurology 29:978–983, 1979

Horan JM, Kurt TL, Landrigan PJ, et al: Neurologic dysfunction from exposure to 2-t-Butylazo-2-hydroxy-5-Methylhexane (BHMH): a new occupational neuropathy. Am J Public Health 75:513–517, 1985

Hurlbut KM, Bernstein JN, Burgess JL, et al: Bell's palsy and frontal lobe functional deficit from ethylene oxide exposure (abstract). Vet Hum Toxicol 34:357, 1992

Kelafant GA, Berg RA, Schleenbaker R: Toxic encephalopathy due to 1,1,1-trichloroethane exposure. Am J Ind Med 25:439–446, 1994

Klees JE, Lash A, Bowler RM, et al: Neuropsychologic "impairment' in a cohort of hospital workers chronically exposed to ethylene oxide. Clin Toxicol 28:21–28, 1990

Lauwerys R, Herbrand J, Buchet JP, et al: Health surveillance of workers exposed to tetrachloroethylene in dry-cleaning shops. Int Arch Occup Environ Health 52: 69–77, 1983

Maroni M, Bulgheroni C, Cassitto MG, et al: A clinical, neurophysiological and behavioral study of female workers exposed to 1,1,1-trichloroethane. Scand J Work Environ Health 3:16–22, 1977

Morrow LA, Callender T, Lottenberg S, et al: PET and neurobehavioral evidence of tetrabromoethane encephalopathy. Journal of Neuropsychiatry 2:431–435, 1990

Ohi G, Wegman SH: Transcutaneous ethylene glycol monomethyl ether poisoning in the work setting. J Occup Med 20:675–676, 1978

Parsons CE, Parsons MEM: Toxic encephalopathy and "granulopenic anemia" due to volatile solvents in industry: report of two cases. Journal of Industrial Hygiene and Toxicology 20:124–133, 1938

Passero S, Battistini N, Cioni R, et al: Toxic polyneuropathy of shoe workers in Italy: a clinical, neurophysiological and follow-up study. Ital J Neurol Sci 4:463–472, 1983

Patch PC, Hartlage LC: Neurological and emotional sequelae of exposure to ethylene oxide. Int J Neurosci 106:101–107, 2001

Ristow GE, Cornelius D: The neurological manifestations of chronic ethylene oxide exposure (abstract). Ann Neurol 20:136, 1986

Seeber A: Neurobehavioral toxicity of long-term exposure to tetrachloroethylene. Neurotoxicol Teratol 11:579–583, 1989

Sherman JE: Inherently dangerous industry approach, in Chemical Exposure and Disease: Diagnostic and Investigative Techniques. Edited by Sherman JD. New York, Van Nostrand Reinhold, 1988, pp 72–96

Sobaszek A, Hache JC, Frimat P, et al: Working conditions and health effects of ethylene oxide exposure at hospital sterilization sites. J Occup Environ Med 41:492–499, 1999

Spencer PS, Beaubernard CM, Bischoff-Fenton MC, et al: Clinical and experimental neurotoxicity of 2-t-butylazo-2-hydroxy-5-methylhexane. Ann Neurol 17:28–32, 1985

Stevens H, Forster FM: Effect of carbon tetrachloride on the nervous system. AMA Archives of Neurology and Psychiatry 70:635–649, 1953

Stewart RD, Hake CL, Wu A, et al: Effects of Perchloroethylene/Drug Interaction on Behavior and Neurological Function (Final Report: Contract No CDC 201-75-0059). Washington, DC, U.S. Government Printing Office, 1977

Tariot PN: Delirium resulting from methylene chloride exposure: case report. J Clin Psychiatry 44:340–342, 1983

White RF, Feldman RG, Proctor SP: Neurobehavioral effects of toxic exposures, in Clinical Syndromes in Adult Neuropsychology: The Practitioner's Handbook. Edited by White RF. Amsterdam, Elsevier, 1992, pp 1–51

White RF, Feldman RG, Moss MB, et al: Magnetic resonance imaging (MRI), neurobehavioral testing, and toxic encephalopathy: two cases. Environ Res 61:117–123, 1998

Yeragani VK, Pohl R, Balon R: Panic attacks and exposure to chemical agents (letter). Am J Psychiatry 145:532, 1988

Zavon MR: Methyl cellosolve intoxication. Am Ind Hyg Assoc J 24:36–41, 1963

Solvent Abuse

Gasoline

Bartlett S, Tapia F: Glue and gasoline "sniffing," the addiction of youth. Mo Med 63:270–272, 1966

Bethell MF: Toxic psychosis caused by inhalation of petrol fumes. BMJ 2:276–277, 1965

Black PD: Mental illness due to the voluntary inhalation of petrol vapour. Med J Aust 2:70–71, 1967

Daniels AM, Latcham RW: Petrol sniffing and schizophrenia in a Pacific island paradise (letter). Lancet 1:389, 1984

Duggal HS, Sinha BN, Nizamie SH: Gasoline inhalation dependence and bipolar disorder. Aust N Z J Psychiatry 34:531–532, 2000

Durden WD Jr, Chipman DW: Gasoline sniffing complicated by acute carbon tetrachloride poisoning. Arch Intern Med 119:371–374, 1967

Easson WM: Gasoline addiction in children. Pediatrics 29:250–254, 1962

Edwards RV: A case report of gasoline sniffing. Am J Psychiatry 117:555–557, 1960

Faucett RL, Jensen RA: Addiction to the inhalation of gasoline fumes in a child. J Pediatr 41:364–368, 1952

Glaser FB: Inhalation psychosis and related states. Arch Gen Psychiatry 14:315–322, 1966

Gold N: Self-intoxication by petrol vapour inhalation. Med J Aust 2:582–584, 1963

Goodheart RS, Dunne JW: Petrol sniffer's encephalopathy. Med J Aust 160:178–181, 1994

Grant WB: Inhalation of gasoline fumes by a child. Psychiatr Q 36:555–557, 1962

Lawton JJ, Malmquist CP: Gasoline addiction in children. Psychiatr Q 35:555–561, 1961

Nitsche CJ, Robinson JF: A case of gasoline addiction. Am J Orthopsychiatry 29:417–419, 1959

Nurcombe B, Bianchi GN, Money J, et al: A hunger for stimuli: the psychosocial background of petrol inhalation. Br J Med Psychol 43:367–374, 1970

Oldham W: Deliberate self-intoxication with petrol vapour. BMJ 2:1687–1688, 1961

Quintanilla J: Gasoline sniffing. Texas State Journal of Medicine 57:570–571, 1961

Shah R, Vankar GK, Upadhyaya HP: Phenomenology of gasoline intoxication and withdrawal symptoms among adolescents in India: a case series. American Journal of Addiction 8:254–257, 1999

Tolan IJ, Lingl FA: "Model psychosis" produced by inhalation of gasoline fumes. Am J Psychiatry 120:757–761, 1964

Glue

Allison WM, Jerrom DWA: Glue sniffing: a pilot study of the cognitive effects of long-term use. International Journal of the Addictions 19:453–458, 1984

Allister C, Lush M, Oliver JS, et al: Status epilepticus caused by solvents (letter). BMJ 283:1156, 1981

Channer KS, Stanley S: Persistent visual hallucinations secondary to chronic solvent encephalopathy: case report and review of the literature. J Neurol Neurosurg Psychiatry 46:83–86, 1983

Dodds J, Santostefano S: A comparison of the cognitive functioning of glue-sniffers and nonsniffers. J Pediatr 64:565–570, 1964

Ehyai A, Freemon FR: Progressive optic neuropathy and sensorineural hearing loss due to chronic glue sniffing. J Neurol Neurosurg Psychiatry 46:349–351, 1983

Glaser HH, Massengale ON: Glue-sniffing in children. JAMA 181:300–303, 1962

Gonzalez EG, Downey JA: Polyneuropathy in a glue sniffer. Arch Phys Med Rehabil 53:333–337, 1972

Keeler MH, Reifler CB: The occurrence of glue sniffing on a university campus. Journal of the American College Health Association 16:69–70, 1967

Massengale ON, Glaser HH, LeLievre RE, et al: Physical and psychologic factors in glue sniffing. N Engl J Med 269:1340–1344, 1963

Merry J, Zachariadis N: Addiction to glue sniffing (letter). BMJ 2:1448, 1962

Trites RL, Suh M, Offord D, et al: Neuropsychologic and psychosocial antecedents and chronic effects of prolonged use of solvents and methamphetamine, part 1: group profiles. Psychiatric Journal of the University of Ottawa 1:14–20, 1976

Wiedmann KD, Power KG, Wilson JT, et al: Recovery from chronic solvent abuse. J Neurol Neurosurg Psychiatry 50:1712–1713, 1987

Paint

Kelly TW: Prolonged cerebellar dysfunction associated with paint-sniffing. Pediatrics 56:605–606, 1975

Tsushima WT, Towne WS: Effects of paint sniffing on neuropsychological test performance. J Abnorm Psychol 86:402–407, 1977

Toluene

Boor JW, Hurtig HI: Persistent cerebellar ataxia after exposure to toluene. Ann Neurol 2:440–442, 1977

Byrne A, Kirby B: Solvent abuse psychosis (letter). Br J Psychiatry 155:132, 1989

Byrne A, Kirby B, Zibin T, et al: Psychiatric and neurological effects of chronic solvent abuse. Can J Psychiatry 36:735–738, 1991

Caldemeyer KS, Pascuzzi RM, Moran CC, et al: Toluene abuse causing reduced MR signal intensity in the brain. American Journal of Radiology 161:1259–1261, 1993

Caldemeyer KS, Armstrong SW, George KK, et al: The spectrum of neuroimaging abnormalities in solvent abuse and their clinical correlation. J Neuroimaging 6:167–173, 1996

Faillace LA, Guynn RW: Abuse of organic solvents. Psychosomatics 17:188–189, 1976

Filley CM, Heaton RK, Rosenberg NL: White matter dementia in chronic toluene abuse. Neurology 40:532–534, 1990

Fornazzari L, Carlen PL, Wilkinson DA: Functional but not morphological recovery in a chronic solvent abuser (abstract). Can J Neurol Sci 10:14, 1983a

Fornazzari L, Wilkinson DA, Kapur BM, et al: Cerebellar, cortical and functional impairment in toluene abusers. Acta Neurol Scand 67:319–329, 1983b

Grabski DA: Toluene sniffing producing cerebellar degeneration. Am J Psychiatry 118: 461–462, 1961

Hirai H, Ikeuchi Y: [MRI of chronic toluene intoxication] (English abstract). Rinsho Shinkeigaku 33:552–555, 1993

Hormes JT, Filley CM, Rosenberg NL: Neurologic sequelae of chronic solvent vapor abuse. Neurology 36:698–702, 1986

Ikeda M, Tsukagoshi H: Encephalopathy due to toluene sniffing. Eur Neurol 30:347–349, 1990

King MD: Neurological sequelae of toluene abuse. Hum Toxicol 1:281–287, 1982

King MD, Day RE, Oliver JS, et al: Solvent encephalopathy. BMJ 283:663–665, 1981

Knox WJ, Nelson JR: Permanent encephalopathy from toluene inhalation. N Engl J Med 275:1494–1496, 1966

Kojima S, Hirayama K, Furumoto H, et al: [Magnetic resonance imaging in chronic toluene abuse, and volitional hyperkinesia] (English abstract). Rinsho Shinkeigaku 33:477–482, 1993

Komiyama M, Yamanaka K: Chronic misuse of paint thinners. J Neurol Neurosurg Psychiatry 67:247, 1999

Lazar RB, Sam UH, Melen O, et al: Multifocal central nervous system damage caused by toluene abuse. Neurology 33:1337–1340, 1983

Lewis JD, Moritz D, Mellis LP: Long-term toluene abuse. Am J Psychiatry 138:368–370, 1981

Malm G, Lying-Tunell U: Cerebellar dysfunction related to toluene sniffing. Acta Neurol Scand 62:188–190, 1980

Ohnuma A, Kimura I, Saso S: MRI in chronic paint-thinner intoxication. Neuroradiology 37:445–446, 1995

Rosenberg NL, Kleinschmidt-Demasters BK, Davis KA, et al: Toluene abuse causes diffuse central nervous system white matter changes. Ann Neurol 23:611–614, 1988a

Rosenberg NL, Spitz MC, Filley CM, et al: Central nervous system effects of chronic toluene abuse—clinical, brainstem evoked response and magnetic resonance imaging studies. Neurotoxicol Teratol 10:489–495, 1988b

Sasa M, Igarashi S, Miyazaki T, et al: Equilibrium disorders with diffuse brain atrophy in long-term toluene sniffing. Archives of Otorhinolaryngology 221:163–169, 1978

Schikler KN, Seitz K, Rice JF, et al: Solvent abuse associated cortical atrophy. Journal of Adolescent Health Care 3:37–39, 1982

Streicher HZ, Gabow PA, Moss AH, et al: Syndromes of toluene sniffing in adults. Ann Intern Med 94:758–762, 1981

Suzuki K, Wakayama Y, Takada H, et al: [A case of chronic toluene intoxication with abnormal MRI findings: abnormal intensity areas in cerebral white matter, basal ganglia, internal capsule, brain stem and middle cerebellar peduncle] (English abstract). Rinsho Shinkeigaku 32:84–87, 1992

Tarsh MJ: Schizophreniform psychosis caused by sniffing toluene. Journal of Social and Occupational Medicine 29:131–133, 1979

Uitti RJ, Snow BJ, Shinotoh H, et al: Parkinsonism induced by solvent abuse. Ann Neurol 35:616–619, 1994

Unger E, Alexander A, Fritz T, et al: Toluene abuse: physical basis for hypointensity of the basal ganglia on T2-weighted MR images. Radiology 193:473–476, 1994

Weisenberger BL: Toluene habituation. J Occup Med 19:569–570, 1977
Xiong L, Matthes JD, Li J, et al: MR imaging of "spray heads": toluene abuse via aerosol paint inhalation. AJNR Am J Neuroradiol 14:1195–1199, 1993
Yamanouchi N, Okada S, Kodama K, et al: White matter changes caused by chronic solvent abuse. AJNR Am J Neuroradiol 16:1643–1649, 1995

Trichloroethylene

Harenko A: Two peculiar instances of psychotic disturbance in trichloroethylene poisoning. Acta Neurol Scand Suppl 31:139–140, 1967

Other

Ackerly WC, Gibson G: Lighter fluid "sniffing." Am J Psychiatry 120:1056–1061, 1964
Berry GJ, Heaton RK, Kirby MW: Neuropsychological deficits of chronic inhalant abusers, in Management of the Poisoned Patient. Edited by Rumack BH, Temple AR. Princeton, NJ, Science Press, 1977, pp 9–29
Berry GJ, Heaton RK, Kirby MW: Neuropsychological assessment of chronic inhalant abusers: a preliminary report, in Voluntary Inhalation of Industrial Solvents. Edited by Sharp CW, Carroll LT. Rockville, MD, U.S. Government Printing Office, 1978, pp 111–136
Biggs SJ, Bender MP, Foreman J: Are there psychological differences between persistent solvent-abusing delinquents and delinquents who do not abuse solvents? J Adolesc 6:71–86, 1983
Bigler ED: Neuropsychological evaluation of adolescent patients hospitalized with chronic inhalant abuse. Clinical Neuropsychology 1:8–12, 1979
Boothroyd LJ, Kirmayer LJ, Spreng S, et al: Completed suicides among the Inuit of northern Quebec, 1982–1996: a case-control study. CMAJ 165:749–755, 2001
Bowen SE, Daniel J, Balster RL: Deaths associated with inhalant abuse in Virginia from 1987 to 1996. Drug Alcohol Depend 53:239–245, 1999
Chadwick O, Yule W, Anderson R: The examination attainments of secondary school pupils who abuse solvents. Br J Educ Psychol 60:180–191, 1990
Comstock BS: A review of psychological measures relevant to central nervous system toxicity, with specific reference to solvent inhalation. Clin Toxicol 11:317–324, 1977
Comstock BS: Psychological measurements in long-term chronic inhalant abusers, in Voluntary Inhalation of Industrial Solvents. Edited by Sharp CW, Carroll LT. Rockville, MD, U.S. Government Printing Office, 1978, pp 159–176
Comstock EG, Comstock BS: Medical evaluation of inhalant abusers, in Review of Inhalants: Euphoria to Dysfunction. Edited by Sharp CW, Brehm ML. Washington, DC, U.S. Government Printing Office, 1977, pp 54–80
Dinwiddie SH, Zorumski CF, Rubin EH: Psychiatric correlates of chronic solvent abuse. J Clin Psychiatry 48:334–337, 1987
Dinwiddie SH, Reich T, Cloninger CR: Solvent use and psychiatric morbidity. British Journal of Addiction 85:1647–1656, 1990
Escobar A, Aruffo C: Chronic thinner intoxication: clinico-pathologic report of a human case. J Neurol Neurosurg Psychiatry 43:986–994, 1980
Gutierrez FDLG, Hernandez IM, Rabago S Psychological, familial, and social study of 32 patients using inhalants, in Voluntary Inhalation of Industrial Solvents. Edited by Sharp CW, Carroll LT. Rockville, MD, U.S. Department of Health, Education, and Welfare, 1978, pp 75–89
Hes JP, Cohn DF, Streifler M: Ethyl chloride sniffing and cerebellar dysfunction (case report). Israeli Annals of Psychiatry and Related Disciplines 17:122–125, 1979
Jacobs AM, Ghodse AH: Depression in solvent abusers. Soc Sci Med 24:863–866, 1987

Jones NP: Self-enucleation and psychosis. Br J Ophthalmol 74:571–573, 1990

Korman M, Trimboli F, Semler I: A psychiatric emergency room study of inhalant use, in Voluntary Inhalation of Industrial Solvents. Edited by Sharp CW, Carroll LT. Rockville, MD, U.S. Government Printing Office, 1978, pp 137–158

Korman M, Trimboli F, Semler I: A comparative evaluation of 162 inhalant users. Addict Behav 5:143–152, 1980

Korman M, Matthews RW, Lovitt R: Neuropsychological effects of abuse of inhalants. Percept Mot Skills 53:547–553, 1981

Kramer RA, Pierpaoli P: Hallucinogenic effects of propellant components of deodorant sprays. Pediatrics 48:322–323, 1971

Kurtzman TL, Otsuka KN, Wahl RA: Inhalant abuse by adolescents. J Adolesc Health 28:170–180, 2001

Lemmen CA, Holden CE, Benedek EP: Criminal responsibility and solvent exposure. New Dir Ment Health Serv 69:59–66, 1996

Mackesy-Amiti ME, Fendrich M: Inhalant use and delinquent behavior among adolescents: a comparison of inhalant users and other drug users. Addiction 94:555–564, 1999

Mahmood Z: Cognitive functioning of solvent abusers. Scott Med J 28:276–280, 1983

Nordin C, Rosenqvist M, Hollstedt C: Sniffing of ethyl chloride—an uncommon form of abuse with serious mental and neurological symptoms. International Journal of the Addictions 23:623–627, 1988

Skuse D, Burrell S: A review of solvent abusers and their management by a child psychiatric out-patient service. Hum Toxicol 1:321–329, 1982

Sodeyama N, Orimo S, Okiyama R, et al: [A case of chronic thinner intoxication developing hyperkinesie volitionnelle three years after stopping thinner abuse] (English abstract). Rinsho Shinkeigaku 33:213–215, 1993

Westermeyer J: The psychiatrist and solvent-inhalant abuse: recognition, assessment, and treatment. Am J Psychiatry 144:903–907, 1987

Zur J, Yule W: Chronic solvent abuse, 1: cognitive sequelae. Child Care Health Dev 16:1–20, 1990

Anesthetics

Aono J, Mamiya K, Manabe M: Preoperative anxiety is associated with a high incidence of problematic behavior on emergence after halothane anesthesia in boys. Acta Anaesthesiol Scand 43:542–544, 1999

Gozal D, Gozal Y: Behavior disturbances with repeated propofol sedation in a child (letter). J Clin Anesth 11:499, 1999

Iwata K, O'Keefe GB, Karanas A: Neurologic problems associated with chronic nitrous oxide abuse in a non-healthcare worker. Am J Med Sci 322:173–174, 2001

McNeely JK, Buczulinski B, Rosner DR: Severe neurological impairment in an infant after nitrous oxide anesthesia. Anesthesiology 93:1549–1550, 2000

Meyer RE: Anesthesia hazards to animal workers. Occup Med 14:225–234, 1999

Moore NN, Bostwick JM: Ketamine dependence in anesthesia providers. Psychosomatics 40:356–359, 1999

Rich JB, Yaster M, Brandt J: Anterograde and retrograde memory in children anesthetized with propofol. J Clin Exp Neuropsychol 21:535–546, 1999

Schneider U, Bevalacqua C, Jacobs R, et al: Effects of fentanyl and low doses of alcohol on neuropsychological performance in healthy subjects. Neuropsychobiology 39:38–43, 1999

Wells LT, Rasch DK: Emergence "delirium" after sevoflurane anesthesia: a paranoid delusion? Anesth Analg 88:1308–1310, 1999

V

Toxic Gases

14

Carbon Monoxide

EPIDEMIOLOGY

Writing from the Government Hospital for the Insane in Washington, DC, in 1912, O'Malley described the delayed psychiatric symptoms of carbon monoxide (CO) poisoning first reported in the 1800s by European physicians (Glaister and Logan 1914). Also in 1912, a second study described neuropsychiatric symptoms that developed after a period of complete recovery from acute CO poisoning (McConnell and Spiller 1912). As twentieth-century industry flourished with the aid of organic fuels such as coal, oil, and gas, CO poisoning soon accounted for more deaths than did other chemicals (Hitchcock 1918; Marzella and Myers 1986; Norkool and Kirkpatrick 1985; Penney and White 1994). Many deaths occurred from "town gas," or natural gas used for lighting and heating. With newer energy sources, CO poisonings decreased but remain a significant source of morbidity and mortality.

Ten million workers risk CO exposure in the occupations listed in Table 14–1 (Anger and Johnson 1985). CO also constitutes the major toxic risk from fires. Most persons who die from smoke inhalation have lethal CO blood concentrations (Terrill et al. 1978). Some of the unexpected sources of poisoning include dynamite blasting and

TABLE 14–1. Occupations at risk for carbon monoxide poisoning

Bakers and cooks	Linotypists
Fire fighters	Miners
Formaldehyde workers	Paper/pulp mill workers
Garage workers (home and work)	Petroleum refinery workers
Gasoline-powered forklift operators	Welders
Iron and steel foundry workers	

propane-fueled ice-surfacing machines used in indoor skating areas (Gosselin et al. 1984; Hamilton and Hardy 1974).

SIGNS AND SYMPTOMS OF CARBON MONOXIDE POISONING

Signs and symptoms of CO poisoning range from headache and fatigue to death (Table 14–2). The only controversy pertaining to CO poisoning concerns the required dose and length of exposure to cause symptoms. Victims frequently complain of headache, fatigue, and dizziness, except in the most severe and rapid poisonings, when coma and death occur without a progression of symptoms. Individuals exposed to the same poisoning event will develop varying degrees of disability (Dunham and Johnstone 1999).

Youth, not age, imparts vulnerability to CO poisoning, possibly from children's higher basal metabolic rate and lower hemoglobin concentration. Children show more gastrointestinal symptoms when poisoned. Young adults experience more depressed mood and CO absorption than do the elderly (Gemelli and Cattani 1985; Groll-Knapp et al. 1982; Harbin et al. 1988). Table 14–3 lists genetic or physical conditions that increase susceptibility to CO poisoning. These individuals could develop symptoms more quickly or at lower doses than others (Calabrese 1978, 1991).

PSYCHIATRIC SIGNS AND SYMPTOMS ATTRIBUTED TO CARBON MONOXIDE POISONING

Table 14–4 lists the psychiatric manifestations of CO poisoning. Survivors can experience chronic and progressive neurological and psychiatric deterioration (Roohi et al. 2001). Persons with severe poisoning may completely recover only to develop a neuropsychiatric syn-

TABLE 14–2. Signs and symptoms of carbon monoxide poisoning

Acute or chronic	
Gastrointestinal	Nausea, vomiting, elevated liver enzymes
Respiratory	Tachypnea, respiratory failure
Cardiac	Palpitations, tachycardia, hypotension, arrhythmias
Neurological	Headache, light-headedness, weakness, decreased exercise tolerance, visual disturbances, dilated pupils, pyramidal tract signs, blindness, deafness, decerebrate posturing, coma, seizures, death
Other	Fever, sweating, pink to cherry skin color, leukocytosis, albuminuria, retinal hemorrhages
Delayed	
Cardiac	Cardiac abnormalities
Neurological	Electroencephalogram changes, seizures, pyramidal signs, extrapyramidal signs, blindness, deafness, apraxia, aphasia, miscellaneous neurological signs, peripheral neuropathy, disorientation, muscular rigidity, gait disturbance, fecal and urinary incontinence, coma
Other	Cutaneous changes, compartmental syndrome/ myonecrosis

TABLE 14–3. Genetic and physical conditions with increased risk for carbon monoxide poisoning

Genetic	Sickle cell anemia and trait, hemoglobin M, glucose-6-phosphate dehydrogenase deficiency
Physical	Vitamin C deficiency, heart disease, pregnancy

drome 2–4 weeks later (Marzella and Myers 1986). Comas lasting 1–2 days often precede the delayed symptoms (Ginsberg 1985). These patients consistently develop memory loss, inappropriate and sometimes violent behavior, symptoms of delirium, and cognitive and mood changes. Death frequently follows delayed symptoms. Medical providers without initial contact with the onset of poisoning may not recognize the delayed symptoms, and some mistake the psychiatric impairments for functional disorders. The mechanism of the delayed neuropsychiatric symptoms remains elusive. Recent theories suggest that membrane damage from hypoxia-induced free radical formation causes the delayed reaction (Penney and White 1994). Magnetic resonance imaging (MRI) of the brains of victims with delayed symptoms demonstrates that demyelination precedes neuronal necrosis (Murata et al. 2001; Roohi et al. 2001).

TABLE 14–4. Psychiatric signs and symptoms attributed to carbon monoxide poisoning

Mood	Irritability, depression, anxiety, mood changes, excitement
Behavior	Agitation, apathy, restlessness, inappropriate laughter, crying, singing, shouting, mania, violence/homicide, poor hygiene, odd behavior, hyperreligiosity, impulsivity
Cognitive	Memory loss, amnesia, confabulation, loss of concentration, dementia, delirium
Perceptual	Delusions, hallucinations, paranoia
Other	Echolalia, learning problems (children), paraphilias, insomnia, loss of libido, fatigue, Gilles de la Tourette's syndrome, Klüver-Bucy syndrome, astasia-abasia

DIAGNOSIS AND TREATMENT OF CARBON MONOXIDE POISONING

CO poisoning can result from a variety of unusual sources of poisoning, and physicians frequently overlook the diagnosis (Barret et al. 1985; Broome et al. 1988; Buckley 1984; "Carbon Monoxide" 1981). Sources include exposure to methylene chloride, a paint stripper ingredient that metabolizes to CO (Norkool and Kirkpatrick 1985). Poisonings also can occur from improperly used or defective wood stoves, kerosene heaters, charcoal heaters, gas water heaters, gas stoves, and other gas appliances. "Winter headache" may suggest "occult poisonings" that pose diagnostic challenges (Heckerling 1987; Heckerling et al. 1990). Symptoms of mild CO poisoning such as headache, nausea, and fatigue mimic influenza and gastroenteritis (Barret et al. 1985; Buckley 1984; "Carbon Monoxide" 1981; Fisher and Rubin 1982). More severe poisonings appear as pneumonia, myocardial infarction, cholecystitis, epilepsy, cerebral disease, migraine, food poisoning, and other drug intoxications (Barret et al. 1985; Fisher and Rubin 1982; Grace and Platt 1981). Preexisting psychiatric conditions leading to suicide attempts with CO complicate the diagnostic picture.

Table 14–5 lists the four CO-induced disorders recognized by DSM-IV-TR (American Psychiatric Association 2000). Table 14–5 includes "symptoms of dementia" that are attributed by DSM-IV-TR to CO poisoning. The diagnostic workup should rule out CO poisoning for frank neuropsychiatric syndromes or vague somatic complaints, especially if they occur during cold weather (Dolan 1985). The evaluation should include measurement of carboxyhemoglobin. This test does not always correlate with clinical severity. Table 14–6 lists diagnostic tests of value in CO poisoning (Dolan 1985; Marzella and Myers 1986).

TABLE 14–5. DSM-IV-TR diagnoses attributed to carbon monoxide poisoning

Substance-induced psychotic disorder
Substance-induced anxiety disorder
Substance-induced delirium
Substance-induced persisting amnestic disorder
Symptoms of dementia

TABLE 14–6. Diagnostic tests for carbon monoxide poisoning

Carboxyhemoglobin level
Drug screening (to rule out other intoxications)
Liver function tests (delayed elevation)
Serum glucose (hyperglycemia)
Complete blood count (leukocytosis)
Electrocardiogram (evidence of myocardial infarction or arrhythmias)
Brain computed tomography or magnetic resonance imaging
Electroencephalogram

The diagnosis of CO poisoning may be aided by radiological findings of brain injury. Computed tomography (CT) of the brain, in cases of coma with resulting neuropsychiatric changes followed by death or slow recovery, often shows cerebral atrophy, periventricular white matter degeneration, and bilateral low-density areas in the basal ganglia (Kim et al. 1980; Taylor and Holgate 1988; Zeiss and Brinker 1988). Several studies found that prognosis correlates more with severity of white matter changes than with basal ganglia lesions (Miura et al. 1985; Penney and White 1994). Positron emission tomography, single photon emission computed tomography, and MRI correlate with CT, neuropsychological, and clinical findings (Chang et al. 1992; Choi et al. 1995; DeReuck et al. 1992; Hopkins et al. 1993; O'Donnell et al. 2000; Pavese et al. 1999; Vion-Dury et al. 1987). Single photon emission computed tomography, MRI, and quantitative MRI have shown hippocampal atrophy, cortical atrophy, cortical necrosis, enlarged ventricle-to-brain ratio, and frontal and temporal lobe hypoperfusion in poisoning victims with neuropsychological changes (Gale et al. 1999; Muller and Gruber 2001). In severe cases, electroencephalogram findings are often abnormal and not directly correlated with severity.

Medical treatment of acute and delayed symptoms consists of immediate 100% oxygen followed by hyperbaric oxygen (Myers et al. 1985). Rapid treatment with hyperbaric oxygen frequently prevents neuropsychiatric sequelae (Norkool and Kirkpatrick 1985). Psychiatric treatment in acute settings includes assessment for suicidality. The patient also may need assistance to remain calm to minimize oxygen use. Sedatives that reduce respiratory effort should be avoided unless dangerous agitation requires them. The possibility of delayed symptoms requires follow-up over a period of weeks for monitoring. One study found dextroamphetamine effective in shortening the delayed effects of cognitive and motor deficits (Smallwood and Murray 1999). Electroconvulsive therapy may mask the onset of delayed neuropsychiatric symptoms or worsen their severity.

REFERENCES

American Psychiatric Association: Diagnostic and Statistical Manual of Mental Disorders, 4th Edition, Text Revision. Washington, DC, American Psychiatric Association, 2000

Anger WK, Johnson BL: Chemicals affecting behavior, in Neurotoxicity of Industrial and Commercial Chemicals, Vol 1. Edited by O'Donoghue JL. Boca Raton, FL, CRC Press, 1985, pp 51–148

Barret L, Danel V, Faure J: Carbon monoxide poisoning, a diagnosis frequently overlooked. Clin Toxicol 23:309–313, 1985

Broome JR, Pearson RR, Skrine H: Carbon monoxide poisoning: forgotten, not gone! British Journal of Hospital Medicine 39:298–305, 1988

Buckley AR: Still forgotten (letter). Lancet 1:165–166, 1984

Calabrese EJ: Pollutants and High-Risk Groups: The Biological Basis of Increased Human Susceptibility to Environmental and Occupational Pollutants. New York, Wiley-Interscience, 1978

Calabrese EJ: Genetic predisposition to occupationally related diseases: current status and future directions, in Ecogenetics: Genetic Predisposition to the Toxic Effects of Chemicals. Edited by Grandjean P. London, Chapman & Hall, 1991, pp 21–55

Carbon monoxide, an old enemy forgot (editorial). Lancet 2:75–76, 1981

Chang KH, Han MH, Kim HS, et al: Delayed encephalopathy after acute carbon monoxide intoxication: MR imaging features and distribution of cerebral white matter lesions. Radiology 184:117–122, 1992

Choi IS, Kim SK, Lee SS, et al: Evaluation of outcome of delayed neurologic sequelae after carbon monoxide poisoning by technetium-99m hexamethylpropyleneamine oxime brain single photon emission computed tomography. Eur Neurol 35:137–142, 1995

DeReuck J, Decoo D, Vienne J, et al: Significance of white matter lucencies in posthypoxic-ischemic encephalopathy: comparison of clinical status and of computed and positron emission tomographic findings. Eur Neurol 32:334–339, 1992

Dolan MC: Carbon monoxide poisoning. Canadian Medical Association Journal 133: 392–399, 1985

Dunham MD, Johnstone B: Variability of neuropsychological deficits associated with carbon monoxide poisoning: four case reports. Brain Inj 13:917–925, 1999

Fisher J, Rubin KP: Occult carbon monoxide poisoning (letter). Arch Intern Med 142: 1270–1271, 1982

Gale SD, Hopkins RO, Weaver LK, et al: MRI, quantitative MRI, SPECT, and neuropsychological findings following carbon monoxide poisoning. Brain Inj 13:229–243, 1999

Gemelli F, Cattani R: Carbon monoxide poisoning in childhood (letter). BMJ 291:1197, 1985

Ginsberg MD: Carbon monoxide intoxication: clinical features, neuropathology and mechanisms of injury. Clin Toxicol 23:281–288, 1985

Glaister J, Logan DD: Gas Poisoning in Mining and Other Industries. Edinburgh, E & S Livingstone, 1914

Gosselin RE, Smith RP, Hodge HC, et al: Clinical Toxicology of Commercial Products. Baltimore, MD, Williams & Wilkins 1984

Grace TW, Platt FW: Subacute carbon monoxide poisoning: another great imitator. JAMA 246:1698–1700, 1981

Groll-Knapp E, Haider M, Jenkner H, et al: Moderate carbon monoxide exposure during sleep: neuro- and psychophysiological effects in young and elderly people. Neurobehavioral Toxicology and Teratology 4:709–716, 1982

Hamilton A, Hardy HL: Carbon monoxide, in Industrial Toxicology. Acton, MA, Publishing Sciences Group, 1974, pp 239–258

Harbin TJ, Benignus VA, Muller KE, et al: The effects of low level carbon monoxide exposure upon evoked cortical potentials in young and elderly men. Neurotoxicol Teratol 10:93–100, 1988

Heckerling PS: Occult carbon monoxide poisoning: a cause of winter headache. Am J Emerg Med 5:201–204, 1987

Heckerling PS, Leikin JB, Terzian CG, et al: Occult carbon monoxide poisoning in patients with neurologic illness. Clin Toxicol 28:29–44, 1990

Hitchcock CW: Carbon monoxide poisoning: its nervous and mental symptoms. JAMA 71:257–260, 1918

Hopkins RO, Weaver LK, Kesner RP: Long term memory impairments and hippocampal magnetic resonance imaging in carbon monoxide poisoned patients (abstract). Undersea Hyperb Med 20:15, 1993

Kim KS, Weinberg PE, Suh JH, et al: Acute carbon monoxide poisoning: computed tomography of the brain. AJNR Am J Neuroradiol 1:399–402, 1980

Marzella L, Myers RAM: Carbon monoxide poisoning. Am Fam Physician 34:186–194, 1986

McConnell JW, Spiller WG: A clinicopathologic study of carbon monoxide poisoning. JAMA 59:2122–2126, 1912

Miura T, Mitomo M, Kawai R, et al: CT of the brain in acute carbon monoxide intoxication: characteristic features and prognosis. AJNR Am J Neuroradiol 6:739–742, 1985

Muller NG, Gruber O: High-resolution magnetic resonance imaging reveals symmetric bitemporal cortical necrosis after carbon monoxide intoxication. J Neuroimaging 11:322–325, 2001

Murata T, Kimura H, Kado H, et al: Neuronal damage in the interval form of CO poisoning determined by serial diffusion weighted magnetic resonance imaging plus 1H-magnetic resonance spectroscopy. J Neurol Neurosurg Psychiatry 71:250–253, 2001

Myers RAM, Snyder SK, Emhoff TA: Subacute sequelae of carbon monoxide poisoning. Ann Emerg Med 14:1163–1167, 1985

Norkool DM, Kirkpatrick JN: Treatment of acute carbon monoxide poisoning with hyperbaric oxygen: a review of 115 cases. Ann Emerg Med 14:1168–1171, 1985

O'Donnell P, Buxton PJ, Pitkin A, et al: The magnetic resonance imaging appearances of the brain in acute carbon monoxide poisoning. Clin Radiol 55:273–280, 2000

O'Malley M: Carbon monoxide poisoning with acute symptoms, relapse with psychotic symptoms, and complete recovery (abstract). JAMA 59:1540–1541, 1912

Pavese N, Napolitano A, De Iaco G, et al: Clinical outcome and magnetic resonance imaging of carbon monoxide intoxication: a long-term follow-up study. Ital J Neurol Sci 20:171–178, 1999

Penney DG, White SR: The neural and behavioral effects of carbon monoxide, in The Vulnerable Brain and Environmental Risks, Vol 3: Toxins in Air and Water. Edited by Isaacson RL, Jensen KF. New York, Plenum, 1994, pp 123–152

Roohi F, Kula RW, Mehta N: Twenty-nine years after carbon monoxide intoxication. Clin Neurol Neurosurg 103:92–95, 2001

Smallwood P, Murray GB: Neuropsychiatric aspects of carbon monoxide poisoning: a review and single case report suggesting a role for amphetamines. Ann Clin Psychiatry 11:21–27, 1999

Taylor R, Holgate RC: Carbon monoxide poisoning: asymmetric and unilateral changes on CT. AJNR Am J Neuroradiol 9:975–977, 1988

Terrill JB, Montgomery RR, Reinhardt CF: Toxic gases from fires. Science 200:1343–1347, 1978

Vion-Dury J, Jiddane M, Van Bunnen Y, et al: Sequelae of carbon monoxide poisoning: an MRI study of two cases. AJNR Am J Neuroradiol 14:60–65, 1987

Zeiss J, Brinker R: Role of contrast enhancement in cerebral CT of carbon monoxide poisoning. J Comput Assist Tomogr 12:341–343, 1988

ADDITIONAL READINGS

Barrowcliff DF, Knell AJ: Cerebral damage due to endogenous chronic carbon monoxide poisoning caused by exposure to methylene chloride. Journal of Social and Occupational Medicine 29:12–14, 1979

Binder JW, Roberts RJ: Carbon monoxide intoxication in children. Clin Toxicol 16: 287–295, 1980

Boon GPG, Winship WS: Carbon monoxide poisoning (letter). S Afr Med J 66:125, 1984

Borman M: Carbon monoxide poisoning: mental and neurological changes in a case of acute carbon monoxid [sic] poisoning with partial recovery. Am J Psychiatry 83: 135–143, 1926

Bourgeois JA: Amnesia after carbon monoxide poisoning (letter). Am J Psychiatry 157: 1884–1885, 2000

Burney RE, Wu S-C, Nemiroff MJ: Mass carbon monoxide poisoning: clinical effects and results of treatment in 184 victims. Ann Emerg Med 11:394–399, 1982

Carlesimo GA, Fadda L, Turriziani P, et al: Selective sparing of face learning in a global amnesic patient. J Neurol Neurosurg Psychiatry 71:340–346, 2001

Chalupa B, Synkova J, Sevcik M: The assessment of electroencephalographic changes and memory disturbances in acute intoxications with industrial poisons. British Journal of Industrial Medicine 17:238–241, 1960

Choi IS: Delayed neurologic sequelae in carbon monoxide intoxication. Arch Neurol 40:432–435, 1983

Choi IS, Cheon HY: Delayed movement disorders after carbon monoxide poisoning. Eur Neurol 42:141–144, 1999

Dancey TE, Reed GE: Mental disease following carbon monoxide poisoning. Canadian Medical Association Journal 35:47–49, 1936

Davis PL: The magnetic resonance imaging appearances of basal ganglia lesions in carbon monoxide poisoning. Magn Reson Imaging 4:489–490, 1986

Dutra FR: Cerebral residua of acute carbon monoxide poisoning. Am J Clin Pathol 22: 925–935, 1952

French LR, Schuman LM, Mortimer JA, et al: A case-control study of dementia of the Alzheimer type. Am J Epidemiol 121:414–421, 1985

Garland H, Pearce J: Neurological complications of carbon monoxide poisoning. Q J Med 36:445–455, 1967

Gilbert GJ, Glaser GH: Neurologic manifestations of chronic carbon monoxide poisoning. N Engl J Med 261:1217–1220, 1959

Ginsburg R, Romano J: Carbon monoxide encephalopathy: need for appropriate treatment. Am J Psychiatry 133:317–320, 1976

Gordon EB: Carbon-monoxide encephalopathy (letter). BMJ 1:1232, 1965

Gottfried JA, Chatterjee A: Carbon monoxide–mediated hippocampal injury. Neurology 57:17, 2001

Hawkins M, Harrison J, Charters P: Severe carbon monoxide poisoning: outcome after hyperbaric oxygen therapy. Br J Anaesth 84:584–586, 2000

Henke K, Kroll NE, Behniea H, et al: Memory lost and regained following bilateral hippocampal damage. J Cogn Neurosci 11:682–697, 1999

Horowitz AL, Kaplan R, Sarpel G: Carbon monoxide toxicity: MR imaging in the brain. Radiology 162:787–788, 1987

Hsu YK, Ch'eng YL: Cerebral subcortical myelinopathy in carbon monoxide poisoning. Brain Journal of Neurology 61:384–392, 1938

Hurley RA, Hopkins RO, Bigler ED, et al: Applications of functional imaging to carbon monoxide poisoning. J Neuropsychiatry Clin Neurosci 13:157–160, 2001

Jaeckle RS, Nasrallah HA: Major depression and carbon monoxide-induced parkinsonism: diagnosis, computerized axial tomography, and response to L-dopa. J Nerv Ment Dis 173:503–508, 1985

Jefferson JW: Subtle neuropsychiatric sequelae of carbon monoxide intoxication: two case reports. Am J Psychiatry 133:961–964, 1976

Hurley RA, Hopkins RO, Bigler ED, et al: Applications of functional imaging to carbon monoxide poisoning. J Neuropsychiatry Clin Neurosci 13:157–160, 2001

Kesler SR, Hopkins RO, Blatter DD, et al: Verbal memory deficits associated with fornix atrophy in carbon monoxide poisoning. J Int Neuropsychol Soc 7:640–646, 2001

Klees M, Heremans M, Dougan S: Psychological sequelae to carbon monoxide intoxication in the child. Sci Total Environ 44:165–176, 1985

Kobayashi K, Isaki K, Fukutani Y, et al: CT findings of the interval form of carbon monoxide poisoning compared with neuropathological findings. Eur Neurol 23:34–43, 1984

Lacey DJ: Neurologic sequelae of acute carbon monoxide intoxication. American Journal of Diseases of Children 135:145–147, 1981

Lennox MA, Peterson PB: Electroencephalographic findings in acute carbon monoxide poisoning. Electroencephalogr Clin Neurophysiol 10:63–68, 1958

Lindgren SA: A study of the effect of protracted occupational exposure to carbon monoxide. Acta Medical Scandinavica Supplmentum 356:1–77, 1961

Mann J: EEG changes and psychiatric findings in suicidal carbon-monoxide poisoning. Diseases of the Nervous System 26:508–511, 1965

Mathieu D, Nolf M, Durocher A, et al: Acute carbon monoxide poisoning risk of late sequelae and treatment by hyperbaric oxygen. Clin Toxicol 23:315–324, 1985

Menninger WC: Psychotic reaction in carbon monoxide poisoning. Bull Menninger Clin 1:29–32, 1936

Min SK: A brain syndrome associated with delayed neuropsychiatric sequelae following acute carbon monoxide intoxication. Acta Psychiatr Scand 73:80–86, 1986

Moore ME, Finestone AJ: The case of the disappearing headache (letter). N Engl J Med 278:1216, 1968

Myers RAM, Snyder SK, Emhoff TA: Subacute sequelae of carbon monoxide poisoning. Ann Emerg Med 14:1163–1167, 1985

Nardizzi LR: Computerized tomographic correlate of carbon monoxide poisoning. Arch Neurol 36:38–39, 1979

Norkool DM, Kirkpatrick JN: Treatment of acute carbon monoxide poisoning with hyperbaric oxygen: a review of 115 cases. Ann Emerg Med 14:1168–1171, 1985

Norris CR Jr, Trench JM, Hook R: Delayed carbon monoxide encephalopathy: clinical and research implications. J Clin Psychiatry 43:294–295, 1982

Plum F, Posner JB, Hain RF: Delayed neurological deterioration after anoxia. Arch Intern Med 110:56–62, 1962

Prockop LD, Naidu KA: Brain CT and MRI findings after carbon monoxide toxicity. J Neuroimaging 9:175–181, 1999

Pulst SM, Walshe TM, Romero JA: Carbon monoxide poisoning with features of Gilles de la Tourette's syndrome. Arch Neurol 40:443–444, 1983

Quilliam S: Encephalopathy four weeks after carbon monoxide poisoning (letter). Lancet 2:408, 1984

Raskin N, Mullaney OC: The mental and neurological sequelae of carbon monoxide asphyxia in a case observed for fifteen years. J Nerv Ment Dis 92:640–659, 1940

Remick RA, Miles JE: Carbon monoxide poisoning: neurologic and psychiatric sequelae. Canadian Medical Association Journal 117:654–657, 1977

Richardson JC, Chambers RA, Heywood PM: Encephalopathies of anoxia and hypoglycemia. AMA Archives of Neurology 1:178–190, 1959

Sandson TA, Lilly RB, Sodkol M: Kluver-Bucy syndrome associated with delayed post-anoxic leucoencephalopathy following carbon monoxide poisoning (letter). J Neurol Neurosurg Psychiatry 51:139–141, 1988

Sawa GM, Watson CPN, Terbrugge K, et al: Delayed encephalopathy following carbon monoxide intoxication. Journal Canadien des Sciences Neurologiques 8:77–79, 1981

Sawada Y, Ohashi N, Maemura K, et al: Computerized tomography as an indication of long-term outcome after acute carbon monoxide poisoning. Lancet 1:783–784, 1980

Shi Y, Pan F, Li H, et al: Role of carbon monoxide and nitric oxide in newborn infants with postasphyxial hypoxic-ischemic encephalopathy. Pediatrics 106:1447–1451, 2000

Shillito FH, Drinker CK, Shaughnessy TJ: The problem of nervous and mental sequelae in carbon monoxide poisoning. JAMA 106:669–674, 1936

Smith JS, Brandon S: Acute carbon monoxide poisoning—3 years' experience in a defined population. Postgrad Med J 46:65–70, 1970

Smith JS, Brandon S: Morbidity from acute carbon monoxide poisoning at three-year follow-up. BMJ 1:318–321, 1973

Smith JS, Mellick RS: Neuropsychiatric relapse following acute carbon monoxide poisoning—the contribution of electroconvulsive therapy. Med J Aust 1:465–468, 1975

Smith JS, Brierley H, Brandon S: Akinetic mutism with recovery after repeated carbon monoxide poisoning. Psychol Med 1:172–177, 1971

Sohn YH, Jeong Y, Kim HS, et al: The brain lesion responsible for parkinsonism after carbon monoxide poisoning. Arch Neurol 57:1214–1218, 2000

Strecker EA, Taft AE, Willey GF: Mental sequelae of carbon monoxide poisoning with reports of autopsy in two cases. Archives of Neurology and Psychiatry 17:552–555, 1927

Swain DG: Late sequelae of carbon monoxide poisoning (letter). Lancet 2:637, 1984

Thorpe M: Chronic carbon monoxide poisoning (letter). Can J Psychiatry 39:59–61, 1994

Tuchman RF, Moser FG, Moshe SL: Carbon monoxide poisoning: bilateral lesions in the thalamus on MR imaging of the brain. Pediatr Radiol 20:478–479, 1990

Werner B, Back W, Akerblom H, et al: Two cases of acute carbon monoxide poisoning with delayed neurological sequelae after a "free" interval. Clin Toxicol 23:249–265, 1985

Winter A, Shatin L: Hyperbaric oxygen in reversing carbon monoxide coma: neurologic and psychologic study. New York State Journal of Medicine 70:880–884, 1970

Zimmerman SS, Truxal B: Carbon monoxide poisoning. Pediatrics 68:215–224, 1981

15

Hydrogen Sulfide

EPIDEMIOLOGY

The earliest reports of hydrogen sulfide poisoning occurred in sewer workers in 1700 (Glass 1990). During the Texas "oil boom" in the 1920s, hydrogen sulfide poisonings from "sour gas," or natural gas containing sulfur, became a serious problem (National Research Council, Committee on Medical and Biologic Effects of Environmental Pollutants, Subcommittee on Hydrogen Sulfide 1979). Exposures also occurred in the viscose rayon and shale oil industries (Glass 1990). "Spinner's eye" from hydrogen sulfide exposure became a recognized illness in the rayon industry (Glass 1990). A major industrial disaster occurred in Mexico when 22 persons died and 320 required hospitalization after an industrial leak of hydrogen sulfide (Goldsmith 1986; World Health Organization 1981). Hydrogen sulfide remains a hazard in many occupations and environmental settings (Table 15–1).

SYMPTOMS OF HYDROGEN SULFIDE POISONING

At toxic levels, hydrogen sulfide has the peculiar ability to paralyze the olfactory nerve and cause anosmia, or inhibition of smelling.

TABLE 15–1. Occupational and environmental sources placing individuals at increased risk for hydrogen sulfide exposure

Coke ovens	Rayon
Farms	Refining
Fish or offal decay	Roofing (asphalt)
Heavy water	Rubber
Hospitals	Septic tanks
Iron smelters	Sewer treatment
Manure	Sewers
Mining	Shale oil
Mixing acidic and basic drain cleaners	Sugar beet processing
Natural gas	Sulfur
Oil drilling	Sulfur springs
Pesticides	Swine containment
Propane tanks	Tanneries
Pulp and paper mills	Volcanic gas

Victims may not detect its well-known "rotten eggs" odor. Exposed workers can experience "knockdowns," or losses of consciousness, described by observers as resembling "turning off the switch of a mechanical doll" (Guidotti 1994). "Oil patch" folklore held that after a few "knockdowns," victims became "simple in the head" (Guidotti 1994).

Table 15–2 lists symptoms associated with hydrogen sulfide poisoning. Many of these symptoms may never appear if victims develop rapid unconsciousness followed by death. Recovery often involves slow resolution of pulmonary and neurological problems (Gosselin et al. 1984). Endogenous levels of sulfide in the brain may influence susceptibility to poisoning. An estimated 10% of the population cannot metabolize organosulfides (Guidotti 1994).

PSYCHIATRIC SIGNS AND SYMPTOMS ATTRIBUTED TO HYDROGEN SULFIDE POISONING

Table 15–3 lists psychiatric signs and symptoms associated with hydrogen sulfide poisoning. Many sequelae probably result from the anoxia during loss of consciousness, but no formal studies exist to support this notion.

TABLE 15–2. Signs and symptoms of hydrogen sulfide poisoning

Eyes	Conjunctivitis, photophobia, lacrimation, corneal opacity
Skin	Erythema, pain, sweating
Respiratory	Rhinitis, anosmia, bronchitis, pulmonary edema, tachypnea
Cardiac	Palpitations, tachycardia, arrhythmias
Gastrointestinal	Salivation, nausea, vomiting, diarrhea
Neurological	Headache, vertigo, giddiness, weakness, cramps, amnesia, confusion, unconsciousness, death

TABLE 15–3. Psychiatric signs and symptoms attributed to hydrogen sulfide exposure

Mood	Nervousness, depression, anxiety, irritability
Behavior	Mania, violence, personality change
Cognitive	Dementia, poor concentration, poor memory, amnesia
Perceptual	Hallucinations, delusions
Other	Insomnia, nightmares, somnolence, fatigue, decreased libido

DIAGNOSIS AND TREATMENT OF HYDROGEN SULFIDE POISONING

Diagnosis is based primarily on history. Blood nitrites may indicate exposure if measured immediately after exposure (Reiffenstein et al. 1992). Treatment consists primarily of supportive measures. Some protocols call for managing symptoms with atropine, amyl nitrite, sodium nitrite, or hyperbaric oxygen (Gosselin et al. 1984; Reiffenstein et al. 1992). The efficacy of these treatments is unclear.

REFERENCES

Glass DC: A review of the health effects of hydrogen sulphide exposure. Ann Occup Hyg 34:323–327, 1990

Goldsmith JR: The 20-minute disaster; hydrogen sulfide spill at Poza Rica, in Environmental Epidemiology: Epidemiological Investigation of Community Environmental Health Problems. Edited by Goldsmith JR. Boca Raton, FL, CRC Press, 1986, pp 65–71

Gosselin RE, Smith RP, Hodge HC, et al Clinical Toxicology of Commercial Products. Baltimore, MD, Williams & Wilkins, 1984

Guidotti TL: Occupational exposure to hydrogen sulfide in the sour gas industry: some unresolved issues. Int Arch Occup Environ Health 66:153–160, 1994

National Research Council, Committee on Medical and Biologic Effects of Environmental Pollutants, Subcommittee on Hydrogen Sulfide: Hydrogen Sulfide. Baltimore, MD, University Park Press, 1979

Reiffenstein RJ, Hulbert WC, Roth SH: Toxicology of hydrogen sulfide. Annu Rev Pharmacol Toxicol 32:109–134, 1992

World Health Organization: Hydrogen Sulfide: Environmental Health Criteria 19. Geneva, World Health Organization, 1981

ADDITIONAL READINGS

Ahlborg G: Hydrogen sulfide poisoning in shale oil industry. AMA Archives of Industrial Hygiene and Occupational Medicine 3:247–266, 1951

Arnold IMF, Dufresne RM, Alleyne BC, et al: Health implication of occupational exposures to hydrogen sulfide. J Occup Med 27:373–376, 1985

Gaitonde UB, Sellar RJ, O'Hare AE: Long term exposure to hydrogen sulphide producing subacute encephalopathy in a child (letter). BMJ 294:614, 1987

Hanninen H: Psychological picture of manifest and latent carbon disulphide poisoning. British Journal of Industrial Medicine 28:374–381, 1971

Hoidal CR, Hall AH, Robinson MD, et al: Hydrogen sulfide poisoning from toxic inhalations of roofing asphalt fumes. Ann Emerg Med 15:826–830, 1986

Jaakkola JJK, Marttila O, Vilkka V, et al: The South Karelia Air Pollution Study: the quantitative effect of malodorous sulfur compounds on daily symptoms: a longitudinal study (abstract). Am Rev Respir Dis 141 (suppl):A75, 1990

Kemper FD: A near-fatal case of hydrogen sulfide poisoning. Canadian Medical Association Journal 94:1130–1131, 1966

Legator MS, Singleton CR, Morris DL, et al: Health effects from chronic low-level exposure to hydrogen sulfide. Arch Environ Health 56:123–131, 2001

Matsuo F, Cummins JW: Neurological sequelae of massive hydrogen sulfide inhalation (letter). Arch Neurol 36:451–452, 1979

Milby TH, Baselt RC: Hydrogen sulfide poisoning: clarification of some controversial issues. Am J Ind Med 35:192–195, 1999

Poda GA: Hydrogen sulfide can be handled safely. Arch Environ Health 12:795–800, 1966

Singer R: Neurotoxicity Guidebook. New York, Van Nostrand Reinhold, 1990

Snyder JW, Safir EF, Summerville GP, et al: Occupational fatality and persistent neurological sequelae after mass exposure to hydrogen sulfide. Am J Emerg Med 13: 199–203, 1995

Stine RJ, Slosberg B, Beacham BE: Hydrogen sulfide intoxication: a case report and discussion of treatment. Ann Intern Med 85:756–758, 1976

Thoman M: Sewer gas: hydrogen sulfide intoxication. Clin Toxicol 2:383–386, 1969

Tvedt B, Edland A, Skyberg K, et al: Delayed neuropsychiatric sequelae after acute hydrogen sulfide poisoning: affection of motor function, memory, vision, and hearing. Acta Neurol Scand 84:348–351, 1991a

Tvedt B, Skyberg K, Aaserud O, et al: Brain damage caused by hydrogen sulfide: a follow-up study of six patients. Am J Ind Med 20:91–101, 1991b

Wasch HH, Estrin WJ, Yip P, et al: Prolongation of the P-300 latency associated with hydrogen sulfide exposure. Arch Neurol 46:902–904, 1989

Wiglesworth J: Remarks on two cases of insanity caused by inhalation of sulphuretted hydrogen. BMJ 2:124–125, 1892

VI

Other Chemicals and Syndromes

16

Polybrominated Biphenyls and Polychlorinated Biphenyls

EPIDEMIOLOGY

Polybrominated biphenyls (PBBs) came to public awareness in the early 1970s after Firemaster BP-6, a PBB fire retardant, contaminated Michigan dairy cattle and other farm animals (Anderson et al. 1978). The catastrophe resulted in the mandatory destruction of thousands of animals and their products. By 1978, most residents of Michigan probably had detectable levels of PBB in their body fat (Anderson et al. 1978). Before the incident, most physicians knew little about PBB or polychlorinated biphenyl (PCB) toxicity. Literature concerning PBB neurotoxicity appeared only in the 1970s and early 1980s following the Michigan incident.

The first cases of PCB toxicity occurred in the 1930s (George et al. 1988). PCBs gained notoriety in 1968 and again in 1978 when PCB-contaminated rice oil poisoned thousands of Japanese and Taiwanese, respectively (Seegal and Shain 1992). Also, during 1978 in North Carolina, illegal "moonlight" dumping of PCBs along roadways exposed unsuspecting citizens (Brown 1979). In 1999, 500 tons of PCB- and dioxin-contaminated feed were distributed to animal farms in Belgian and other European countries (van Larebeke et al. 2001).

PBBs and PCBs were used in a variety of electrical and chemical applications, especially capacitors, transformers, machine oils, plastics, carbonless copy paper, and sealants (George et al. 1988; Seegal and Shain 1992). In 1975, an estimated 12,000 occupational exposures, primarily dermal, occurred (George et al. 1988). Leaks, fires, or explosions of electrical devices containing PCBs caused most of the PCB poisonings in the 1980s. Since the U.S. Environmental Protection Agency banned further production of PCBs and PBBs in 1977, few occupations today have inherent PCB exposure risks, except for fire fighting. When transformers from the PCB era burn, they pose significant exposure risks. Table 16–1 lists industries engaged in PCB use before the production ban.

Most environmental exposures involve "background" levels of PCBs in food. The continued appearance of studies of the neurotoxic potential of PCBs in humans results from the stability and persistence of PCBs in the environment and their tendency to accumulate in human tissues (Chase et al. 1982; Gray 1996; Jacobson and Jacobson 1996). In the United States, this includes studies of low-level in utero exposure to PCBs in offspring of mothers who ate contaminated fish from Lake Michigan (Jacobson and Jacobson 1996) or of mothers in North Carolina with "background" exposures (Gladen and Rogan 1991). Similar studies took place in the Netherlands (Jacobson et al. 1985) and the Faroe Islands (Weihe et al. 1996).

TABLE 16–1. Past industrial uses of polychlorinated biphenyls

Coolant for transformers and capacitors
Dedusting agents, adhesives, pesticide extenders
Hydraulic fluids, heat transfer fluids, high-pressure lubricants
Ink and dye carriers
Insulation for electrical wires, cables, and condensers
Microencapsulation of dyes for carbonless duplicating papers
Paint additives, ink dyes, plasticizers
Protective coats for low flammable woods

SIGNS AND SYMPTOMS OF PBB AND PCB POISONING

Table 16–2 lists the manifestations of PBB and PCB exposure. Exposed individuals in the Michigan PBB incident had detectable PBB serum levels in conjunction with subjective neurological, gastrointestinal, cutaneous, and musculoskeletal complaints. Objective measures did not indicate abnormalities that correlated with the subjective complaints (Stross et al. 1981).

The symptoms of PCB poisoning were described in several industrial accidents and the so-called Yusho and Yu-cheng poisoning epidemics in Japan and Taiwan, respectively (Reggiani and Bruppacher 1985). Numerous persistent dermatological, ocular, neurological, and respiratory manifestations resulted from these exposures. More than 80% of the victims usually developed dermatological and ocular symptoms—notably, chloracne, pigmentation, and eye discharges (Reggiani and Bruppacher 1985).

Certain genetic and physical factors predispose individuals to greater sensitivity to PCBs (Table 16–3). Individuals who do not detoxify and excrete PCBs rapidly have the greatest risk (Calabrese 1978). Numerous studies of the development of infants exposed to background PCB suggest that immature enzyme detoxification systems render young persons susceptible to PCB neurotoxicity.

TABLE 16–2. Signs and symptoms attributed to polybrominated biphenyl and polychlorinated biphenyl poisoning

Polybrominated biphenyls	
Gastrointestinal	Irregular bowels, abdominal pain
Skin	Rashes
Neurological	Weakness, fatigue, arthralgias, myalgias, poor coordination
Other	Frequent infections, psychiatric complaints
Polychlorinated biphenyls	
Pulmonary	Chronic bronchitis
Gastrointestinal	Vomiting, diarrhea
Skin	Jaundice, dark skin pigmentation, rashes, itching, sweating
Neurological	Visual disturbance, hearing problems, headache
Other	Eye discharge; elevated serum triglycerides; irregular menstrual cycles; variety of fetal abnormalities, including sensory/motor conduction abnormalities; psychiatric complaints

TABLE 16–3. Genetic and physical conditions with polychlorinated biphenyl susceptibility

Embryos, fetuses, and neonates to age 2–3 months
Crigler-Najjar syndrome
Gilbert's syndrome
Vitamin A deficiency
Liver disease (Reggiani and Bruppacher 1985)
Alcohol and drug use

PSYCHIATRIC SIGNS AND SYMPTOMS ATTRIBUTED TO PBB AND PCB POISONING

Psychiatric symptoms attributed to PBBs and PCBs are summarized in Table 16–4.

Polybrominated Biphenyls

The literature does not support a direct neurotoxic effect of PBBs of psychiatric importance. Most authors attribute the depression experienced by Michigan farm families to the financial losses inflicted by the disaster. Adult exposures occurred only during a 4-year period from 1977 to 1981, and their evaluations contained no objective measures of neurotoxic injury. Studies of exposed workers in PBB plants have been done, but their exposures were primarily dermal, not by ingestion, as experienced by the Michigan residents.

TABLE 16–4. Psychiatric symptoms attributed to polybrominated biphenyls and polychlorinated biphenyls

Polybrominated biphenyls	
Mood	Irritability, nervousness
Cognitive	Poor concentration and memory
Other	Fatigue, somnolence, decreased libido, somatic complaints
Polychlorinated biphenyls	
Mood	Irritability, nervousness, depression
Cognitive	Poor concentration and memory
Other	Fatigue, somnolence, insomnia, decreased libido, impotence, somatic complaints, various developmental delays in infants

Polychlorinated Biphenyls

Children poisoned in the Yusho and Yu-cheng events were described as dull, apathetic, and of low intelligence. These findings agreed with those of studies in the United States (Seegal and Shain 1992; Tilson and Harry 1994). Some authors concluded that other chlorinated aromatic hydrocarbons, including dibenzofurans, also contaminated the Yusho and Yu-cheng victims and could not be ruled out as the cause of symptoms (Schantz 1996a; Seegal and Shain 1992). The most recent opinions suggest that although mental retardation or other serious impairments do not result from exposure, PCBs may cause subtle defects in memory and attention in both children and adults (Boersma and Lanting 2000; Darvill et al. 2000; Grandjean et al. 2001; Kilburn 2000; Jacobson and Jacobson 1994; Ribas-Fito et al. 2001; Schantz et al. 2001). Animal studies that show altered serotonin metabolism in the brains of exposed rats support the notion of PCB neurotoxicity (Morse et al. 1996). The effect of PCBs on children's development remains a lively debate (Schantz 1996b). Several issues are unresolved, including methodological problems, poor control for highly toxic heat-degradation products present in PCBs, and lack of exposure indices relative to symptoms (Middaugh and Egeland 1997; Schantz 1996a).

Occupational studies of the psychiatric effects of PCBs appeared in the 1970s and 1980s. The most recent reports described psychiatric symptoms in firefighters exposed to burning PCBs. Trauma and litigation concurrent with the firemen's vague somatic symptoms made it difficult to determine whether symptoms resulted from stress, malingering, or PCB exposure (Fitzgerald et al. 1989). Two lines of evidence support the claim that PCBs caused the symptoms. First, the frequent reports of sleepiness or somnolence in exposed adults may equate to the dull and apathetic symptoms in PCB-poisoned children. Second, victims of the Yu-cheng incident had abnormal electroencephalogram findings but complained of only dizziness, headache, or pain. PCBs could cause neurotoxic injury subjectively manifested by vague somatic complaints (Chia and Chu 1984).

DIAGNOSIS AND TREATMENT OF PBB AND PCB POISONING

Serum measurements of PBBs and PCBs indicate exposure, but levels do not correlate with clinical severity (Lu and Wong 1984; Stross et al. 1981).

No specific instructions guide the treatment of PBB and PCB poisoning. During the Yu-cheng incident, various treatments with vitamins and antibiotics had limited success (Lu and Wong 1984). Some individuals in Taiwan responded to a "fasting cure" consisting of mostly vegetables and fruits (Imamura and Tung 1984). Firemen with neuropsychological symptoms after inhalational exposure at a transformer fire experienced improved neuropsychological test scores with supervised diets, exercise, and sauna (Kilburn et al. 1989). Whether treatment was effective more from reducing the body burden of PCB or from the relaxing "spa"-like experience remains unknown, but treatment with exercise and sauna has biological plausibility. PCB is highly lipophilic and accumulates in liver and adipose tissue (George et al. 1988). Effective treatments would increase fat metabolism and sweating to reduce the PCB burden (Kilburn et al. 1989). The reduction of serotonin in the frontal cortex and hippocampus of animals exposed to PCBs suggests that selective serotonin reuptake inhibitors also may help psychiatric symptoms from poisoning (Morse et al. 1996; Seegal et al. 1986).

REFERENCES

Anderson HA, Lilis R, Selikoff IJ, et al: Unanticipated prevalence of symptoms among dairy farmers in Michigan and Wisconsin. Environ Health Perspect 23:217–226, 1978

Boersma ER, Lanting CI: Environmental exposure to polychlorinated biphenyls (PCBs) and dioxins: consequences for long-term neurological and cognitive development of the child lactation. Adv Exp Med Biol 478:271–287, 2000

Brown M: Laying Waste: The Poisoning of America by Toxic Chemicals. New York, Pantheon, 1979

Calabrese EJ: Pollutants and High-Risk Groups: The Biological Basis of Increased Human Susceptibility to Environmental and Occupational Pollutants. New York, Wiley-Interscience, 1978

Chase KH, Wong O, Thomas D, et al: Clinical and metabolic abnormalities associated with occupational exposure to polychlorinated biphenyls (PCBs). J Occup Med 24:109–114, 1982

Chia L-G, Chu F-L: Neurological studies on polychlorinated biphenyl (PCB)–poisoned patients. Am J Ind Med 5:117–126, 1984

Darvill T, Lonky E, Reihman J, et al: Prenatal exposure to PCBs and infant performance on the Fagan test of infant intelligence. Neurotoxicology 21:1029–1038, 2000

Fitzgerald EF, Weinstein AL, Youngblood LG, et al: Health effects three years after potential exposure to the toxic contaminants of an electrical transformer fire. Arch Environ Health 44:214–221, 1989

George CJ, Bennett GF, Simoneaux D, et al: Polychlorinated biphenyls—a toxicological review. Journal of Hazardous Materials 18:113–144, 1988

Gladen BC, Rogan WJ: Effects of perinatal polychlorinated biphenyls and dichlorodiphenyl dichloroethene on later development. J Pediatr 119:58–63, 1991

Grandjean P, Weihe P, Burse VW, et al: Neurobehavioral deficits associated with PCB in 7-year-old children prenatally exposed to seafood neurotoxicants. Neurotoxicol Teratol 23:305–317, 2001

Gray LE Jr: Comments on "developmental neurotoxicity of PCBs in humans: what do we know and where do we go from here?" Neurotoxicol Teratol 18:243–245, 1996
Imamura M, Tung T-C: A trial of fasting cure for PCB-poisoned patients in Taiwan. Am J Ind Med 5:147–153, 1984
Jacobson JL, Jacobson SW: The effects of perinatal exposure to polychlorinated biphenyls and related contaminants, in Prenatal Exposure to Toxicants: Developmental Consequences. Edited by Needleman HL, Bellinger D. Baltimore, MD, Johns Hopkins University Press, 1994, pp 130–147
Jacobson JL, Jacobson SW: Intellectual impairment in children exposed to polychlorinated biphenyls in utero. N Engl J Med 335:783–789, 1996
Jacobson SW, Fein GG, Jacobson JL, et al: The effect of intrauterine PCB exposure on visual recognition memory. Child Dev 56:853–860, 1985
Kilburn KH, Warsaw RH, Shields MG: Neurobehavioral dysfunction in firemen exposed to polychlorinated biphenyls (PCBs): possible improvement after detoxification. Arch Environ Health 44:345–350, 1989
Kilburn KH: Visual and neurobehavioral impairment associated with polychlorinated biphenyls. Neurotoxicology 21:489–499, 2000
Lu Y-C, Wong P-N: Dermatological, medical, and laboratory findings of patients in Taiwan and their treatments. Am J Ind Med 5:81–115, 1984
Middaugh JP, Egeland GM: Intellectual function of children exposed to polychlorinated biphenyls in utero (letter). N Engl J Med 336:660–661, 1997
Morse DC, Seegal RF, Brosch KO, et al: Long-term alterations in regional brain serotonin metabolism following maternal polychlorinated biphenyl exposure in the rat. Neurotoxicology 17:631–638, 1996
Reggiani G, Bruppacher R: Symptoms, signs and findings in humans exposed to PCBs and their derivatives. Environ Health Perspect 60:225–232, 1985
Ribas-Fito N, Sala M, Kogevinas M, et al: Polychlorinated biphenyls (PCBs) and neurological development in children: a systematic review. J Epidemiol Community Health 55:537–546, 2001
Schantz SL: Developmental neurotoxicity of PCBs in humans: what do we know and where do we go from here? Neurotoxicol Teratol 18:217–227, 1996a
Schantz SL: Response to commentaries. Neurotoxicol Teratol 18:271–276, 1996b
Schantz SL, Gasior DM, Polverejan E, et al: Impairments of memory and learning in older adults exposed to polychlorinated biphenyls via consumption of Great Lakes fish. Environ Health Perspect 109:605–611, 2001
Seegal RF, Shain W: Neurotoxicity of polychlorinated biphenyls, in The Vulnerable Brain and Environmental Risks, Vol 2: Toxins in Food. Edited by Isaacson RL, Jensen KF. New York, Plenum, 1992, pp 169–195
Seegal RF, Brosch KO, Bush B: Regional alterations in serotonin metabolism induced by oral exposure of rats to polychlorinated biphenyls. Neurotoxicology 7:155–165, 1986
Stross JK, Smokler IA, Isbister J, et al: The human health effects of exposure to polybrominated biphenyls. Toxicol Appl Pharmacol 58:145–150, 1981
Tilson HA, Harry GJ: Developmental neurotoxicology of polychlorinated biphenyls and related compounds, in The Vulnerable Brain and Environmental Risks, Vol 3: Toxins in Air and Water. Edited by Isaacson RL, Jensen KF. New York, Plenum, 1994, pp 267–279
van Larebeke N, Hens L, Schepens P, et al: The Belgian PCB and dioxin incident of January–June 1999: exposure data and potential impact on health. Environ Health Perspect 109:265–273, 2001
Weihe P, Grandjean P, Debes F, et al: Health implications for Faroe Islanders of heavy metals and PCBs from pilot whales. Sci Total Environ 186:141–148, 1996

ADDITIONAL READINGS

Polybrominated Biphenyls

Anderson HA, Wolff MS, Lilis R, et al: Symptoms and clinical abnormalities following ingestion of polybrominated-biphenyl-contaminated food products. Ann N Y Acad Sci 320:684–701, 1979

Brown GG, Nixon RK: Exposure to polybrominated biphenyls: some effects on personality and cognitive functioning. JAMA 242:523–527, 1979

Brown GG, Preisman RC, Anderson MD, et al: Memory performance of chemical workers exposed to polybrominated biphenyls. Science 212:1413–1415, 1981

Lilis R, Anderson HA, Valciukas JA, et al: Comparison of findings among residents on Michigan dairy farms and consumers of produce purchased from these farms. Environ Health Perspect 23:105–109, 1978

Meester WD, McCoy DJ: Human toxicology of polybrominated biphenyls, in Management of the Poisoned Patient. Edited by Rumack BH, Temple AR. Princeton, NJ, Science Press, 1977, pp 32–60

Schwartz EM, Rae WA: Effect of polybrominated biphenyls (PBB) on developmental abilities in young children. Am J Public Health 73:277–281, 1983

Seagull E: Developmental abilities of children exposed to polybrominated biphenyls (PBB). Am J Public Health 73:281–285, 1983

Stross JK, Nixon RK, Anderson MD: Neuropsychiatric findings in patients exposed to polybrominated biphenyls. Ann N Y Acad Sci 320:368–372, 1979

Valciukas JA, Lilis R, Wolff MS, et al: Comparative neurobehavioral study of a polybrominated biphenyl–exposed population in Michigan and a nonexposed group in Wisconsin. Environ Health Perspect 23:199–210, 1978

Valciukas JA, Lilis R, Anderson HA, et al: The neurotoxicity of polybrominated biphenyls: results of a medical field survey. Ann N Y Acad Sci 320:337–367, 1979

Weil WB, Spencer M, Benjamin D, et al: The effect of polybrominated biphenyls on infants and young children. J Pediatr 98:47–51, 1981

Polychlorinated Biphenyls

Aoki Y: Polychlorinated biphenyls, polychlorinated dibenzo-p-dioxins, and polychlorinated dibenzofurans as endocrine disrupters—what we have learned from Yusho disease. Environ Res 86:2–11, 2001

Chen Y-CJ, Hsu C-C: Effects of prenatal exposure to PCBs on the neurological function of children: a neuropsychological and neurophysiological study. Dev Med Child Neurol 36:312–320, 1994

Chen Y-CJ, Guo Y-L, Hsu C-C, et al: Cognitive development of Yu-Cheng ("oil disease") children prenatally exposed to heat-degraded PCBs. JAMA 268:3213–3218, 1992

Chen Y-CJ, Yu M-LM, Rogan WJ, et al: A 6-year follow-up of behavior and activity disorders in the Taiwan Yu-cheng children. Am J Public Health 84:415–421, 1994

Fischbein A, Wolff MS, Lilis R, et al: Clinical findings among PCB-exposed capacitor manufacturing workers. Ann N Y Acad Sci 320:703–715, 1979

Gladen BC, Rogan WJ, Hardy P, et al: Development after exposure to polychlorinated biphenyls and dichlorodiphenyl dichloroethene transplacentally and through human milk. J Pediatr 113:991–995, 1988

Golka K, Kiesswetter E, Kieper H, et al: Psychological effects upon exposure to polyhalogenated debenzodioxins and dibenzofurans. Chemosphere 40:1271–1275, 2000

Guo YL, Yu ML, Hsu CC, et al: Chloracne, goiter, arthritis, and anemia after polychlorinated biphenyl poisoning: 14-year follow-up of the Taiwan Yucheng cohort. Environ Health Perspect 107:715–719, 1999

Halperin W, Landrigan PJ, Altman R, et al: Chemical fire at toxic waste disposal plant: epidemiologic study of exposure to smoke and fumes. The Journal of the Medical Society of New Jersey 78:591–594, 1981

Houck P, Nebel D, Milham S: Organic solvent encephalopathy: an old hazard revisited. Am J Ind Med 22:109–115, 1992

Hsu S-T, Ma C-I, Hsu SKH, et al: Discovery and epidemiology of PCB poisoning in Taiwan: a four-year followup. Environ Health Perspect 59:5–10, 1985

Huisman M, Koopman-Esseboom C, Fidler V, et al: Perinatal exposure to polychlorinated biphenyls and dioxins and its effect on neonatal neurological development. Early Hum Dev 41:111–127, 1995a

Huisman M, Koopman-Esseboom C, Lanting CI, et al: Neurological condition in 18-month-old children perinatally exposed to polychlorinated biphenyls and dioxins. Early Hum Dev 43:165–176, 1995b

Jacobson JL, Jacobson SW, Schwartz PM, et al: Prenatal exposure to an environmental toxin: a test of the multiple effects model. Dev Psychol 20:523–532, 1984

Jacobson JL, Jacobson SW, Humphrey HEB: Effects of exposure to PCBs and related compounds on growth and activity in children. Neurotoxicol Teratol 12:319–326, 1990a

Jacobson JL, Jacobson SW, Humphrey HEB: Effects of in utero exposure to polychlorinated biphenyls and related contaminants on cognitive functioning in young children. J Pediatr 116:38–45, 1990b

Jacobson JL, Jacobson SW, Padgett RJ, et al: Effects of prenatal PCB exposure on cognitive processing efficiency and sustained attention. Dev Psychol 28:297–306, 1992

Jacobson SW, Ko HC, Yao BL, et al: Preliminary findings confirming effects of prenatal PCB exposure on infant memory (abstract). Neurotoxicol Teratol 16:315, 1994

Koopman-Esseboom C, Weisglas-Kuperus N, de Ridder MAJ, et al: Effects of polychlorinated biphenyl/dioxin exposure and feeding type on infants' mental and psychomotor development. Pediatrics 97:700–706, 1996

Lai TJ, Guo YL, Guo NW, et al: Effect of prenatal exposure to polychlorinated biphenyls on cognitive development in children: a longitudinal study in Taiwan. Br J Psychiatry 40:49–52, 2001

Patandin S, Lanting CI, Mulder PG, et al: Effects of environmental exposure to polychlorinated biphenyls and dioxins on cognitive abilities in Dutch children at 42 months of age. J Pediatr 134:33–41, 1999

Rice DC: Behavioral impairment produced by low-level postnatal PCB exposure in monkeys. Environ Res 80 (2 pt 2):S113–S121, 1999

Rice DC: Parallels between attention deficit hyperactivity disorder and behavioral deficits produced by neurotoxic exposure in monkeys. Environ Health Perspect 108 (suppl 3):405–408, 2000

Rogan WJ, Gladen BC: PCBs, DDE, and child development at 18 and 24 months. Ann Epidemiol 1:407–413, 1991

Rogan WJ, Gladen BC, McKinney JD, et al: Neonatal effects of transplacental exposure to PCBs and DDE. J Pediatr 109:335–341, 1986

Rogan WJ, Gladen BC, Hung K-L, et al: Congenital poisoning by polychlorinated biphenyls and their contaminants in Taiwan. Science 241:334–336, 1988

Schecter A, Tiernan T: Occupational exposure to polychlorinated dioxins, polychlorinated furans, polychlorinated biphenyls, and biphenylenes after an electrical panel and transformer accident in an office building in Binghamton, NY. Environ Health Perspect 60:305–313, 1985

Schell JD Jr, Budinsky RA, Wernke MJ: PCBs and neurodevelopmental effects in Michigan children: an evaluation of exposure and dose characterization. Regul Toxicol Pharmacol 33:300–312, 2001

Singer R: Methodology of forensic neurotoxicity evaluation: PCB case. Toxicology 49: 403–408, 1988

Stewart P, Reihman J, Lonky E, et al: Prenatal PCB exposure and neonatal behavioral assessment scale (NBAS) performance. Neurotoxicol Teratol 22:21–29, 2000

17

Miscellaneous Elements, Chemicals, and Syndromes

BORON

Boron, an element, occurs in many compounds, including borax, borates, boric acid, and carboxyboranes used in glass, ceramics, detergents, bleaches, fire retardants, disinfectants, alloys, specialty metals, preservatives, pesticides, and fertilizers (Mastromatteo and Sullivan 1994). Boron compounds also constitute an important group of "dopants" in the semiconductor industry. Dopants alter crystalline substrates' electrical conductivities in the manufacturing of diodes, transistors, and capacitors (Lewis 1986).

Following the introduction of the boron hydrides in the 1940s as rocket fuels, the neurotoxic properties of diborane, pentaborane, and decaborane became known (Yarbrough et al. 1985). Diborane, a gas, produces mostly pulmonary symptoms. Pentaborane, a liquid, and decaborane, a solid, cause severe cardiac and neurological damage.

Table 17–1 lists neurological signs and symptoms of decaborane and pentaborane poisoning. Other symptoms include hepatic injury and metabolic acidosis (Yarbrough et al. 1985). Table 17–2 lists psychiatric signs and symptoms of decaborane and pentaborane poisoning. In the 1980s, an industrial accident in Virginia involving the release of pentaborane caused neurotoxic injury, in some cases fatal, to workers and rescue personnel. Six of the 12 victims of accidental exposure had abnormal brain computed tomography findings (Hart et al. 1984). The exposed persons had significantly increased central nervous system neurotransmitter metabolite levels and mean ventricular brain ratios compared with control subjects (Silverman et al. 1985). These findings contradicted earlier reports suggesting that symptoms of boron exposure resolved in a few days.

TABLE 17–1. Neurological signs and symptoms of decaborane and pentaborane poisoning

Blurred vision	Electroencephalogram changes
Cortical blindness	Myoclonic jerks
Deafness	Quadriplegia
Death	Seizures
Dizziness	Slurred speech
Drowsiness	Tremors

TABLE 17–2. Psychiatric signs and symptoms attributed to decaborane and pentaborane poisoning

Mood	Euphoria, anxiety, depression
Behavior	Personality change, inappropriate behavior, agitation, restlessness, sleepwalking
Cognitive	Memory loss, poor concentration, confusion
Perceptual	Hallucinations
Other	Somnolence, derealization, insomnia, nightmares

CARBON DIOXIDE

Inhalation of 5% carbon dioxide can induce panic in certain adults and children who are hypersensitive to carbon dioxide (CO_2) (Kent et al. 2001; Pine et al. 2000). This suggests that CO_2-hypersensitive persons in occupations or environments with high levels of CO_2 exposure could have panic attacks, but there is no literature to support this notion. The only case report of occupational CO_2 exposure described a 31-year-old dry-ice packer who lost consciousness from exposure (Perez and Silverman 1981). He developed intense hate or attraction, agitation, anger, and irritability followed by violence toward his nurses. He was talkative 7 months later, with tedious, pressured speech, decreased concentration, poor memory, and abnormal electroencephalogram findings.

COPPER

In 1912, S.A.K. Wilson described "progressive lenticular degeneration, . . . a familial nervous disease associated with cirrhosis of the liver" (p. 296). Later known as Wilson's disease, the disorder included features of "emotionalism." Resulting from a recessively inherited disorder of copper metabolism, symptoms of Wilson's disease arise from copper deposits in organs, including the eyes, liver, and brain. Several reviews describe the numerous psychiatric symptoms that include impairments in thought, mood, behavior, and cognition (Akil and Brewer 1995; Akil et al. 1991; Dening 1985; Dening and Berrios 1989a, 1989b; Medalia et al. 1988). Treatment consists of chelation with penicillamine, although the literature recommends zinc sulfate or acetate (Brewer and Yuzbasiyan-Gurkan 1992; Hartard et al. 1993; Modai et al. 1985).

A lack of neurotoxicity from copper ingestion contrasts the psychiatric picture of Wilson's disease. Inhalation of copper particles by inhalant abusers who "sniff" metallic paint results in pulmonary deposits of copper but no apparent neurotoxicity (Wilde 1975). Acute poisoning causes "nervous excitation followed by depression," but no other central nervous system symptoms appear, even after massive ingestions (Gosselin et al. 1984; Yelin et al. 1987). The same lack of neurotoxicity applies to chronic exposures (Gosselin et al. 1984).

SILICONE

A link between silicone and health problems remains controversial. One study performed a retrospective study of 131 litigants for alleged problems from silicone breast implants. The litigants claimed the implants caused cognitive and memory problems, but the study attributed the complaints to nonneurological causes, including depression and anxiety (Rosenberg 1996). A more recent cohort study of women with silicone breast implants found no association between implants and neurological disease (Winther et al. 2001). Emerging literature generally supports the lack of association between silicone implants and connective tissue diseases (Kjoller et al. 2001; Laing et al. 2001; Wolfe and Anderson 1999). Other studies found an excess of suicide and fibromyalgia in implant recipients (Brinton et al. 2001; Wolfe and Anderson 1999).

VANADIUM

Vanadium, a metal, has many applications in the steel, automotive, and chemical industries. It constitutes a significant portion of exhaust from fuels. Cleaners of oil-fired power plant burners have high urinary vanadium excretion (Maroni et al. 1987). A description of Australian boiler cleaners included trembling, headache, blindness, "nervous troubles," and "psychic derangement" (Thomas and Stiebris 1956). The earliest reports of vanadiumism in the twentieth century described symptoms of "hysteria and melancholia" accompanied by tremor, vertigo, headache, neuroretinitis, and amaurosis (Dutton 1911).

Some evidence supports an association of vanadium with mania or bipolar disorder. Vanadium poisoning alters levels of neurotransmitters in rat brains, and two studies correlated elevated vanadium with mania. One study placed manic, depressed, and individuals without such symptoms on a low-vanadium diet. Most of the manic and depressed patients improved (Naylor and Smith 1981). Another study failed to find an association of vanadium with mania (Kumar et al. 1989).

VINYL CHLORIDE

Vinyl chloride, the base for polyvinyl chloride (PVC), is important in the plastics industry. Also called chloroethane or chloroethylene, vinyl chloride's past uses included propellants for pesticides and reagents in trichloroethylene production. PVC also has uses in apparel, building and construction, electrical components, homes, packaging, recreation, transportation, and numerous other aspects of modern society (Warren et al. 1978). Vinyl chloride, a toxic gas, causes numerous physical symptoms (see Table 17–3). Table 17–4 lists psychiatric symptoms attributed to vinyl chloride exposures.

OTHER CHEMICALS OR ELEMENTS

Table 17–5 lists case reports or epidemiological studies of other miscellaneous substances with psychiatric importance.

TABLE 17–3. Physical signs and symptoms of vinyl chloride poisoning

Cardiovascular	Hypotension, hypertension, vascular occlusions, varices, Raynaud's disease
Gastrointestinal	Liver disease, cholestasis, splenomegaly, Banti's syndrome
Skin	Scleroderma-like changes, dermatitis, formication, thickening of skin, skin nodules, fissuration of elastic fibers
Bone	Pseudoclubbing of fingers, acro-osteolysis
Blood	Thrombocytopenia, leukopenia, reticulocytosis

TABLE 17–4. Psychiatric signs and symptoms attributed to vinyl chloride poisoning

Mood	Nervousness, euphoria, irritability, depression
Behavior	Singing, whistling, sardonic or careless laughter (acute)
Cognitive	Memory loss
Perceptual	Hallucinations
Other	Insomnia, somnolence, loss of libido, fatigue, "psychic disturbances or astheno-autonomic syndrome" (older European literature)

GEOPHAGIA

Geophagia consists of eating dirt or clay, although early descriptions from the West Indies included charcoal, chalk, dried mortar, mud, sand, shells, rotten wood, cloth, paper, and hair (Cragin 1835). During the nineteenth century, many believed that geophagia stopped vomiting, cured constipation and syphilis, and improved fetal posture (Edwards et al. 1959). More recent literature describes individuals who consume cornstarch, flour, soot, and baking soda (Edwards et al. 1954). Some attribute the behavior to hookworm infestation or iron deficiency; the former is not supported by epidemiological research (Dickins and Ford 1942). Geophagia meets the DSM-IV-TR criteria for a culture-bound syndrome (American Psychiatric Association 2000). In the United States, geophagia is practiced primarily by African American women in southern communities who have the cultural belief that to resist cravings for a given substance during pregnancy "marks the unborn" (Edwards et al. 1954). Some individuals bake and eat substances before, with, or after meals. They become

TABLE 17–5. Case reports or epidemiological studies of other substances with psychiatric importance

Nitrous oxide	
Brodsky and Zuniga 1975	Case report of 32-year-old dentist: daily inhalant abuse of nitrous oxide for 6 months; developed paranoid delusions and hallucinations; resolved rapidly with hospitalization.
Carbon tetrachloride	
Stevens and Forster 1953	Literature review: one report of mania with 7 months' hospitalization; case report of social drinker who consumed carbon tetrachloride while cleaning a gun: on day 18, patient had neurological signs and hallucinations; on day 84, patient had confusion, personality change, memory loss, euphoria. Summary of 15 cases of poisoning often associated with alcohol intake that worsens symptoms of confusion, disorientation, and impaired mental function.
Dimethylaminopropionitrile (DMAPN)	
Keogh et al. 1980	Epidemic exposure of 141 workers: compared with control subjects, exposed group had greater impotence, insomnia, and irritability.
Acrylamide	
Igisu et al. 1975	Family poisoned by acrylamide in well water: one case with neurological signs, confusion, hallucinations, poor memory; second case with euphoria, poor memory, and hallucinations for 1 week; third case with hallucinations, sleepiness, and poor memory; children sleepy and showing peculiar behavior.
Cesium	
Ali et al. 1985	Study of 25 depressed individuals: decreased levels of cesium that increased during recovery compared with control subjects.
Kumar et al. 1989	Study of groups of depressed, manic, recovered, and "normal" individuals: no differences in hair, whole blood, serum, or urine levels of cesium.
Tellurium	
Blackadder and Manderson 1975	Two case reports of laboratory exposure: symptoms of somnolence with garlic breath and bluish black discoloration of webs of fingers; streaks on face and neck.

anxious when unable to eat the substance, and they eat the substance when upset (Edwards et al. 1959). Some men also engage in the behavior (Edwards et al. 1959). Infants of clay-eating women often have "coatings" at birth (Edwards et al. 1954). Geophagia places an individual at risk for consuming neurotoxic naturally occurring elements or chemicals contaminating the soil. One case report described lead nephropathy from eating contaminated garden soil (Grandjean 1993).

REFERENCES

Akil M, Brewer GJ: Psychiatric and behavioral abnormalities in Wilson's disease. Adv Neurol 65:171–178, 1995

Akil M, Schwartz JA, Dutchak D, et al: The psychiatric presentations of Wilson's disease. Journal of Neuropsychiatry 3:377–382, 1991

Ali SA, Peet M, Ward NI: Blood levels of vanadium, caesium, and other elements in depressive patients. J Affect Disord 9:187–191, 1985

American Psychiatric Association: Diagnostic and Statistical Manual of Mental Disorders, 4th Edition, Text Revision. Washington, DC, American Psychiatric Association, 2000

Blackadder ES, Manderson WG: Occupational absorption of tellurium: a report of two cases. British Journal of Industrial Medicine 32:59–61, 1975

Brewer GJ, Yuzbasiyan-Gurkan V: Wilson disease. Medicine 71:139–164, 1992

Brinton LA, Lubin JH, Burich MC, et al: Mortality among augmentation mammoplasty patients. Epidemiology 12:321–326, 2001

Brodsky L, Zuniga J: Nitrous oxide: a psychotogenic agent. Compr Psychiatry 16:185–188, 1975

Cragin FW: Observations on cachexia Africana or dirt-eating. Am J Med Sci 17:356–364, 1835

Dening TR: Psychiatric aspects of Wilson's disease. Br J Psychiatry 147:677–682, 1985

Dening TR, Berrios GE: Wilson's disease: a prospective study of psychopathology in 31 cases. Br J Psychiatry 155:206–213, 1989a

Dening TR, Berrios GE: Wilson's disease: psychiatric symptoms in 195 cases. Arch Gen Psychiatry 46:1126–1134, 1989b

Dickins D, Ford RN: Geophagy (dirt eating) among Mississippi Negro school children. American Sociological Review 7:59–65, 1942

Dutton WF: Vanadiumism (abstract). JAMA 56:1648, 1911

Edwards CH, McSwain H, Haire S: Odd dietary practices of women. J Am Diet Assoc 30:976–981, 1954

Edwards CH, McDonald S, Mitchell JR, et al: Clay- and cornstarch-eating women. J Am Diet Assoc 35:810–815, 1959

Gosselin RE, Smith RP, Hodge HC: Copper, in Clinical Toxicology of Commercial Products. Edited by Gosselin RE, Smith RP, Hodge HC. Baltimore, MD, Williams & Wilkins, 1984, pp 120–123

Grandjean P: Application of neurobehavioral methods in environmental and occupational health. Environ Res 60:57–61, 1993

Hart RP, Silverman JJ, Garrettson LK, et al: Neuropsychological function following mild exposure to pentaborane. Am J Ind Med 6:37–44, 1984

Hartard C, Weisner B, Dieu C, et al: Wilson's disease with cerebral manifestation: monitoring therapy by CSF copper concentration. J Neurol 241:101–107, 1993

Igisu H, Goto I, Kawamura Y, et al: Acrylamide encephaloneuropathy due to well water pollution. J Neurol Neurosurg Psychiatry 38:581–584, 1975

Kent JM, Papp LA, Martinez JM, et al: Specificity of panic response to CO_2 inhalation in panic disorder: a comparison with major depression and premenstrual dysphoric disorder. Am J Psychiatry 158:58–67, 2001

Keogh JP, Pestronk A, Wertheimer D, et al: An epidemic of urinary retention caused by dimethylaminopropionitrile. JAMA 243:746–749, 1980

Kjoller K, Friis S, Mellemkjaer L, et al: Connective tissue disease and other rheumatic conditions following cosmetic breast implantation in Denmark. Arch Intern Med 161:973–979, 2001

Kumar R, Wright I, Naylor GJ, et al: Caesium levels in manic depressive psychosis. J Affect Disord 17:17–19, 1989

Laing TJ, Schottenfeld D, Lacey JV Jr, et al: Potential risk factors for undifferentiated connective tissue disease among women: implanted medical devices. Am J Epidemiol 154:610–617, 2001

Lewis DR: Dopant materials used in the microelectronics industry. State of the Art Reviews in Occupational Medicine 1:35–47, 1986

Maroni M, Colombi A, Buratti M, et al: Human exposure to vanadium and nickel from fuel-oil combustion residues, in Heavy Metals in the Environment, Vol 2. Edited by Lindberg SE, Hutchinson TC. Edinburgh, CEP Consultants, 1987, pp 101–103

Mastromatteo E, Sullivan F: Summary: International Symposium on the Health Effects of Boron and Its Compounds. Environ Health Perspect 102 (suppl 7):139–141, 1994

Medalia A, Isaacs-Glaberman K, Scheinberg IH: Neuropsychological impairment in Wilson's disease. Arch Neurol 45:502–504, 1988

Modai I, Karp L, Liberman UA, et al: Penicillamine therapy for schizophreniform psychosis in Wilson's disease. J Nerv Ment Dis 173:698–701, 1985

Naylor GJ, Smith AHW: Vanadium: a possible aetiological factor in manic depressive illness. Psychol Med 11:249–256, 1981

Perez EL, Silverman M: CO_2 intoxication. Psychiatric Journal of the University of Ottawa 6:226–228, 1981

Pine DS, Klein RG, Coplan JD, et al: Differential carbon dioxide sensitivity in childhood anxiety disorders and non-ill comparison group. Arch Gen Psychiatry 57:960–967, 2000

Rosenberg NL: The neuromythology of silicone breast implants. Neurology 46:308–314, 1996

Silverman JJ, Hart RP, Garrettson LK, et al: Posttraumatic stress disorder from pentaborane intoxication: neuropsychiatric evaluation and short-term follow-up. JAMA 254:2603–2608, 1985

Stevens H, Forster FM: Effect of carbon tetrachloride on the nervous system. AMA Archives of Neurology and Psychiatry 70:635–649, 1953

Thomas DLG, Stiebris K: Vanadium poisoning in industry. Med J Aust 1:607–609, 1956

Warren HS, Huff JE, Gerstner HB: Vinyl Chloride: A Review 1835–1975; An Annotated Literature Collection 1835–1975; A Literature Compilation 1976–1977. Oak Ridge, TN, Oak Ridge National Laboratory, 1978

Wilde C: Aerosol metallic paints: deliberate inhalation: a study of inhalation and/or ingestion of copper and zinc particles. International Journal of the Addictions 10:127–134, 1975

Wilson SAK: Progressive lenticular degeneration: a familial nervous disease associated with cirrhosis of the liver. Brain 34:295–509, 1912

Winther JF, Friis S, Bach FW, et al: Neurological disease among women with silicone breast implants in Denmark. Acta Neurol Scand 103:93–96, 2001

Wolfe F, Anderson J: Silicone filled breast implants and the risk of fibromyalgia and rheumatoid arthritis. J Rheumatol 26:2025–2028, 1999

Yarbrough BE, Garrettson LK, Zolet DI, et al: Severe central nervous system damage and profound acidosis in persons exposed to pentaborane. Clin Toxicol 23:519–536, 1985

Yelin G, Taff ML, Sadowski GE: Copper toxicity following massive ingestion of coins. Am J Forensic Med Pathol 8:78–85, 1987

ADDITIONAL READINGS

Langauer-Lewowicka H, Kurzbauer H, Byczkowska Z, et al: Vinyl chloride disease—neurological disturbances. Int Arch Occup Environ Health 52:151–157, 1983

Lowe HJ, Freeman G: Boron hydride (borane) intoxication in man. AMA Archives of Industrial Hygiene and Occupational Medicine 16 523–533, 1957

Mindrum G: Pentaborane intoxication. Arch Intern Med 114:364–374, 1964

Rozendaal HM: Clinical observations on the toxicology of boron hydrides. AMA Archives of Industrial Hygiene and Occupational Medicine 4:257–260, 1951

Styblova V, Lambl V, Chumcal O, et al: Neurological changes in vinyl chloride-exposed workers. Journal of Hygiene, Epidemiology, Microbiology and Immunology 25:233–243, 1981

Suciu I, Prodan L, Ilea E, et al: Clinical manifestations in vinyl chloride poisoning. Ann N Y Acad Sci 246:53–69, 1975

Veltman G, Lange C-E, Juhe S, et al: Clinical manifestations and course of vinyl chloride disease. Ann N Y Acad Sci 246:6–17, 1975

18

Sensitivity Syndromes

MULTIPLE CHEMICAL SENSITIVITY

An allergist, Theron Randolph, proposed the concept of multiple chemical sensitivities (MCS) 40 years ago when he theorized that food allergies cause fatigue, irritability, and behavior problems in children (Randolph 1947). He hospitalized patients and treated them with "comprehensive environmental control," during which they stayed in special units with no exposure to drugs, cosmetics, perfumes, or other chemicals (Miller and Ashford 1992; Randolph 1962). Over a period of 4–7 days, patients "withdrew" from chemicals, after which they were said to develop a sense of well-being. A challenge with low-level chemical exposures then tested their reactions to exposure (Miller and Ashford 1992). Frequently, patients showed sensitivity to a few chemicals, only to have a "spreading" of their reactions to broad categories of chemicals. The recommended treatment often involved living in specially constructed dwellings in reclusive lifestyles to avoid all levels of chemical exposure. Other treatments included "neutralization procedures," megadoses of vitamins, antimycotic drugs, enemas, and sweating cures (Wolf 1994). The field became known as "clinical ecology" ("Clinical Ecology" 1976) but never gained acceptance by mainstream medicine.

The Controversy

Table 18–1 lists the various names given to MCS. The most recent name for MCS is "idiopathic environmental intolerances," or IEI (Bornschein et al. 2001). The variety of names reflects the unresolved definition of MCS. A survey of physicians familiar with MCS proposed six characteristics of MCS, as listed in Table 18–2 (Bartha et al. 1999). Table 18–3 lists the most frequent symptoms. MCS symptoms often overlap with symptoms of chronic fatigue syndrome and fibromyalgia (Jason et al. 2000; Nawab et al. 2000). Prevalence of MCS in community surveys and occupational health clinics was found to be 6.3% and 23.0%, respectively (Kreutzer et al. 1999; Kutsogiannis and Davidoff 2001).

TABLE 18–1. Other names for multiple chemical sensitivities

Allergic to everything	Environmentally induced disease
Allergic toxemia	Environment-related malabsorption
Autointoxication	Food and chemical sensitivities
Candida hypersensitivity syndrome	Idiopathic environmental intolerance
Cerebral allergy	Immune dysregulation syndrome
Chemical acquired immunodeficiency syndrome	Multiple chemical intolerance
	Panallergy
Chemical hypersensitivity disease	Systemic candidiasis
Chemical multiple sensitivity	Total allergy syndrome
Chemical-induced immune dysregulation	Total environmental allergy
	Twentieth-century disease
Ecological illness	Universal allergy
Environmental illness or disease	Yeast disease
Environmental somatization disorder	

TABLE 18–2. Six common characteristics of multiple chemical sensitivities

1. Symptoms reoccur with exposure.
2. The condition is chronic.
3. Low-level exposures result in symptoms.
4. Symptoms resolve after removal from chemicals.
5. Responses occur with multiple, unrelated chemicals.
6. Symptoms involve several organ systems.

TABLE 18–3. Most frequent symptoms of multiple chemical sensitivities

Central nervous system	Lack of energy, trouble concentrating, depression, memory loss, weakness, dizziness, headache, abnormal sleep, fainting, impaired speech
Gastrointestinal	Fullness, flatulence, diarrhea, constipation, abdominal pain, heartburn
Other	Heat intolerance, joint pain, muscle pain, skin problems, irritation of the ocular mucosa and upper respiratory tract

Source. Lax and Henneberger 1995; Wolf 1996.

Proponents and opponents of MCS agree on two epidemiological characteristics of the multiple chemical sensitivity syndrome. Individuals said to have MCS usually are 35- to 50-year-old white women who are employed primarily in manufacturing or services jobs and who have serious personal and social impairments (Keplinger 1994; Lax and Henneberger 1995; Rosenthal and Cameron 1991; Wilson 1994). The controversy over MCS focuses on the cause and treatment of the impairments. Proponents of MCS describe a mechanism of pathogenesis consisting of "stages," shown in Table 18–4. Several professional societies, including the American Academy of Allergy and Immunology, the American College of Physicians, the American Medical Association Council on Scientific Affairs (1992), the American College of Occupational and Environmental Medicine (1999), the Alberta Implementation Committee for Health, and the California Medical Association, found no scientific basis for these proposed stages of MCS (Anderson et al. 1986; California Medical Association Scientific Board Task Force on Clinical Ecology 1986; Kurt 1995; Perry 1995). A survey of the physician members of the Association of Occupational and Environmental Clinics found that 83% believed that MCS result from combined psychiatric and physical factors, 62% believed that psychiatric factors play a greater role, 9% viewed physical factors as more important, and 25% had no opinion (Rest 1992).

Opponents of MCS argue that behavioral and stress-mediated mechanisms control the symptoms. They claim that MCS most likely represents the overlapping of primary psychiatric disorders, misdiagnosed medical disorders, and classical conditioning. One study found significantly increased prevalence of the panic disorder–associated cholecystokinin B receptor allele 7 in subjects with MCS (Binkley et al. 2001). Three opposing interpretations of MCS are that

TABLE 18–4. Stages of multiple chemical sensitivity

Stage 1	"Adaptation" begins with "alarm" or awareness that exposure causes symptoms.
Stage 2	Development of "tolerance" or "masking" of symptoms.
Stage 3	Maladaptation to exposure, leading to end-organ failure over 20–30 years, including coronary artery disease and lung failure.
Bipolarity	Bipolarity occurs in any stage; a two-step process of immune and enzyme reactions to toxins; during the first part, the exposed person develops "addiction" to pollutants, causing "highs" and "withdrawal"; "junk food addiction" prevents withdrawal; second phase involves impairment of detoxification and metabolic processes.
Spreading	As the person becomes chemically sensitive, the sensitivity "spreads" to other chemicals that did not originally cause symptoms.
Switching	Symptoms of sensitivity "switch" from one organ system to another, causing multiple symptoms.

Source. Data gathered from Rea 1992, 1994.

1) MCS results from chemical exposures, but the sensitivity is stress mediated or is a classically conditioned response; 2) MCS represents misdiagnosed physical or psychiatric problems; or 3) MCS is a culturally shaped illness belief system (Simon 1994; Sparks et al. 1994a). Regardless of mechanism, the opposing consensus holds that disagreement over etiology does not prohibit treatment of an individual's symptoms (Sparks et al. 1994a). Symptoms, critics say, respond to conventional treatments that avoid the disabling social and occupational withdrawal recommended by clinical ecologists.

Table 18–5 lists diagnostic and treatment approaches with the greatest success according to scientific consensus. Individuals with the belief that their symptoms result from chemical exposure have poorer treatment outcomes than those without such beliefs (Black et al. 2000; Gupta and Horne 2001). Evaluations of patients with MCS should include a full medical examination, including exposure history and consultations with occupational and psychiatric specialists (Sparks et al. 1994b). Adrenal insufficiency, seizures, and certain classes of medications can decrease the olfactory detection threshold and must be ruled out in complaints of MCS (Scott 1989). One case report described an individual with MCS found to have an occipital lobe meningioma. Removal of the tumor did not resolve the MCS symptoms (Moorhead and Suruda 2000).

TABLE 18–5. Diagnostic and treatment considerations for alleged multiple chemical sensitivity

- In many cases, multiple chemical sensitivity symptoms result from classical conditioning. An initial exposure causes emotional reactions during or after the exposure; odor acts as a future "trigger" or "conditioned stimulus" for symptoms. Symptoms result from autonomic hyperactivity from fear of exposure (Amundsen et al. 1996; Bolla-Wilson et al. 1988; Schottenfeld 1987; Shusterman and Dager 1991).
- No scientifically validated test substantiates the diagnosis of multiple chemical sensitivities. The diagnosis of multiple chemical sensitivities may "perpetuate illness, prolong disability, and delay therapy" (Sparks et al. 1994b).
- The importance of thorough medical examination cannot be overemphasized in the assessment of symptoms attributed to chemical exposure. Overlap of direct toxic effects of chemicals can occur with posttraumatic stress symptoms; odor may act as the reminder of a life-threatening event.
- Individuals with multiple chemical sensitivities may have undiagnosed psychiatric illnesses or histories of physical and sexual abuse presenting as illness from chemicals (Black 1993; Friedman 1994; Staudenmayer et al. 1992).
- Rather than recommend withdrawal from the environment and society, appropriate treatment includes tolerance of the environment through stress reduction through marriage, physical therapy, prayer, guided imagery with music, group and individual therapy, meditation, regular exercise, biofeedback, behavior desensitization, and increased social activity. Avoidance reinforces the learned connection between exposure and symptoms; increased exposure establishes symptom control (Guglielmi et al. 1994; Haller 1993; Simon 1994; Sparks et al. 1994b).
- Patients who deny the role of stress have a poorer prognosis (Sparks et al. 1994b).
- Formal testing does not substantiate cognitive deficits claimed by patients with multiple chemical sensitivities (Fiedler et al. 1994).

Unresolved Issues

Three issues in the area of chemical susceptibility need further research. First, the medical literature contains reports not associated with MCS ideology that describe individuals with enhanced sensitivities to chemical exposures after initial exposures (Dille and Smith 1964; Tabershaw and Cooper 1966). These reactions could result from posttraumatic stress disorder, in which later exposures to odors induce recurrent symptoms. The role of odor in evoking the symptoms of posttraumatic stress disorder needs further study. Second, a growing body of literature supports the notion that some persons have enhanced genetic susceptibility to low doses of chemicals (Calabrese 1978, 1991; Stokinger and Mountain 1967). This does not equate to a physiological basis of MCS but does represent an opportunity to identify individuals who may develop unexpected toxic responses. Third, toxicological and epidemiological information is lacking for women who may have a sex-based sensitivity to certain chemical classes (Calabrese 1986; Zielhuis et al. 1984).

FOOD ADDITIVES AND CHILDHOOD BEHAVIOR DISORDERS

In the 1970s, Feingold proposed that food additives, especially colors and flavors, caused hyperactivity and other childhood behavior disorders. He further claimed that instituting a special diet lacking these substances would treat the conditions (Feingold 1974, 1975a, 1975b, 1976, 1978, 1982).

The putative association between additives and behavior came to the public's attention and gained popularity before well-controlled studies tested the theory. In some families, the belief in "food allergies" resulted in bizarre lifestyles and diets, referred to as an "allergic form of Munchausen by proxy" (Crook 1974). Adverse medical outcomes also occurred when physicians misdiagnosed food allergies when there were serious medical conditions (Robertson et al. 1988). Several investigations that used placebo-controlled, double-blind crossover experiments did not confirm the association. Similar findings ruled out any effect of sugar on children's behavior (Milich et al. 1986). Several groups issued consensus opinions rejecting the effectiveness of the Feingold diet (Consensus Conference 1982; Singh et al. 1998; U.S. Interagency Collaborative Group on Hyperkinesis 1975; Wender and Lipton 1980). The Consensus Conference of the National Institutes of Health (NIH) (Consensus Conference 1982) provided clear recommendations that stood the test of more recent clinical studies.

Table 18–6 summarizes the NIH recommendations, which also state that a small number of children may benefit from a diet without additives. The basis for the benefit remains unclear, but studies that used placebo-controlled, double-blind techniques substantiated the idea (Boris and Mandel 1994; Carter et al. 1993; Kaplan et al. 1989; Rowe 1988; Rowe and Rowe 1994). The effect may be limited and may occur only if high doses of additives are initially being con-

TABLE 18–6. Evaluation and treatment recommendations for children's hyperactivity attributed to food additives

- Controlled studies of hyperactivity in children on defined diets produce inconsistent results.
- Defined diets should not be used universally for treating childhood hyperactivity.
- A small group of individuals who cannot be identified beforehand may show improvement with a defined diet. Dietary treatment in these cases may be warranted.
- A defined diet should not be initiated without thorough evaluation of the child and family, consideration of traditional treatment, and evaluation of cultural, ethnic, and socioeconomic factors involved in implementing the diet.

sumed (Warner 1997). The plausibility of the concept extends from recognition that of the thousands of food additives, some may pose problems for a few individuals with specific sensitivities (Concon 1988; Weiss 1984). Certain adults may exhibit sensitivities to foods and food additives (Ledochowski et al. 2000; Smith et al. 2001).

SICK BUILDING SYNDROME

Building-related illnesses range from life-threatening illnesses that need immediate medical treatment to sick building syndrome, a serious but less urgent condition. Building-related illness is known by several names (Table 18–7) and can be confused with mass hysteria and multiple chemical sensitivity. Building-related illnesses emerged in the 1970s and 1980s following the energy crisis that forced more buildings to have high-efficiency insulation and central mechanical ventilation (Kreiss 1989). To further conserve energy, the recommended minimum of indoor air exchange was reduced by 50% (Bardana Jr. et al. 1988). These circumstances produced emergent infectious diseases, including legionnaires' disease from *Legionella pneumophila,* an organism isolated from air conditioning systems; Pontiac fever, the nonpneumonic form of legionnaires' disease; and Q fever, caused by airborne transmission of *Coxiella burnetii* in certain buildings (Bardana Jr. et al. 1988; Seltzer 1994). An assortment of new diseases, listed in Table 18–8, appeared, sometimes in remarkable circumstances. One instance involved a federal building with an air conditioning system that generated 83,000 fungal spores per cubic meter of air (Bardana Jr. et al. 1988).

TABLE 18–7. Names applied to building-related illness

Tight building syndrome	Indoor air pollution
Problem building	Sick building syndrome
Closed building problem	Building-associated illness
Building-related illness	Transient office-related annoyance
New building syndrome	Transient office-related irritation
Crisis building	Idiopathic building intolerance

TABLE 18–8. Building-related illnesses and their causes

Illness	**Cause**
Hypersensitivity pneumonitis	Fungi, bacteria, protozoa in heating and cooling systems
Humidifier fever	Various infectious agents
Asthma and allergic rhinitis	Dust mites and fungi
Infectious diseases	Legionnaires' disease, Pontiac fever, Q fever
Building-related dermatitis	Fibrous glass, mineral wool
Corneal lacerations	Fibrous glass, mineral wool
Sick building syndrome	Multifactorial

Source. Data collected from Bardana Jr. 1992; Bardana Jr. et al. 1988; Colligan 1981.

The U.S. Public Health Service estimates that most building-related complaints result from poor ventilation, with smaller percentages of complaints from combinations of indoor air contaminants, outside contaminants, humidity, building fabrics, tobacco smoke, noise, or illumination (Bardana Jr. et al. 1988). Indoor pollutants include chemicals from duplicating, signature, and blueprint machines; pesticides; boiler additives; rug shampoos; tobacco smoke; and combustion gases from cafeterias and laboratories (Letz 1990). Cigarette smoke plays a major role in causing many symptoms (Bardana Jr. 1992). In smaller buildings and homes, improperly installed wood stoves may explain symptoms (Montanaro and Bardana Jr. 1992). Outdoor pollutants found in buildings include vehicle exhausts from indoor parking garages, contaminants from nearby construction and renovation projects, and gasoline leaks from underground tanks (Letz 1990). The World Health Organization estimated that 30% of new or remodeled buildings show indications of building-related complaints affecting 10%–30% of the occupants (Lyles et al. 1991).

Symptoms and Treatment of Sick Building Syndrome

Sick building syndrome constitutes a type of building-related illness with several subjective symptoms, listed in Table 18–9. General symptoms include complaints of fatigue and sleep and mood problems. In the absence of objective findings of disease, the literature supports a multifactorial cause of sick building syndrome that includes elements of mass hysteria and somatization. Organizational dysfunction, poor communications with workers, and personality factors may enhance subjective complaints (Berglund and Gunnarsson 2000; Thorn 2000). Causes of sick building syndrome include chemical odors that act as "triggers" of autonomic arousal. Employees then attribute their workplace psychological problems to chemical exposures. Table 18–10 summarizes the numerous factors associated with outbreaks of sick building syndrome. When diagnosing sick building syndrome, the clinician should not discount a fever or other indication of infectious or other disease. Treatment of sick building syndrome should follow recommendations described for multiple chemical sensitivities and mass hysteria.

TABLE 18–9. Common symptoms of sick building syndrome

Chest tightness	Nasal obstruction and complaints
Decreased concentration and memory	Ocular complaints, including dry eyes
Depression	Odd tastes
Dizziness	Oropharyngeal complaints, dryness
Epistaxis	Palpitations
Fatigue, headache, myalgias	Skin complaints

Formaldehyde

Half the formaldehyde produced is used to make insulation and particleboard. The remainder contributes to 13 other chemical classes and more than 25 consumer product classes that require more than 75 occupational classes to manufacture (Feinman 1988a; Lilis 1992). Cigarette smoke also contains formaldehyde. During the energy crisis of the 1970s, many homeowners heavily insulated their homes with urea-formaldehyde foam insulation. People attributed various health complaints, including sick building syndrome, to the new insulation. Symptoms attributed to formaldehyde included headache, nausea, memory loss, anorexia, indigestion, insomnia, and depression.

TABLE 18–10. Factors associated with outbreaks of sick building syndrome

Psychosocial	Female sex; poor workplace cooperation; preexisting psychological problems; dissatisfaction with job, superiors, or colleagues; high school education or less; boring job category; work stress; excessive layers of clothing
Environmental	Uncomfortable humidity and temperature; cigarette smoke; photocopiers and video display terminals; handling carbonless paper; chilled, humidified air from mechanical ventilation; level of lighting; odor complaints; organic debris/volatile organic compounds
Medical	Atopy

The debate over the association of formaldehyde with health complaints overlapped the controversies over multiple chemical sensitivities and sick building syndrome.

Acute, and sometimes fatal, complications of pulmonary, metabolic, renal, and hepatic functions result from formaldehyde intoxication (Feinman 1988b; Gosselin et al. 1984). No strong evidence links formaldehyde to significant and consistent neurotoxicity (Bardana and Montanaro 1987).

REFERENCES

American College of Occupational and Environmental Medicine: Multiple chemical sensitivities: idiopathic environmental intolerance. J Occup Environ Med 41: 940–942, 1999

American Medical Association Council on Scientific Affairs: Clinical ecology. JAMA 268:3465–3467, 1992

Amundsen MA, Hanson NP, Bruce BK, et al: Odor aversion or multiple chemical sensitivities: recommendation for a name change and description of successful behavioral medicine treatment. Regul Toxicol Pharmacol 24:S116–S118, 1996

Anderson JA, Chai H, Claman HN, et al: Position statements: clinical ecology. J Allergy Clin Immunol 78:269–271, 1986

Bardana EJ, Montanaro A: The formaldehyde fiasco: a review of the scientific data. Immunology and Allergy Practice 9:11–24, 1987

Bardana EJ Jr: Building-related illness, in Occupational Asthma. Edited by Bardana EJ Jr, Montanaro A, O'Hollaren MT. Philadelphia, PA, Hanley & Belfus, 1992, pp 237–254

Bardana EJ Jr, Montanaro A, O'Hollaren MT: Building-related illness: a review of available scientific data. Clinical Reviews in Allergy 6:61–89, 1988

Bartha L, Baumzweiger W, Buscher D, et al: Multiple chemical sensitivity: a 1999 consensus. Arch Environ Health 54:147–149, 1999

Berglund B, Gunnarsson AG: Relationships between occupant personality and the sick building syndrome explored. Indoor Air 10:152–169, 2000

Binkley K, King N, Poonai N, et al: Idiopathic environmental intolerance: increased prevalence of panic-disorder-associated cholecystokinin B receptor allele 7. J Allergy Clin Immunol 107:887–890, 2001
Black DW: Environmental illness and misdiagnosis—a growing problem. Regul Toxicol Pharmacol 18:23–31, 1993
Black DW, Okiishi C, Schlosser S: A nine-year follow-up of people diagnosed with multiple chemical sensitivities. Psychosomatics 41:253–261, 2000
Bolla-Wilson K, Wilson RJ, Bleecker ML: Conditioning of physical symptoms after neurotoxic exposure. J Occup Med 30:684–686, 1988
Boris M, Mandel FS: Foods and additives are common causes of the attention deficit hyperactive disorder in children. Ann Allergy 72:462–468, 1994
Bornschein S, Forstl H, Zilker T: Idiopathic environmental intolerances (formerly multiple chemical sensitivity): psychiatric perspectives. J Intern Med 250:309–321, 2001
Calabrese EJ: Pollutants and High-Risk Groups: The Biological Basis of Increased Human Susceptibility to Environmental and Occupational Pollutants. New York, Wiley-Interscience, 1978
Calabrese EJ: Editorial: sex differences in susceptibility to toxic industrial chemicals. British Journal of Industrial Medicine 43:577–579, 1986
Calabrese EJ: Genetic predisposition to occupationally related diseases: current status and future directions, in Ecogenetics: Genetic Predisposition to the Toxic Effects of Chemicals. Edited by Grandjean P. London, Chapman & Hall, 1991, pp 21–55
California Medical Association Scientific Board Task Force on Clinical Ecology: Clinical ecology—a critical appraisal. West J Med 144:239–245, 1986
Carter CM, Urbanowicz M, Hemsley R, et al: Effects of a few food diet in attention deficit disorder. Arch Dis Child 69:564–568, 1993
Clinical Ecology. Springfield, IL, Charles C Thomas, 1976
Colligan MJ: The psychological effects of indoor air pollution. Bull N Y Acad Med 57: 1014–1026, 1981
Concon JM: Food Toxicology. New York, Marcel Dekker, 1988
Consensus Conference: Defined diets and childhood hyperactivity. JAMA 248:290–292, 1982
Crook WG: An alternate method of managing the hyperactive child (letter). Pediatrics 54:656, 1974
Dille JR, Smith PW: Central nervous system effects of chronic exposure to organophosphate insecticides. Aerospace Medicine 35:475–478, 1964
Feingold BF: Why Your Child Is Hyperactive. New York, Random House, 1974
Feingold BF: Adverse reactions to food additives with special reference to hyperkinesis and learning difficulty (H-LD), in The Man/Food Equation. Edited by Steele F, Bourne A. London, Academic, 1975a, pp 215–234
Feingold BF: Hyperkinesis and learning disabilities linked to artificial food flavors and colors. Am J Nurs 75:797–803, 1975b
Feingold BF: Hyperkinesis and learning disabilities linked to the ingestion of artificial food colors and flavors. J Learn Disabil 9:19 (551)–27 (559), 1976
Feingold BF: Dietary management of juvenile delinquency. International Journal of Offender Therapy and Comparative Criminology 22:73–84, 1978
Feingold BF: The role of diet in behavior. Ecology of Disease 1:153–165, 1982
Feinman SE: Exposure to formaldehyde, in Formaldehyde Sensitivity and Toxicity. Edited by Feinman SE. Boca Raton, FL, CRC Press, 1988a, pp 18–36
Feinman SE: Formaldehyde toxicity, in Formaldehyde Sensitivity and Toxicity. Edited by Feinman SE. Boca Raton, FL, CRC Press, 1988b, pp 156–166
Fiedler N, Kipen H, DeMarco J, et al: Neuropsychology and psychology of MCS. Toxicol Ind Health 10:545–554, 1994
Friedman MJ: Neurobiological sensitization models of PTSD: their possible relevance to multiple chemical sensitivity syndrome. Toxicol Ind Health 10:449–462, 1994

Gosselin RE, Smith RP, Hodge HC, et al: Clinical Toxicology of Commercial Products. Baltimore, MD, Williams & Wilkins, 1984

Guglielmi RS, Cox DJ, Spyker DA: Behavioral treatment of phobic avoidance in multiple chemical sensitivity. J Behav Ther Exp Psychiatry 25:197–209, 1994

Gupta K, Horne R: The influence of health beliefs on the presentation and consultation outcome in patients with chemical sensitivities. J Psychosom Res 50:131–137, 2001

Haller E: Successful management of patients with "multiple chemical sensitivities" on an inpatient psychiatric unit. J Clin Psychiatry 54:196–199, 1993

Jason LA, Taylor RR, Kennedy CL: Chronic fatigue syndrome, fibromyalgia, and multiple chemical sensitivities in a community-based sample of persons with chronic fatigue syndrome–like symptoms. Psychosom Med 62:655–663, 2000

Kaplan BJ, McNicol J, Conte RA, et al: Dietary replacement in preschool-aged hyperactive boys. Pediatrics 83:7–17, 1989

Keplinger H: Patient statement: chemically sensitive. Toxicol Ind Health 10:313–317, 1994

Kreiss K: The epidemiology of building-related complaints and illness. Occup Med 4:575–592, 1989

Kreutzer R, Neutra RR, Lashuay N: Prevalence of people reporting sensitivities to chemicals in a population-based survey. Am J Epidemiol 150:1–12, 1999

Kurt TL: Multiple chemical sensitivities—a syndrome of pseudotoxicity manifest as exposure perceived symptoms. J Toxicol Clin Toxicol 33:101–105, 1995

Kutsogiannis DJ, Davidoff AL: A multiple center study of multiple chemical sensitivity syndrome. Arch Environ Health 56:196–207, 2001

Lax MB, Henneberger PK: Patients with multiple chemical sensitivities in an occupational health clinic: presentation and follow-up. Arch Environ Health 50:425–431, 1995

Ledochowski M, Widner B, Bair H, et al: Fructose- and sorbitol-reduced diet improves mood and gastrointestinal disturbances in fructose malabsorbers. Scand J Gastroenterol 35:1048–1052, 2000

Letz GA: Sick building syndrome: acute illness among office workers—the role of building ventilation, airborne contaminants and work stress. Allergy Proceedings 11:109–116, 1990

Lilis R: Diseases associated with exposure to chemical substances: organic compounds, in Public Health and Preventive Medicine. Edited by Last JM, Wallace RB. Norwalk, CT, Appleton & Lange, 1992, pp 403–454

Lyles WB, Greve KW, Bauer RM, et al: Sick building syndrome. South Med J 84:65–71, 1991

Milich R, Wolraich M, Lindgren S: Sugar and hyperactivity: a critical review of empirical findings. Clin Psychol Rev 6:493–513, 1986

Miller CS, Ashford NA: Allergy and multiple chemical sensitivities distinguished, in Multiple Chemical Sensitivities: Addendum to Biologic Markers in Immunotoxicology. Edited by Board on Environmental Studies and Toxicology. Washington, DC, National Academy Press, 1992, pp 47–63

Montanaro A, Bardana EJ Jr: The chemically sensitive patient, in Occupational Asthma. Edited by Bardana EJ Jr, Montanaro A, O'Hollaren MT. Philadelphia, PA, Hanley & Belfus, 1992, pp 255–266

Moorhead JF, Suruda AJ: Occipital lobe meningioma in a patient with multiple chemical sensitivities. Am J Ind Med 37:443–446, 2000

Nawab SS, Miller CS, Dale JK, et al: Self-reported sensitivity to chemical exposures in five clinical populations and healthy controls. Psychiatry Res 95:67–74, 2000

Perry S: Tech-brief from the Alberta Implementation Committee for Health Technology Assessment. Int J Technol Assess Health Care 11:623–639, 1995

Randolph TG: Allergy as a causative factor of fatigue, irritability, and behavior problems of children. J Pediatr 31:560–572, 1947

Randolph TG: Human Ecology and Susceptibility to the Chemical Environment. Springfield, IL, Charles C Thomas, 1962

Rea WJ: Chemical Sensitivity. Boca Raton, FL, Lewis Publishers, 1992

Rea WJ: Chemical Sensitivity: Sources of Total Body Load. Boca Raton, FL, Lewis Publishers, 1994

Rest KM: A survey of AOEC physician practices and attitudes regarding multiple chemical sensitivity. Toxicol Ind Health 8:51–65, 1992

Robertson DAF, Ayres RCS, Smith CL, et al: Adverse consequences arising from misdiagnosis of food allergy. BMJ 297:719–720, 1988

Rosenthal NE, Cameron CL: Exaggerated sensitivity to an organophosphate pesticide (letter). Am J Psychiatry 148:270, 1991

Rowe KS: Synthetic food colourings and "hyperactivity": a double-blind crossover study. Australian Paediatric Journal 24:143–147, 1988

Rowe KS, Rowe KJ: Synthetic food coloring and behavior: a dose response effect in a double-blind, placebo-controlled, repeated-measures study. J Pediatr 125:691–698, 1994

Schottenfeld RS: Workers with multiple chemical sensitivities: a psychiatric approach to diagnosis and treatment. Occup Med 2:739–753, 1987

Scott AE: Clinical characteristics of taste and smell disorders. Ear Nose Throat J 68: 297–315, 1989

Seltzer JM: Building-related illnesses. J Allergy Clin Immunol 94:351–362, 1994

Shusterman DJ, Dager SR: Prevention of psychological disability after occupational respiratory exposures. Occup Med 6:11–27, 1991

Simon GE: Psychiatric symptoms in multiple chemical sensitivity. Toxicol Ind Health 10:487–496, 1994

Singh NN, Ellis CR, Mulich JA, et al: Vitamin, mineral and dietary treatments, in Psychotropic Medication and Developmental Disabilities. Edited by Reiss S, Aman M. Columbus, Nisonger Center, Ohio State University, 1998, pp 311–320

Smith JD, Terpening CM, Schmidt SO, et al: Relief of fibromyalgia symptoms following discontinuation of dietary excitotoxins. Ann Pharmacother 35:702–706, 2001

Sparks PJ, Daniell W, Black DW, et al: Multiple chemical sensitivity syndrome: a clinical perspective, I: case definition, theories of pathogenesis, and research needs. J Occup Med 36:718–730, 1994a

Sparks PJ, Daniell W, Black DW, et al: Multiple chemical sensitivity syndrome: a clinical perspective, II: evaluation, diagnostic testing, treatment, and social considerations. J Occup Med 36:731–737, 1994b

Staudenmayer H, Selner ME, Selner JC: Adult sequelae of childhood abuse presenting as environmental illness. Ann Allergy 71:538–546, 1992

Stokinger HE, Mountain JT: Progress in detecting the worker hypersusceptible to industrial chemicals. J Occup Med 9:537–542, 1967

Tabershaw IR, Cooper WC: Sequelae of acute organic phosphate poisoning. J Occup Med 8:5–20, 1966

Thorn A: Emergence and preservation of a chronically sick building. J Epidemiol Community Health 54:552–556, 2000

U.S. Interagency Collaborative Group on Hyperkinesis: First Report of the Preliminary Findings and Recommendations of the Interagency Collaborative Group on Hyperkinesis. U.S. Department of Health, Education and Welfare, 1975

Warner JO: Behavior and adverse food reactions, in Food Allergy: Adverse Reactions to Foods and Food Additives. Edited by Metcalfe DD, Sampson HA, Simon RA. Cambridge, UK, Blackwell Science, 1997, pp 511–518

Weiss B: Food additive safety evaluation: the link to behavioral disorders in children, in Advances in Clinical Child Psychology. Edited by Lahey BB, Kazdin AE. New York, Plenum, 1984, pp 221–251

Wender EH, Lipton MA: National Advisory Committee on Hyperkinesis and Food Additives: Final Report to the Nutrition Foundation. New York, Nutrition Foundation, 1980

Wilson C: Patient statement: chemical sensitivity—one victim's perspective. Toxicol Ind Health 10:319–321, 1994

Wolf C: Multiple chemical sensitivities: is there a scientific basis? Int Arch Occup Environ Health 66:213–216, 1994

Wolf C: Multiple chemical sensitivity (MCS): idiopathic environmental intolerances (IEI). Environmental Science and Pollution Research International 3:139–143, 1996

Zielhuis RL, Stijkel A, Verbeck MM, et al: Health Risks to Female Workers in Occupational Exposure to Chemical Agents. Berlin, Springer-Verlag, 1984

ADDITIONAL READINGS

Multiple Chemical Sensitivity—Generally Supportive of a Physiological Cause

Bell IR, Schwartz GE, Peterson JM, et al: Possible time-dependent sensitization to xenobiotics: self-reported illness from chemical odors, foods, and opiate drugs in an older adult population. Arch Environ Health 48:315–327, 1993a

Bell IR, Schwartz GE, Peterson JM, et al: Self-reported illness from chemical odors in young adults without clinical syndromes or occupational exposures. Arch Environ Health 48:6–13, 1993b

Bell IR, Schwartz GE, Peterson JM, et al: Symptom and personality profiles of young adults from a college student population with self-reported illness from foods and chemicals. J Am Coll Nutr 12:693–702, 1993c

Bell IR, Schwartz GE, Amend D, et al: Psychological characteristics and subjective intolerance for xenobiotic agents of normal young adults with trait shyness and defensiveness: a parkinsonian-like personality type. J Nerv Ment Dis 182:367–374, 1994a

Bell IR, Schwartz GE, Amend D, et al: Sensitization to early life stress and response to chemical odors in older adults. Biol Psychiatry 35:857–863, 1994b

Bell IR, Peterson JM, Schwartz GE: Medical histories and psychological profiles of middle-aged women with and without self-reported illness from environmental chemicals. J Clin Psychiatry 56:151–160, 1995

Bell IR, Bootzin RR, Ritenbaugh C, et al: A polysomnographic study of sleep disturbance in community elderly with self-reported environmental chemical odor intolerance. Biol Psychiatry 40:123–133, 1996a

Bell IR, Miller CS, Schwartz GE, et al: Neuropsychiatric and somatic characteristics of young adults with and without self-reported chemical odor intolerance and chemical sensitivity. Arch Environ Health 51:9–21, 1996b

Davidoff AL, Fogarty L, Keyl PM: Psychiatric inferences from data on psychologic/psychiatric symptoms in multiple chemical sensitivities syndrome. Arch Environ Health 55:165–175, 2000

Fernandez M, Bell IR, Schwartz GE: EEG sensitization during chemical exposure in women with and without chemical sensitivity of unknown etiology. Toxicol Ind Health 15:305–312, 1999

Gupta K, Horne R: The influence of health beliefs on the presentation and consultation outcome in patients with chemical sensitivities. J Psychosom Res 50:131–137, 2001

King DS: Can allergic exposure provoke psychological symptoms? A double-blind test. Biol Psychiatry 16:3–19, 1981

Meggs WJ, Bloch RM, Goodman PE, et al: Prevalence and nature of allergy and chemical sensitivity in a general population. Arch Environ Health 51:275–282, 1996

Miller CS, Mitzel HC: Chemical sensitivity attributed to pesticide exposure versus remodeling. Arch Environ Health 50:119–129, 1995

Miller CS, Gammage RB, Jankovic JT: Exacerbation of chemical sensitivity: a case study. Toxicol Ind Health 15:398–402, 1999

Persson R, Osterberg K, Karlson B, et al: Influence of personality traits on neuropsychological test performance in toxic encephalopathy cases and healthy referent subjects. Neurotoxicology 21:667–675, 2000

Woolf A: A 4-year-old girl with manifestations of multiple chemical sensitivities. Environ Health Perspect 108:1219–1223, 2000

Multiple Chemical Sensitivity—Generally Not Supportive of a Physiological Cause

Altenkirch H: Multiple chemical sensitivity (MCS)—differential diagnosis in clinical neurotoxicology: a German perspective. Neurotoxicology 21:589–597, 2000

Binkley KE, Kutcher S: Panic responses to sodium lactate infusion in patients with multiple chemical sensitivity syndrome. J Allergy Clin Immunol 99:570–574, 1997

Black DW: Environmental illness and misdiagnosis—a growing problem. Regul Toxicol Pharmacol 18:23–31, 1993

Black DW: The relationship of mental disorders and idiopathic environmental intolerance. Occup Med 15:557–570, 2000

Black DW, Rathe A, Goldstein RB: Environmental illness: a controlled study of 26 subjects with "20th century disease." JAMA 264:3166–3170, 1990

Black DW, Rathe A, Goldstein RB: Measures of distress in 26 "environmentally ill" subjects. Psychosomatics 34:131–138, 1993

Black DW, Okiishi C, Gabel J, et al: Psychiatric illness in the first-degree relatives of persons reporting multiple chemical sensitivities. Toxicol Ind Health 15:410–414, 1999

Bolla KI: Neurobehavioral performance in multiple chemical sensitivities. Regul Toxicol Pharmacol 24:S52–S54, 1996a

Bolla KI: Neuropsychological evaluation for detecting alterations in the central nervous system after chemical exposure. Regul Toxicol Pharmacol 24:S48–S51, 1996b

Bolla-Wilson K, Wilson RJ, Bleecker ML: Conditioning of physical symptoms after neurotoxic exposure. J Occup Med 30:684–686, 1988

Brodsky CM: Allergic to everything: a medical subculture. Psychosomatics 24:731–742, 1983

Brown-DeGane AM, McGlone J: Multiple chemical sensitivity: a test of the olfactory-limbic model. J Occup Environ Med 41:366–377, 1999

Caccappolo E, Kipen H, Kelly-McNeil K, et al: Odor perception: multiple chemical sensitivities, chronic fatigue, and asthma. J Occup Environ Med 42:629–638, 2000

Cone JE, Harrison R, Reiter R: Patients with multiple chemical sensitivities: clinical diagnostic subsets among an occupational health clinic population. Occup Med 2:721–738, 1987

Dalton P: Cognitive influences on health symptoms from acute chemical exposures. Health Psychol 18:579–590, 1999

Doty RL: Olfaction and multiple chemical sensitivity. Toxicol Ind Health 10:359–368, 1994

Fiedler N, Maccia C, Kipen H: Evaluation of chemically sensitive patients. J Occup Med 34:529–538, 1992

Fiedler N, Kipen HM, Deluca J, et al: A controlled comparison of multiple chemical sensitivities and chronic fatigue syndrome. Psychosom Med 58:38–49, 1996

Giardino ND, Lehrere PM: Behavioral conditioning and idiopathic environmental intolerance. Occup Med 15:519–528, 2000

Goodman M: Illness as lifestyle. Can Fam Physician 41:267–270, 1995

Guglielmi RS, Cox DJ, Spyker DA: Behavioral treatment of phobic avoidance in multiple chemical sensitivity. J Behav Ther Exp Psychiatry 25:197–209, 1994

Haller E: Successful management of patients with "multiple chemical sensitivities" on an inpatient psychiatric unit. J Clin Psychiatry 54:196–199, 1993

Hotopf M: Seasonal affective disorder, environmental hypersensitivity and somatisation. Br J Psychiatry 164:246–248, 1994

Leznoff A: Provocative challenges in patients with multiple chemical sensitivity. J Allergy Clin Immunol 99:438–442, 1997

Leznoff A, Binkley KE: Idiopathic environmental intolerances: results of challenge studies. Occup Med 15:529–537, 2000

Montanaro A, Bardana EJ Jr: The chemically sensitive patient, in Occupational Asthma. Edited by Bardana EJ Jr, Montanaro A, O'Hollaren MT. Philadelphia, PA, Hanley & Belfus, 1992, pp 255–266

Rosenberg SJ, Freedman MR, Schmaling KB, et al: Personality styles of patients asserting environmental illness. J Occup Med 32:678–681, 1990

Seeber A, Demes P, Golka K, et al: Subjective symptoms due to solvent mixtures, dioxin, and toluene: impact of exposure versus personality factors. Neurotoxicology 21:677–684, 2000

Shusterman D, Balmes J, Cone J: Behavioral sensitization to irritants/odorants after acute overexposures. J Occup Med 30:565–567, 1988

Simon GE: Epidemic multiple chemical sensitivity in an industrial setting. Toxicol Ind Health 8:41–46, 1992

Simon GE, Katon WJ, Sparks PJ: Allergic to life: psychological factors in environmental illness. Am J Psychiatry 147:901–906, 1990

Simon GE, Daniell W, Stockbridge H, et al: Immunologic, psychological, and neuropsychological factors in multiple chemical sensitivity: a controlled study. Ann Intern Med 19:97–103, 1993

Spyker DA: Multiple chemical sensitivities—syndrome and solution. J Toxicol Clin Toxicol 33:95–99, 1995

Staudenmayer H: Psychological treatment of psychogenic idiopathic environmental intolerance. Occup Med 15:627–646, 2000

Staudenmayer H, Kramer RE: Psychogenic chemical sensitivity: psychogenic pseudoseizures elicited by provocation challenges with fragrances. J Psychosom Res 47:185–190, 1999

Staudenmayer H, Selner JC: Neuropsychophysiology during relaxation in generalized, universal 'allergic' reactivity to the environment: a comparison study. J Psychosom Res 34:259–270, 1990

Staudenmayer H, Selner JC, Buhr MP: Double-blind provocation chamber challenges in 20 patients presenting with "multiple chemical sensitivity." Regul Toxicol Pharmacol 18:44–53, 1993

Stewart DE, Raskin J: Psychiatric assessment of patients with "20th-century disease" ("total allergy syndrome"). Canadian Medical Association Journal 133:1001–1006, 1985

Terr AI: Environmental illness: a clinical review of 50 cases. Arch Intern Med 146: 145–149, 1986

Terr AI: Clinical ecology in the workplace. J Occup Med 31:257–261, 1989

Food Additives

Adams W: Lack of behavioral effects from Feingold diet violations. Percept Mot Skills 52:307–313, 1981

Brenner A: A study of the efficacy of the Feingold diet on hyperkinetic children. Clin Pediatr 16:652–656, 1977

Chernick E: Effects of the Feingold diet on reading achievement and classroom behavior. Reading Teacher 34:171–174, 1980
Conners CK, Goyette CH, Southwick DA, et al: Food additives and hyperkinesis: a controlled double-blind experiment. Pediatrics 58:154–166, 1976
Conners CK, Goyette CH, Newman EB: Dose-time effect of artificial colors in hyperactive children. J Learn Disabil 13:43–52, 1980
Cook PS, Woodhill JM: The Feingold dietary treatment of the hyperkinetic syndrome. Med J Aust 2:85–90, 1976
David TJ: Reactions to dietary tartrazine. Arch Dis Child 62:119–122, 1987
Egger J, Graham PJ, Carter CM, et al: Controlled trial of oligoantigenic treatment in the hyperkinetic syndrome. Lancet 1:540–545, 1985
Eich WF, Thim EB, Crowder JE: Effect of the Feingold Kaiser Permanente diet in minimal brain dysfunction. Journal of the Medical Association of the State of Alabama 49:16–20, 1979
Gross MD, Tofanelli RA, Butzirus SM, et al: The effect of diets rich in and free from additives on the behavior of children with hyperkinetic and learning disorders. J Am Acad Child Adolesc Psychiatry 26:53–55, 1987
Haavik S, Altman K, Woelk C: Effects of the Feingold diet on seizures and hyperactivity: a single-subject analysis. J Behav Med 2:365–374, 1979
Harley JP, Matthews CG, Eichman PL: Synthetic food colors and hyperactivity in children: a double-blind challenge experiment. Pediatrics 62:975–983, 1978a
Harley JP, Ray RS, Tomasi L, et al: Hyperkinesis and food additives: testing the Feingold hypothesis. Pediatrics 61:818–828, 1978b
Harner IC, Foiles RAL: Effect of Feingold's K-P diet on a residential, mentally handicapped population. J Am Diet Assoc 76:575–580, 1980
Hindle RC, Priest J: The management of hyperkinetic children: a trial of dietary therapy. N Z Med J 88:43–45, 1978
Holborow P, Elkins J, Berry P: The effect of the Feingold diet on "normal" school children. J Learn Disabil 14:143–147, 1981
Hughes EC, Oettinger L, Johnson F, et al: Case report: a chemically defined diet in diagnosis and management of food sensitivity in minimal brain dysfunction. Ann Allergy 42:174–176, 1979
Jewett DL, Fein G, Greenberg MH: A double-blind study of symptom provocation to determine food sensitivity. N Engl J Med 323:429–433, 1990
Levy F, Hobbes G: Hyperkinesis and diet: a replication study. Am J Psychiatry 135: 1559–1560, 1978
Levy F, Dumbrell S, Hobbes G, et al: Hyperkinesis and diet: a double-blind crossover trial with a tartrazine challenge. Med J Aust 1:61–64, 1978
Mattes JA, Gittelman R: Effects of artificial food colorings in children with hyperactive symptoms. Arch Gen Psychiatry 38 714–718, 1981
Mattes JA, Gittelman-Klein R: A crossover study of artificial food colorings in a hyperkinetic child. Am J Psychiatry 135:987–988, 1978
Millman M, Campbell MB, Wright KL, et al: Allergy and learning disabilities in children. Ann Allergy 36:149–160, 1976
O'Banion D, Armstrong B, Cummings RA, et al: Disruptive behavior: a dietary approach. Journal of Autism and Childhood Schizophrenia 8:325–337, 1978
O'Shea JA, Porter SF: Double-blind study of children with hyperkinetic syndrome treated with multi-allergen extract sublingually. J Learn Disabil 14:189–191, 237, 1981
Palmer S, Rapoport JL, Quinn PO: Food additives and hyperactivity. Clin Pediatr 14: 956–959, 1975
Pearson DJ, Rix KJB, Bentley SJ: Food allergy: how much in the mind? A clinical and psychiatric study of suspected food hypersensitivity. Lancet 1:1259–1261, 1983
Pollock I, Warner JO: A follow-up study of childhood food additive intolerance. J R Coll Physicians Lond 21:248–250, 1987

Pollock I, Warner JO: Effect of artificial food colours on childhood behaviour. Arch Dis Child 65:74–77, 1990
Prinz RJ, Roberts WA, Hantman E: Dietary correlates of hyperactive behavior in children. J Consult Clin Psychol 48:760–769, 1980
Rapp DJ: Does diet affect hyperactivity? J Learn Disabil 11:56–62, 1978
Rapp DJ: Food allergy treatment for hyperkinesis. J Learn Disabil 12:42–50, 1979
Rix KJB, Pearson DJ, Bentley SJ: A psychiatric study of patients with supposed food allergy. Br J Psychiatry 145:121–126, 1984
Rose TL: The functional relationship between artificial food colors and hyperactivity. J Appl Behav Anal 11:439–446, 1978
Salzman LK: Allergy testing, psychological assessment and dietary treatment of the hyperactive child syndrome. Med J Aust 2:248–251, 1976
Schoenthaler SJ, Doraz WE, Wakefield JA: The impact of a low food additive and sucrose diet on academic performance in 803 New York City public schools. International Journal of Biosocial and Medical Research 8:185–195, 1986
Spring C, Vermeersch J, Blunden D, et al: Case studies of effects of artificial food colors on hyperactivity. Journal of Special Education 15:361–372, 1981
Stine JJ: Symptom alleviation in the hyperactive child by dietary modification: a report of two cases. Am J Orthopsychiatry 46:637–645, 1976
Swanson JM, Kinsbourne M: Food dyes impair performance of hyperactive children on a laboratory learning test. Science 207:1485–1486, 1980
Thorley G: Pilot study to assess behavioral and cognitive effects of artificial food colours in a group of retarded children. Dev Med Child Neurol 26:56–61, 1984
Tryphonas H, Trites RL: Food allergy in children with hyperactivity, learning disabilities and/or minimal brain dysfunction. Ann Allergy 42:22–27, 1979
Uhlig T, Merkenschlager A, Brandmaier R, et al: Topographic mapping of brain electrical activity in children with food-induced attention deficit hyperkinetic disorder. Eur J Pediatr 156:557–561, 1997
Weiss B, Willaims JH, Margen S, et al: Behavioral responses to artificial food colors. Science 207:1487–1489, 1980
Williams JI, Cram DM, Tausig FT, et al: Relative effects of drugs and diet on hyperactive behaviors: an experimental study. Pediatrics 61:811–817, 1978
Young E, Patel S, Stoneham M, et al: The prevalence of reaction to food additives in a survey population. J R Coll Physicians Lond 21:241–247, 1987

Sick Building Syndrome

Bachmann MO, Myers JE: Influences on sick building syndrome symptoms in three buildings. Soc Sci Med 40:245–251, 1995
Bachmann MO, Turck AV, Myers JE: Sick building symptoms in office workers: a follow-up study before and one year after changing buildings. Occup Med 45:11–15, 1995
Bauer RM, Greve KW, Besch EL, et al: The role of psychological factors in the report of building-related symptoms in sick building syndrome. J Consult Clin Psychol 60:213–219, 1992
Bourbeau J, Brisson C, Allaire S: Prevalence of the sick building syndrome symptoms in office workers before and after being exposed to a building with an improved ventilation system. Occup Environ Med 53:204–210, 1996
Bourbeau J, Brisson C, Allaire S: Prevalence of the sick building syndrome symptoms in office workers before and six months and three years after being exposed to a building with an improved ventilation system. Occup Environ Med 54:49–53, 1997
Burge S, Hedge A, Wilson S, et al: Sick building syndrome: a study of 4373 office workers. Ann Occup Hyg 31:493–504, 1987

Chandrakumar M, Evans J, Arulanantham P: An investigation into sick building syndrome among local authority employees. Ann Occup Hyg 38:789–799, 1994
Chester AC, Levine PH: Concurrent sick building syndrome and chronic fatigue syndrome: epidemic neuromyasthenia revisited. Clin Infect Dis 18 (suppl 1):S43–S48, 1994
Chester AC, Levine PH: The natural history of concurrent sick building syndrome and chronic fatigue syndrome. J Psychiatr Res 31:51–57, 1997
Cone J, Sult TA: Acquired intolerance to solvents following pesticide/solvent exposure in a building: a new group of workers at risk for multiple chemical sensitivities. Toxicol Ind Health 8:29–39, 1992
Donnell HD, Bagby JR, Harmon RG, et al Report of an illness outbreak at the Harry S. Truman State Office Building. Am J Epidemiol 129:550–558, 1989
Finnegan MJ, Pickering CAC, Burge PS: The sick building syndrome: prevalence studies. BMJ 289:1573–1575, 1984
Hodgson MJ, Frohliger J, Permar E, et al: Symptoms and microenvironmental measures in nonproblem buildings. J Occup Med 33:527–533, 1991
Jaakkola JJK, Tuomaala P, Seppanen O: Air recirculation and sick building syndrome: a blinded crossover trial. Am J Public Health 84:422–428, 1994
Martin JR: The sensitive individual and the indoor environment: case study. Am Ind Hyg Assoc J 56:1121–1126, 1995
Menzies R, Tamblyn R, Farant J-P, et al: The effect of varying levels of outdoor-air supply on the symptoms of sick building syndrome. N Engl J Med 328:821–827, 1993
Middaugh DA, Pinney SM, Linz DH: Sick building syndrome: medical evaluation of two work forces. J Occup Med 34:1197–1203, 1992
Norback D, Edling C: Environmental, occupational, and personal factors related to the prevalence of sick building syndrome in the general population. British Journal of Industrial Medicine 48:451–462, 1991
Norback D, Michel I, Widstrom J: Indoor air quality and personal factors related to the sick building syndrome. Scand J Work Environ Health 16:121–128, 1990a
Norback D, Torgen M, Edling C: Volatile organic compounds, respirable dust, and personal factors related to prevalence and incidence of sick building syndrome in primary schools. British Journal of Industrial Medicine 47:733–741, 1990b
Ooi PL, Goh KT: Sick building syndrome: an emerging stress-related disorder? Int J Epidemiol 26:1243–1249, 1997
Shefer A, Dobbins JG, Fukuda K, et al: Fatiguing illness among employees in three large state office buildings, California, 1993: was there an outbreak? J Psychiatr Res 31:31–43, 1997
Skov P, Valbjorn O, Danish Indoor Climate Study Group: The "sick" building syndrome in the office environment: the Danish Town Hall Study. Environment International 13:339–349, 1987
Skov P, Valbjorn O, Pedersen BV: Influence of personal characteristics, job-related factors and psychosocial factors on the sick building syndrome. Scand J Work Environ Health 15:286–295, 1989
Stenberg B, Eriksson N, Hoog J, et al: The sick building syndrome (SBS) in office workers: a case-referent study of personal, psychosocial and building-related risk indicators. Int J Epidemiol 23:1190–1197, 1994
Tavris DR, Field L, Brumback CL: Outbreak of illness due to volatilized asphalt coming from a malfunctioning fluorescent lighting fixture. Am J Public Health 74: 614–615, 1984
Thrasher JD, Madison R, Broughton A, et al: Building-related illness and antibodies to albumin conjugates of formaldehyde, toluene diisocyanate, and trimellitic anhydride. Am J Ind Med 15:187–195, 1989
Welch LS, Sokas R: Development of multiple chemical sensitivity after an outbreak of sick-building syndrome. Toxicol Ind Health 8:47–50, 1992

Formaldehyde

Kilburn KH: Indoor air effects after building renovation and in manufactured homes. Am J Med Sci 320:249–254, 2000

Kilburn KH, Warshaw R: Neurobehavioral effects of formaldehyde and solvents on histology technicians: repeated testing across time. Environ Res 58:134–146, 1992

Kilburn KH, Warshaw R, Boylen CT, et al: Pulmonary and neurobehavioral effects of formaldehyde exposure. Arch Environ Health 40:254–260, 1985

Kilburn KH, Warshaw R, Thornton JC: Formaldehyde impairs memory, equilibrium, and dexterity in histology technicians: effects which persist for days after exposure. Arch Environ Health 42:117–120, 1987

Olsen JH, Dossing M: Formaldehyde induced symptoms in day care centers. Am Ind Hyg Assoc J 43:366–370, 1982

Schenker MB, Weiss ST, Murawski BJ: Health effects of residence in homes with urea formaldehyde foam insulation: a pilot study. Environment International 8:359–363, 1982

Singer R: Neurotoxicity Guidebook. New York, Van Nostrand Reinhold, 1990

Thun MJ, Lakat MF, Altman R: Symptom survey of residents of homes insulated with urea-formaldehyde foam. Environ Res 29:320–334, 1982

Woodbury MA, Zenz C: Formaldehyde in the home environment: prenatal and infant exposures, in Formaldehyde Toxicity. Edited by Gibson JE. Washington, DC, Hemisphere, 1980, pp 203–211

Index

Page numbers printed in **boldface type** refer to tables.